Musculoskeletal Radiology

This book in the *FRCRverse Series* is dedicated to musculoskeletal radiology, following the latest RCR curriculum. Section 1 discusses clinical presentations and imaging strategies to help in daily tasks that radiologists and residents face in reporting rooms and MDTs. Section 2 explores imaging of core pathologies with additional topics such as multisystemic diseases, MSK interventions and sports imaging, along with model SBA questions in each chapter for self-assessment. With more than 280 high-quality images and practical concepts from renowned authors, this book is an excellent preparatory resource for the final FRCR candidate as well as a guide for daily musculoskeletal radiology practice.

FRCRverse
The Ultimate Guide to Passing the Final FRCR

Series Editors: Siddharth Thaker and Harun Gupta

Musculoskeletal Radiology
The Ultimate Guide to Passing the Final FRCR
Edited by Siddharth Thaker and Harun Gupta

Musculoskeletal Radiology

The Ultimate Guide to Passing the Final FRCR

Edited by
Siddharth Thaker and Harun Gupta

CRC Press
Taylor & Francis Group
Boca Raton London New York

CRC Press is an imprint of the
Taylor & Francis Group, an **informa** business

Designed cover image: Siddharth Thaker and Harun Gupta

First edition published 2026
by CRC Press
2385 NW Executive Center Drive, Suite 320, Boca Raton, FL 33431

and by CRC Press
4 Park Square, Milton Park, Abingdon, Oxon, OX14 4RN

CRC Press is an imprint of Taylor & Francis Group, LLC

ISBN: 978-1-032-81528-2 (hbk)
ISBN: 978-1-032-81515-2 (pbk)
ISBN: 978-1-003-50024-7 (ebk)

DOI: 10.1201/9781003500247

Typeset in Palatino
by Apex CoVantage, LLC

Contents

Preface

The final FRCR exam is the prerequisite to obtaining a full licence to practice radiology in the UK as a consultant. The Royal College of Radiologists is constantly revising and improving examination patterns and syllabus to ensure that UK radiology trainees and international medical graduate radiologists are up to date for practising radiology in the UK. All exam-takers must realise that they are attending an examination on clinical radiology with a focus on being a safe radiologist who can deliver high-quality radiology services including on-call commitments, subspecialty-specific input, MDTs, and interventions.

Our book has been written with the aim of providing all FRCR aspirants with factual and to-the-point knowledge about how radiology is routinely practised in the NHS. We have divided the entire series into seven books reflecting seven different specialties, which can help not only with preparing for FRCR exams but also during early years of practice as a consultant radiologist. It can serve as a handy guide covering the various subtopics one may encounter in their routine work. The book has two sections: Section 1 depicts the clinical reasoning behind requested radiological exams and imaging strategies, and Section 2 enumerates imaging findings of core pathologies set by the RCR curriculum. Model questions in the FRCR 2A SBA format, against which readers can assess their understanding and knowledge, have been included at the end of each chapter in Section 2. All the chapters in Section 2 illustrate pathologies with example images covering different modalities. These include ultrasound, MRI including advanced sequences, CT and PET-CT. Charts, illustrations, and flowcharts have been used extensively throughout the book, and each chapter has suggested readings at the end.

We would like to thank all the editors and authors who have contributed to the books and thank the publishers for all their help at every stage of the publication. We would like to particularly thank Balaji Karuppanan, Kanchi Shridhar, and Shivangi Pramanik for their tireless efforts and for putting up with us through the editorial process.

We would like to acknowledge our mentors, colleagues, trainees, and patients who have been the source of knowledge and inspiration.

Dr Siddharth Thaker
Prof Harun Gupta

Editors

Siddharth Thaker MBBS, MD (India), FRCR (UK), CESR (UK) is a Dual Fellowship-trained Consultant Musculoskeletal Radiologist currently working at the University Hospitals of Leicester NHS Trust. He completed his general radiology residency in India, followed by two dedicated musculoskeletal radiology fellowships in India and the UK, an ESOR scholarship in Vienna, and a RNOH clinical attachment.

He enjoys all facets of musculoskeletal radiology including soft tissue sarcoma imaging, musculoskeletal interventions, rheumatology, spinal imaging, and musculoskeletal trauma. He is particularly passionate about musculoskeletal radiology research and education. He regularly contributes to undergraduate, foundation doctor, and registrar teaching at Leicester using various online platforms as well as on an in-person basis. He is a well-published author with an editorship of a book *(Practical Guide for Imaging of Soft Tissue Tumours)* along with Prof Gupta, 10 book chapters, and 31 publications in peer-reviewed indexed journals. He is a reviewer for the *Indian Journal of Radiology and Imaging*, and clinical radiology and tomography journals. He believes in continuous and unhindered propagation of musculoskeletal radiology education and makes constant efforts to achieve this goal.

Harun Gupta MBBS, MD, DNB, MRCP (UK), FRCR (UK) has been a Consultant Musculoskeletal Radiologist at Leeds Teaching Hospitals since 2010. He received his radiology training from Aberdeen and also did out-of-program training in Oxford, which was followed by a one-year MSK Fellowship in Leeds. He is an expert in all aspects of musculoskeletal radiology with subspecialty interests in soft tissue sarcoma and musculoskeletal intervention. He is an elected member of the Council, British Society of Skeletal Radiology; Advisory Editor, MSK Section, *Clinical Radiology Journal*; member of the Ultrasound, Tumour and Intervention Subcommittees, European Society of Skeletal Radiology; member of Refresher Program Promotion and Social Media Committee, International Skeletal Society; international advisory member of the board, MSK Society of India; and Honorary Senior Lecturer, University of Leeds, UK. He was awarded the Musculoskeletal Radiologist of the Year in 2023 and the Prafulla Kumar Ganguli Professorship of the Royal College of Radiologists of the UK in 2024. He is actively involved in training specialist registrars and MSK radiology fellows. He has been the Special Interest Lead for MSK for the Leeds Radiology Academy and Clinical Supervisor for all trainees in the MSK Department. He also helped the RCR with Making Best Use of Radiology Department (iRefer) as the lead for the MSK Sub-Section.

He has written multiple books and book chapters and over 60 publications in peer-reviewed journals. He regularly contributes to teaching through lectures, courses, and webinars at national and international levels. He is also actively involved in research at the NIHR Leeds Biomedical Research Centre.

He is the founder of the MSK radiology learning platforms www.mskteachingroom.com and www.primeradacacdemy.com.

Contributors

Sinan Al-Qassab
Consultant Musculoskeletal Radiologist
The Robert Jones and Agnes Hunt Orthopaedic
    Hospital NHS Foundation Trust
Oswestry, United Kingdom

Rahoz Aziz
Clinical Radiology Resident (Musculoskeletal
    Radiology)
Leeds Radiology Academy
Leeds Teaching Hospitals NHS Trust
Leeds, United Kingdom

Patrick Baker
Clinical Radiology Resident (Musculoskeletal
    Radiology)
NHS Greater Glasgow & Clyde
Glasgow, United Kingdom

James Baren
Consultant Musculoskeletal Radiologist
Leeds Teaching Hospitals NHS Trust
Leeds, United Kingdom

Nishika Bhatt
Medical Student
University College London Medical School
London, United Kingdom

Raj Bhatt
Consultant Musculoskeletal Radiologist
University Hospitals of Leicester NHS Trust
Leicester, United Kingdom

Lenetta Boyce
Consultant Musculoskeletal Radiologist
Liverpool University Hospitals Foundation Trust
Liverpool, United Kingdom

Raj Chari
Consultant Musculoskeletal Radiologist
Oxford University Hospitals NHS Foundation Trust
Oxford, United Kingdom

Saurabh Deore
Clinical Radiology Resident (Musculoskeletal
    Radiology)
Northwest Radiology Academy
Liverpool, United Kingdom

Harun Gupta
Consultant Musculoskeletal Radiologist
Leeds Teaching Hospitals NHS Trust
Leeds, United Kingdom

Moomal Rose Harris
Consultant Radiologist
Department of Radiology
Calderdale and Huddersfield Foundation NHS Trust
Huddersfield, United Kingdom

Ganesh Hegde
Consultant Musculoskeletal Radiologist
Royal National Orthopaedic Hospital NHS
    Trust
Stanmore, United Kingdom

Mohsin AM Hussein
Consultant Musculoskeletal Radiologist
University Hospitals of Leicester NHS Trust
Leicester, United Kingdom

Madhavi K
Associate Professor & Lead of MSK Radiology
    Subunit
Department of Clinical Radiology
CMC Vellore, India

Joseph KT
Consultant Radiologist & Assistant Professor
Department of Clinical Radiology
CMC Vellore, India

Kirran Khalid
Locum Consultant Musculoskeletal Radiologist
Royal National Orthopaedic Hospital NHS
    Trust
Stanmore, United Kingdom

Anand Kirwadi
Consultant Musculoskeletal Radiologist
Manchester University Hospitals Foundation
    Trust
Manchester, United Kingdom

Mark Kong
Clinical Radiology Resident (Musculoskeletal
    Radiology)
Oxford University Hospitals Trust
Oxford, United Kingdom

Kenneth Lupton
Consultant Musculoskeletal Radiologist
NHS Greater Glasgow and Clyde
Glasgow, United Kingdom

Michelle Ooi
Consultant Musculoskeletal Radiologist
Leeds Teaching Hospitals NHS Trust
Leeds, United Kingdom

Radhika Prasad
Consultant Musculoskeletal Radiologist
Liverpool University Hospitals NHS Foundation Trust
Liverpool, United Kingdom

Neel Raja
Clinical Radiology Resident (Musculoskeletal
    Radiology)
University Hospitals of Leicester NHS Trust
Leicester, United Kingdom

Winston J Rennie
Consultant Musculoskeletal Radiologist &
    Professor of Radiology
University Hospitals of Leicester NHS Trust
Loughborough University
Leicester, United Kingdom

Amit Shah
Consultant Musculoskeletal Radiologist
Royal Surrey County Hospital NHS Foundation Trust
Guildford, United Kingdom

Sandeep Singh
Consultant Radiologist
Frimley Health NHS Foundation Trust
Camberley, United Kingdom

Ankit Tandon
Senior Consultant Radiologist & Lead of
    Musculoskeletal Radiology
Department of Diagnostic Radiology
Tan Tock Seng Hospital
Singapore

Joshua Taylor
Clinical Radiology Resident (Musculoskeletal
    Radiology)
Northwest Radiology Academy
Liverpool, United Kingdom

Siddharth Thaker
Consultant Musculoskeletal Radiologist
University Hospitals of Leicester NHS Trust
Leicester, United Kingdom

Phillipa Tyler
Consultant Musculoskeletal Radiologist
Royal National Orthopaedic Hospital NHS
    Trust
Stanmore, United Kingdom

Zoe Winston
Clinical Radiology Resident (Musculoskeletal
    Radiology)
Northwest Radiology Academy
Manchester, United Kingdom

Tsz Shing Joshua Wong
Clinical Radiology Resident (Musculoskeletal
    Radiology)
Leeds Radiology Academy
Leeds Teaching Hospitals NHS Trust
Leeds, United Kingdom

SECTION 1
IMAGING STRATEGIES

This section deals with common presentations to A&E, outpatient clinics, and MDTs. Clinicians frequently require imaging to answer clinical questions or to narrow down differentials. It is crucial to perform appropriate imaging for a particular pathology in the question. Therefore, it is essential for the radiologist to understand the clinician's mind. We will discuss seven common clinical scenarios faced in routine practice. In practice, it is important to follow Trust-defined imaging protocols, as practices vary between hospitals.

Chapter 1.1
Bone Pain

Saurabh Deore and Harun Gupta

LEARNING OBJECTIVES

- To provide a structured radiological approach to evaluating bone pain
- To review key imaging modalities and their role in diagnosis
- To outline common causes of bone pain and their characteristic imaging findings
- To emphasise the importance of multimodality imaging in accurate diagnosis and management

---

IMPORTANCE

Bone pain is a frequent clinical presentation arising from various pathological processes. Radiology plays a vital role in identifying the underlying cause and guiding management. This section provides an overview of the radiological approach to bone pain, emphasising key imaging modalities and differential diagnoses.

Age and clinical history including history of any underlying relevant medical conditions are important in interpreting patients' imaging.

Traumatic fractures as a cause of bone pain will not be covered further in this section. These patients present typically to A&E and fracture clinic departments and sometimes primary care when there has been subacute injury. Briefly, however, the aetiology of bone pain can be classified based on its underlying pathology:

- Traumatic: Stress injuries including stress fractures and traumatic fractures
- Infective: Osteomyelitis and septic arthritis
- Neoplastic: Benign such as osteoid osteoma and malignant such as primary bone tumours (e.g. osteosarcoma, Ewing sarcoma), myeloma, and metastatic disease
- Metabolic: Osteoporosis, osteomalacia, and Paget's disease
- Inflammatory: Rheumatoid arthritis, seronegative spondyloarthropathies
- Vascular: Avascular necrosis (AVN) and sickle cell bone infarction
- Idiopathic: Chronic recurrent multifocal osteomyelitis (CRMO) and complex regional pain syndrome

IMAGING MODALITIES

Plain Radiography

- First-line imaging modality
- Evaluates bone density, cortical integrity, trabecular changes, and periosteal reactions
- Limited in detecting early-stage infections, tumours, and metabolic bone diseases

Computed Tomography (CT)

- Greater cortical bone detail
- Useful for detecting fractures, bone destruction in neoplasia, and sequestrae in osteomyelitis
- Findings: High-resolution depiction of cortical fractures, bone matrix mineralisation patterns, and calcified soft tissue masses

DOI: 10.1201/9781003500247-2

Magnetic Resonance Imaging (MRI)

- Modality of choice for marrow pathology, soft tissue involvement, early stress changes, AVN, infections, neoplasms

- T1-weighted images assess marrow replacement, while T2-weighted fat-saturated (T2 FS)/STIR sequences highlight oedema

- Findings: Marrow signal alterations (low on T1, high on T2 FS/STIR), contrast enhancement in inflammatory or neoplastic conditions and soft tissue involvement

Nuclear Medicine

- Bone scintigraphy (Tc-99m) detects multifocal pathology, including metastases and occult fractures

- PET-CT with FDG is increasingly used for oncological assessment

- Findings: Increased radiotracer uptake in infection, malignancy, or metabolic disease; cold lesions in avascular necrosis

RADIOLOGICAL FEATURES OF COMMON CAUSES OF BONE PAIN

Stress Injuries

Stress fractures are partial or complete and usually result in bones being unable to withstand subthreshold stress applied in a rhythmical and repeated manner. Fractures can be fatigue or insufficiency (Figure 1.1.1).

- **Fatigue fractures** occur from abnormal repetitive stress causing temporal mechanical failure in a normal bone. Fatigue fractures happen in the normal bone due to abnormal repetitive stress and are more frequent in young, suboptimally conditioned individuals who abruptly engage in strenuous activities, military recruits, and athletes who abruptly intensify their training regimen.

- **Insufficiency fractures** happen because of normal stress on an abnormally weakened bone. These generally happen in elderly patients and especially in women with osteoporosis; a fragility fracture following a single minimally traumatic event such as in a woman with osteoporosis is an insufficiency fracture. Atypical femoral fractures are insufficiency fractures occurring in the femoral diaphysis. They are strongly linked to long-term therapy for osteoporosis with bisphosphonates.

- **Pathological fractures** are insufficiency fractures that occur in a bone weakened by a benign or malignant neoplastic lesion affecting its trabecular integrity. By the same definition, fracture through osteomyelitis is regarded as a pathological fracture.

Early radiographs can be normal before periosteal reaction, sclerosis, and faint lucency appear. MRI is the gold standard examination and shows marrow oedema and periosteal and cortical changes in thickening, and these stress changes indicate abnormalities; as these changes progress, an overt fracture line can become visible on T1 imaging, at which time it will constitute an established stress fracture.

Infection

In one infection, osteomyelitis, plain radiographs can initially be normal, as noticeable changes take 2–3 weeks to develop on radiographs. That is, positive radiographs are helpful, but negative study does not exclude osteomyelitis. MRI is the gold standard imaging modality and can reveal marrow oedema, cortical destruction, abscess formation, periosteal reaction, and surrounding soft tissue oedematous changes.

For septic arthritis, findings include joint effusion, periarticular osteopenia, and late-stage bone erosion. MRI shows synovial thickening and enhancement. In acute cases, effusions should be aspirated and the aspirate analysed microbiologically for definitive diagnosis.

Neoplasia

As an example of benign neoplasia, osteoid osteoma patients often have night bone pain that responds to NSAIDs, and CT is the best imaging modality for showing the diagnostic nidus. MRI shows bony changes of periosteal and cortical thickening and oedema. Regarding malignant neoplasia, plain films are mandatory

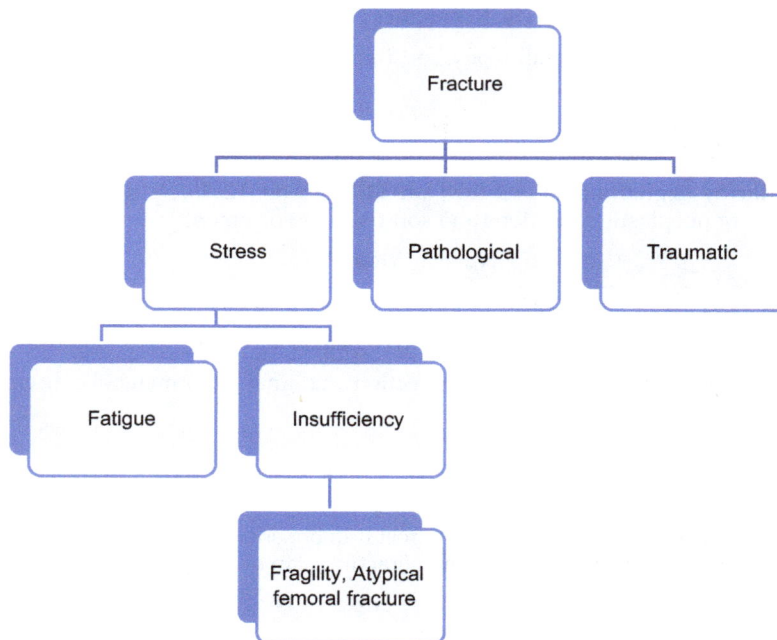

Figure 1.1.1 Types of fractures.

in patients with bone neoplasms and play a significant role in lesion characterisation; MRI is used for local staging and characterisation, and CT is for diagnosed cases for staging.

Aggressive features on imaging include poor zone of transition, cortical destruction, periosteal changes, and extra osseous and multicompartment extension. MRI intrinsic features include lesion heterogenicity on fluid-sensitive sequences, necrosis, and haemorrhage.

PRIMARY BONE MALIGNANCIES

- Osteosarcoma: Aggressive periosteal reaction (Codman's triangle, sunburst pattern), mixed lytic–sclerotic appearance and soft tissue extension on MRI

- Ewing sarcoma: Onion-skin periosteal reaction, permeative bone destruction, and associated soft tissue mass with restricted diffusion on MRI

SECONDARIES/METASTATIC DISEASE

- Lytic expansile (renal, thyroid), sclerotic (prostate, breast) or mixed lesions

Metabolic and Degenerative Conditions

- Osteoporosis: Generalised demineralisation, cortical thinning, vertebral compression fractures with "codfish vertebrae" appearance

- Paget's disease: Cortical thickening, trabecular coarsening, bowing deformities, "cotton wool" skull appearance

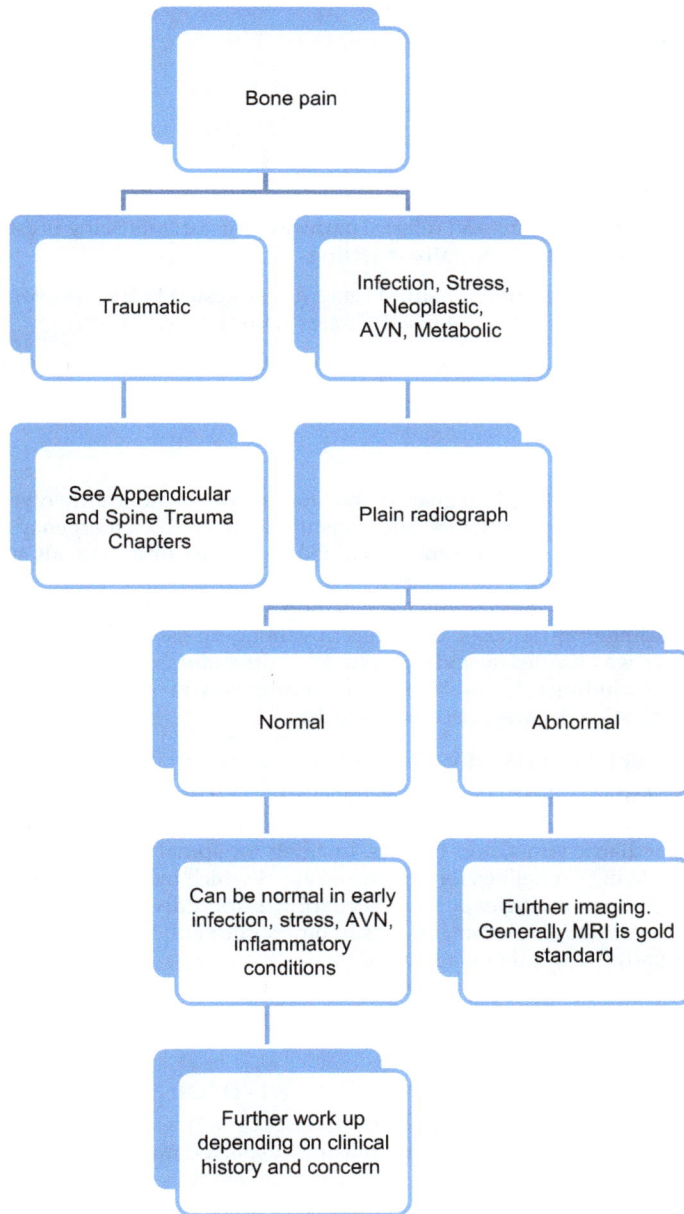

Figure 1.1.2   Aetiologies of bone pain.

CONCLUSION

A systematic radiological approach is crucial for evaluating bone pain. Correlation with clinical history and multimodality imaging ensures accurate diagnosis and optimal management (Figure 1.1.2).

SUGGESTED READING

■ Atraumatic fractures of femur. *British Journal of Radiology*, 2021;94(1121):20201457. https://doi.org/10.1259/bjr.20201457

Chapter 1.2
Joint Pain/Deformity

Siddharth Thaker

LEARNING OBJECTIVES

- To illustrate various presentations and referral pathways for patients being presented to healthcare practitioners in community and specialised settings

- To understand the clinical reasoning behind imaging requested to the radiology department and types of imaging performed for various pathologies leading to joint pain

- To differentiate the types of imaging performed for different pathologies that lead to joint pain

---

IMPORTANCE

The topic is particularly relevant to UK registrars and radiologists who are involved in vetting requests sent by GPs, junior and middle-grade doctors, and consultants from ED (emergency department), fracture clinics, orthopaedic outpatient clinics, and approved allied healthcare professionals such as extended scope physiotherapists and advanced nurse practitioners.

The latter requires approval from both trauma and orthopaedics (T&O) and radiology clinical governance teams to be able to send imaging requests. Until recently, imaging assessment of joint pain/deformity in community/primary care was limited to radiographs and ultrasounds. Recently, the focus has shifted to provide holistic imaging including CTs and MRIs in the community to offload service pressures on specialist hospitals, with the formation of integrated care boards.

GUIDANCE FOR ON-CALL T&O UNDERPINNING IMAGING REQUESTS

National Institute of Clinical Excellence (NICE) has developed various guidelines for specific joints to diagnose causes of joint pain and deformity, including separate guidelines for hip, knee, shoulder, hand and wrist, spine, foot and ankle, paediatric joints, and trauma. Imaging for spinal causes is described in Chapter 1.3. NICE has developed practicing guidelines for individual joints which include reference standards and management outlines for common pathologies such as osteoarthritis for individual joints, as well as joint-specific pathologies such as femoroacetabular impingements in hip, rotator cuff tears for shoulder, and other conditions that call for conservative surgical management.

In secondary care, imaging for joint pain/deformity is requested from two different settings: by ED/fracture clinics in the presence of acute trauma (suspected complex and non-complex fractures) and by orthopaedic clinics seeing insidious-onset joint pain.

IMAGING OF COMPLEX (POLY)TRAUMA PATIENTS WITH JOINT PAIN/DEFORMITIES

- Use whole-body CT (consisting of a vertex-to-toes scanogram followed by CT from vertex to mid-thigh scan) in adults (16 or over) with blunt major trauma and suspected multiple injuries. No repositioning of the patient during the CT. (Polytrauma protocols—Contrast-enhanced scans, biphasic)

- Suspected high-energy pelvic fractures in 16 years and over: CT

- Suspected high-energy pelvic fractures in children below 16 years: CT vs radiograph, depending on suspected abdominal and pelvic injury

- Suspected proximal femur or neck of femur fractures: Radiographs (if clinical suspicion is high and radiographs are negative, consider CT or MRI)

IMAGING OF NON-COMPLEX TRAUMA PATIENTS WITH JOINT PAIN/DEFORMITIES

- Suspected knee and ankle fractures (Ottawa rules positive) and proximal humeral fractures: Radiographs (CT with 3D reconstruction is helpful in surgical planning)

- Shoulder dislocations: AP, Scapular Y view, Axillary or West-point view depending upon patient's comfort

DOI: 10.1201/9781003500247-3

- Suspected elbow, wrist and hand, and foot fractures: Radiographs (2 projections)

- Suspected scaphoid fracture: Scaphoid series, followed by MRI screening if radiographically occult

- Suspected Lisfranc fracture-dislocation: CT

- Any long bone fracture: Radiographs (2 orthogonal projections)

IMAGING OF PATIENTS WITH ATRAUMATIC JOINT PAIN/DEFORMITIES

Any atraumatic joint pain requires discussion between the referring clinical team and radiologists/registrars to formulate appropriate imaging strategy. Such discussions are based on the "surgical sieve" method. Causes of joint pain/deformity include degenerative, post-traumatic, infectious, inflammatory, metabolic (including endocrinal and crystalline disease), and neoplastic causes.

Degenerative (Primary)

- Radiographs in two orthogonal projections such as AP and lateral (first-line imaging); consider weight-bearing radiographs for knees and ankles

- MRI to assess soft tissue and cartilage changes in early OA

- CT to assess bone quality, create patient-specific implant, and intraoperative guidance

- Ultrasound for soft tissue assessment and conservative management such as steroid and hyaluronic acid injection into degenerated joints

Post-Traumatic

- Radiographs (first line) to assess joint changes and deformity

- MRI when ligamentous/soft tissue injuries (ACL or meniscal tear in knee, scapholunate ligament, or TFCC injury in wrist) or post-traumatic osteonecrosis is suspected

- Shoulder dislocations: MR arthrograms vs high-field strength MRI

Infective

- Primary diagnosis is clinical: Symptoms (joint pain, loss of movement, swelling, fever) with biochemical changes (high WBC, CRP, and ESR)

- The role of imaging: (a) To confirm clinical suspicion and early detection; (b) to assess complications such as soft tissue and intraosseous abscesses, osteomyelitis and cartilage degradation, and bony deformities; and (c) to differentiate from mimickers such as inflammatory, crystalline, and metabolic arthropathies

- Radiographs can be normal in early stage

- MRI: Gold standard and sensitive but non-specific

- Ultrasound: Guidance for diagnostic sampling in clinically "dry" taps

Inflammatory

- Clinical decision guided by various criteria and biochemical markers (CRP, rheumatoid factors, different antibodies for various autoimmune/inflammatory disorders) and genetic markers, for example HLA-B27 for axial spondyloarthritis (AxSpA)

- Radiographs (initial imaging) to assess erosions, joint deformities, and calcifications

- Ultrasound with power Doppler imaging to assess synovitis and joint effusion in RA and autoimmune diseases and to detect enthesitis in seronegative spondyloarthritis

- MRI (most sensitive) for erosions, synovitis, tenosynovitis, and bursitis in RA and autoimmune diseases and inflammatory and structural lesions in the spine and SIJs in AxSpA (Chapter 2.13)

Crystalline Arthropathies

- Common: Gout (Monosodium urate), pseudogout (calcium pyrophosphate dihydrate, CPPD, chondro-calcinosis), and hydroxyapatite deposition disease (HADD), each requiring its own imaging strategy:

- Gout: Radiographs (symptomatic joint—extraarticular erosions, soft tissue nodules known as tophi, preserved joint spaces); if in doubt, dual-energy CT, ultrasound, and MRI (less useful). Sometimes, tophi present as sarcoma mimickers—US-guided biopsy vs DECT

- CPPD: Incidental finding in elderly (>80 years) on radiographs and CT

- HADD: May present as septic arthritis; common around tendon insertions; site-specific—shoulder, greater and lesser trochanters, hamstrings. Radiographs (first imaging), followed by CT, ultrasound used for shoulder barbotage (calcific tendinitis), MRI differentiates it from septic arthritis

Metabolic Causes

■ Renal causes: Radiographs for renal osteodystrophy; CT picks up early renal osteodystrophy finding when performed for renal causes; CT and MRI for brown tumours; CT and MRI for amyloid arthropathy in presence of positive biochemical findings (beta2 microglobinemia)

■ Diabetic foot: Serial radiographs for suspected osteomyelitis or treatment response or for neuropathic arthropathy; MRI for non-responding osteomyelitis and complications such as abscess; and digital subtraction angiography for vascular supply before foot preservation surgery or amputation.

Neoplastic Causes (Discussed in Detail in Chapter 1.1)

■ Metastases: Radiographs (for initial diagnosis and fracture risk), followed by MRI (for locoregional spread); staging CT—CT chest, abdomen, and pelvis in most of malignancies; CT head, neck, chest, abdomen, and pelvis in metastatic melanoma; CT neck, chest, abdomen, and pelvis; and PET-CT for lymphoma; bony metastases—bone scan. Full cancer workup depending upon the primary

■ Myeloma: Radiographs and whole-body MRI in presence of biochemical markers

■ Soft tissue and primary bone tumours: Radiographs and ultrasound (triage and biopsy), CT for bone tumour biopsy, MRI for locoregional staging, and staging CT

FURTHER READING

■ NICE/British Orthopaedic Association guidelines for trauma and orthopaedics.

■ RCR major adult trauma radiology guidance.

Chapter 1.3
Back Pain

Siddharth Thaker

LEARNING OBJECTIVES

- To understand various referral pathways through which patients with low back pain present for imaging
- To understand the NICE guidance which underpins the imaging strategies and onwards referral depending upon imaging findings

---

CLINICAL PRESENTATION

Back pain is the most common musculoskeletal complaint presented in primary care and specialist settings. There are numerous referral pathways through which a patient is captured for further imaging and management, including primary care referrals from GPs, advanced-scope physiotherapists, community clinics, and integrated care boards. In addition, patients might seek secondary care or visit specialised institutes for a particular spinal problem. It is important to understand the patient can self-refer to a GP or a physiotherapist or attend an A&E willingly, but the patient CANNOT self-refer oneself for imaging in the NHS. Therefore, MRI request on a patient demand is NOT a valid clinical indication.

The following facts led to the development of NICE guidance for low back pain in adults over 16:

- <5%–10% of all LBP is due to a specific pathology
- The remaining 90%–95% do not indicate a serious cause and should be managed by conservative treatment
- Diagnostic triage can distinguish b/w serious and non-serious causes
- Imaging can do more harm than good when serious conditions are not suspected: Delayed recovery and added cost

NICE guidance and the clinical thinking behind LBP imaging requests are divided according to the treatment setting; imaging will be only helpful when it will affect how the patient will be managed. Although LBP is assessment and imaging strategies differ regionally, the following is one model strategy that could be considered. (We recommend that practising radiologists follow locally agreed guidance and pathways for better outcomes.) Table 1.3.1 gives a number of spine imaging strategies according to their aetiologies.

CLINICAL ASSESSMENT/DIAGNOSTIC TRIAGE

Adult (>16 years) patient with low back pain—Exclude non-spinal causes first

- Hip pathologies
- Referred pain (pancreatitis, pyelonephritis, prostatitis, pancreatic Ca)
- Vascular causes (aortic aneurysm or arterial occlusion)

Adult (>16 years) with specific spinal cause (less than 1%)

- Vertebral fracture/spinal injury
- Suspected malignancy
- Spinal infection
- AxSpA in adults
- Cauda equina syndrome/MSCC

DOI: 10.1201/9781003500247-4

Table 1.3.1 Imaging Criteria for Low Back Pain in Adults by Cause

Suspected Pathology	Demographics/History/Presentation	Imaging/When?
Vertebral fracture	• Older age (>65 years for men, >75 years for women) • Prolonged corticosteroid use • Severe trauma • Presence of contusion or abrasion	Imaging: X-ray or CT Major risk: Immediate Minor risk: Watch and wait
Suspected malignancy	• History of malignancy • Strong clinical suspicion • Unexplained weight loss • >50 years	Imaging: X-ray and MRI followed by staging CT When? 2-week wait
Suspected spinal infection	• Fever or chills • Immune-compromised patient • Pain at rest or at night • Intravenous drug user • Recent injury • Dental or spine procedure	Imaging: X-ray and MRI When? Immediately
Suspected cauda equina syndrome/MSCC (see Chapter 1.6 for details)	• New bowel or bladder dysfunction • Perineal numbness or saddle anaesthesia • Persistent or progressive lower motor neuron changes/neurological deficit at multiple levels	Imaging: MRI (Lumbar spine for ?CES, whole spine for ?MSCC) When? Immediately
Axial spondyloarthritis in over >16 years (See Chapter 2.13 for more details)	• >3 Months back pain, <age 45 OR • Stigmata of inflammatory back pain • <Age 40, insidious, improve with exercise • No improvement with rest, night pain • Peripheral manifestations • Extra-articular manifestations • Family history of AxSpA • Good response to NSAIDs	Imaging: MRI (whole spine and sacroiliac joint MRI in ankylosing spondylitis protocol) + Rheumatology referral

Adults (>16) with radicular symptoms (5%–10%)

- Back pain with leg pain in L4, L5, and S1 distribution

- Positive result on straight leg raise test or crossed straight leg raise twist

- Bilateral buttock, thigh, or leg pain

- Older age

- Pseudoclaudication

Imaging/When?

- Consider MRI in patients who are candidates for surgery

- Defer work until a trial of therapy is completed

Adults (>16 years) with non-specific low back pain (90%–95%)

- Presumed lumbosacral origin of pain

- No tests can reliably detect the source of pain

Recommendations

- Good prognosis and low risk of serious disease

- Immediate imaging is not necessary

- Education and reassurance for self-management

It is important to know the background of the referral and clinical history mentioned in the referral during vetting of such clinical requests. These criteria along with knowledge of locally agreed-on pathways can be used as a generic guide to tackle challenges that arise during daily vetting, reporting, and onwards referral.

SUGGESTED READING

- https://www.nice.org.uk/guidance/NG59

Chapter 1.4
Soft Tissue and Bony Lumps

Siddharth Thaker

LEARNING OBJECTIVES

- To understand sarcoma services in the UK and referral pathways across primary and secondary care services

- To understand the role of imaging in the diagnosis and treatment of sarcomas

---

THE UK SARCOMA SERVICES

Definitive management of all soft tissue and bony sarcomatous lumps happen at specialised sarcoma centres. The UK follows a hub-and-spoke model under which peripheral and community diagnostic sites refer to all suspected sarcomatous cases to a central specialised sarcomatous service. It involves a dedicated sarcoma multidisciplinary team (MDT) consisting of sarcoma surgeons, radiologists, oncologists, pathologists, specialist nurses, and an MDT co-ordinator.

SOFT TISSUE LUMPS

- Most common presentation is a painless enlarging soft tissue mass

- Rare and can occur at any site; deep-seated sarcomas are challenging to diagnose early and have various histological types and grades

- Any soft tissue mass >5 cm associated with pain and enlargement is referred directly to regional sarcoma service

- NICE 2015 guidance for early diagnosis of soft tissue sarcoma in the primary care:
  - Consider 2-week wait ultrasound to assess for soft tissue sarcoma in adults with unexplained lump that is enlarging
  - Consider 2-week wait suspected cancer pathway referral in patients with ultrasound suggestive of soft tissue sarcoma or ultrasound findings are uncertain and clinical suspicion remains high

- Benign lipomas are the most common soft tissue lumps presented to primary care. The British Sarcoma Group has provided specific guidance to primary care and sonographers to provide urgent referrals to the regional sarcoma service.

IMAGING IN A SUSPECTED SOFT TISSUE SARCOMA AT REGIONAL SARCOMA SERVICES

Initial Diagnosis

- Ultrasound: Most frequently employed imaging technique. Works as an effective triage tool and can diagnose certain conditions like cysts, arteriovenous malformations, and benign lipomas with confidence. Can be highly user dependent and uncertain, and MRI is helpful

- MRI: Provides accurate diagnostic information for trunk, extremity, and pelvic sarcomas; helps surgical and diagnostic planning

- X-rays: Limited role in soft tissue sarcomas, detect calcifications, identify bone involvement, and assess fracture risk

- CT: Reserved for intrathoracic and retroperitoneal sarcomas

Staging

- Chest X-ray: Usually sufficient for low-grade sarcoma, low metastatic potential, elderly, or frail patients with low-volume systemic burden and no significant treatment implication

DOI: 10.1201/9781003500247-5

- CT chest: All intermediate- to high-grade sarcoma before definitive treatment
- Staging CT including chest, abdomen, and pelvis: Myxoid liposarcoma, leiomyosarcoma, and all high-grade sarcomas of lower limb

Sarcoma-Specific Additional Imaging for Complete Staging and Follow-Up

- Regional lymph node assessment by US/MRI: Synovial sarcoma, angiosarcoma, clear cell sarcoma, or epithelioid sarcoma
- Chest X-ray follow-up: ALT without features of dedifferentiation
- Staging CT + whole-body MRI: Myxoid liposarcoma
- Contrast CT/MRI of the brain: Alveolar soft tissue sarcoma and clear cell sarcoma
- PET-CT: Ewing's sarcoma and rhabdomyosarcoma in young patients and suspected MPNST in neurofibromatosis type 1 patients

Post-Treatment Follow-Up

- Mostly clinical
- Follow up with localised MRI if any new abnormality at the previously treated site
- CT if the primary site is difficult to follow-up clinically, e.g. intrathoracic or retroperitoneal tumours
- Chest X-ray followed up by CT if any abnormality

BONY LUMP

- Most common presentation is bone pain and/or swelling; uncommonly pathological fracture or neurological symptoms/spinal cord compression in primary spinal tumours.
- Night pain is a red flag; investigate further if present.
- History of recent injury DOES NOT exclude primary bone sarcoma.
- Following clinical history and examination, X-ray of the affected site is the most commonly performed imaging investigation.
- Investigate further if bone destruction, new bone formation, periosteal reaction, or soft tissue swelling.
- Normal X-ray DOES NOT exclude primary bone sarcoma.
- Persistent mass or pain requires MRI +/− bone sarcoma centre referral.
- If the patient is under age 40: X-rays and MRI of the local site with urgent referral to regional bone sarcoma centre.
- If the patient is over 40: Rule out metastasis and myeloma first. Use CT chest, abdomen, and pelvis with contrast, whole-body MRI, isotope bone scan, and myeloma screen to confirm number of lesions/primary tumour. If solitary bone lesion with persistent clinical suspicion of sarcoma, refer to bone tumour centre.
- Primary care GPs should be aware to refer patients with suspected bone sarcoma straight to regional bone sarcoma centre.

IMAGING IN A SUSPECTED PRIMARY BONE SARCOMA AT REGIONAL SARCOMA SERVICES

Initial Diagnosis

- X-rays of the local site in two orthogonal planes
- MRI of the local site: Cover entire involved bone and adjacent joints
- CT to detect microcalcification, periosteal new bone formation, and cortical destruction
- MRI and CT for pelvic tumours
- Dynamic contrast-enhanced MRI in chondrosarcoma to identify biopsy targets

Staging

- CT chest for all bone sarcomas
- Follow-up CT chest for all indeterminate nodules on CT chest
- Whole-body MRI and PET-CT for staging and treatment response in Ewing's sarcoma and osteosarcoma
- Clinical assessment + localised MRI + CT chest for chemotherapy response assessment

Follow-Up

- Low-grade bone sarcomas: Follow-up at intervals of 2–4 months for the first 3 years after completion of therapy, every 6 months for years 4 and 5, and annually thereafter till 10 years; annual X-ray/CT chest surveillance up to 5 years
- Intermediate-grade bone sarcomas: Every 3 months for 2 years and then annually up to 10 years
- High-grade sarcomas: Every 3 months for first 2 years, then every 6 months from years 2 to 5, and annually from years 5 to 10
- Standard imaging follow-up: Chest X-ray + local site X-ray + clinical assessment
- For chordoma/pelvic tumours: MRI of the pelvis

Secondary cancers can occur in survivors of primary bone sarcoma. Secondary leukemia (especially acute myeloid leukemia) can happen within 5 years or later. Consider genetic profiling including whole-genome sequencing, cancer surveillance, and genetic counselling in patients with predisposition syndromes, e.g. Li-Fraumeni syndrome.

SUGGESTED READING

- https://www.england.nhs.uk/commissioning/publication/sarcoma-services-all-ages/

Chapter 1.5
Acute or Chronic Injury of Muscles, Tendons, and Ligaments

Siddharth Thaker

LEARNING OBJECTIVES

- To enumerate common musculoskeletal pathologies encountered in daily practice according to joints

- To understand the use of the most efficient imaging method according to suspected musculoskeletal pathologies

---

Soft tissue injuries are common presentations in both primary and secondary care settings. In primary care, the patient usually presents to GPs, specialised GPs, musculoskeletal triage units, extended-scope physiotherapists, or extended community clinics from secondary care; in secondary care settings, the patient may present to orthopaedic and sports medicine outpatient clinics, fracture clinics, and A&Es.

Patient categories included participants in competitive sports, leisure, or recreational sports activities; persons without appropriate strength training or nutrition; and persons with or without a history of trauma presenting with clinical symptoms of soft tissue injury, e.g. pain, laxity, or lack/reduction in normal movements.

Imaging strategies for soft tissue injuries vary depending upon the patient's demographics, activities, type of injury suspected, and whether or level of sports performance and return-to-play is required or not.

Generally, paediatric injuries to muscles, tendons, and ligaments are less common, as soft tissue structures are more pliable. It makes bone–tendon, bone–muscle, and bone–ligament junction more prone to avulsion-type injuries. X-rays are the initial imaging technique of choice. Ultrasound is used sometimes to detect muscle and tendon injuries in adolescent athlete patients. Ultrasound is also useful in a few selected interventions for performance-related injuries if required.

In adults, acute or chronic injuries to soft tissue are usually diagnosed clinically. Most injuries are low-grade and self-resolving and DO NOT require any additional imaging. However, imaging is usually sought after once symptoms of such injuries start limiting daily activity or performance.

Acute injuries classically present with trauma history, sudden loss of function, and concomitant symptoms; chronic injuries, on the other hand, are repetitive stress and microtrauma related. Clinical history of acute trauma is usually absent. They are difficult to diagnose and treat. Such injuries usually require multidisciplinary treatments—including physiotherapy rehabilitation, image-guided interventions and rarely, surgical treatments. Table 1.5.1 lists common upper limb injuries and imaging investigations, and Table 1.5.2 lists the same for lower limbs.

Table 1.5.1 Common Upper Limb Pathologies and Imaging Strategies

Anatomical Region	Injured Area and Technique
Shoulder	■ Rotator cuff tendons—Ultrasound followed by MRI ■ Glenoid labrum—MRI arthrography/less commonly CT arthrography ■ Long head of biceps tendon (proximal)—US followed by MRI
Elbow	■ Distal biceps tendon—US followed by MRI ■ Traumatic elbow injuries—X-ray/CT followed by MRI ■ Lateral epicondylitis (tennis elbow)—US, less commonly MRI ■ Medial epicondylitis (golfer's elbow)—US, less commonly MRI ■ Triceps injuries (rare)—US/MRI ■ Osteochondral injuries—MR arthrogram

(Continued)

DOI: 10.1201/9781003500247-6

Table 1.5.1 (Continued) Common Upper Limb Pathologies and Imaging Strategies

Anatomical Region	Injured Area and Technique
Wrist	■ Scaphoid fracture—X-rays followed by CT or MRI ■ Scapholunate or lunotriquetral injury—MRI or MR arthrogram ■ TFCC injury—MRI or MR arthrogram ■ Extensor tendon injuries—US followed by MRI ■ Flexor tendon injuries—US followed by MRI
Hand	■ Pulley injuries/trigger finger/thumb—High-resolution US ■ Bony avulsions—X-rays followed by US ■ MRI—depends on image acquisition quality

Table 1.5.2 Common Lower Limb Pathologies and Imaging Strategies

Anatomical Region	Injured Area and Technique
Pelvis	■ Hamstrings/adductors/gluteal tendon injuries—MRI + US for interventions ■ Avulsions at ASIS and AIIS—X-rays followed by MRI ■ Hip labrum—MR arthrogram ■ FAI—X-ray pelvis followed by MRI pelvis
Knee	■ Ligamentous and meniscal injuries—MRI ■ Capsular and corner injuries—MRI ■ Quadriceps and patellar tendon pathologies—US followed by MRI ■ Osteochondral injuries—MRI ■ Intra-articular fractures—MRI or CT ■ Proximal tibiofibular joint instability—MRI
Tibia and fibula	■ Stress fractures/MTSS—X-rays followed by MRI
Ankle	■ High ankle sprain (ligamentous injury)—MRI, less commonly X-rays ■ Low ankle sprain (ATFL injury)—MRI ■ Osteochondral injury—MRI ■ Tibialis posterior tendinopathy/peroneal subluxations/Achilles tendon tendinopathies/Achilles tendon tear/plantar fasciitis—US, uncommonly MRI ■ Metatarsal stress fractures—X-rays followed by MRI ■ Morton's neuroma/Intermetatarsal bursitis—US/MRI

Whenever avulsion fractures or stress fractures are suspected, X-ray followed by MRI is common. Ultrasound is the investigation of choice for interventions for intramuscular haematoma aspiration in muscle injuries; dry needling or platelet-rich plasma injection in chronic tendinopathies; and steroid injections and high-volume saline injection with Achilles tendinopathy.

Chapter 1.6
Symptoms of Cord or Cauda Equina Compression

Siddharth Thaker

LEARNING OBJECTIVES

- To understand the variety of presentations of cord, cauda equina, and nerve root compression in primary care, community services, and emergency (secondary care services)

- To appreciate initial investigation strategies, clinical reasoning, and governance guidelines dictating the urgency of the imaging investigations

---

IMPORTANCE

Most UK radiology registrars and consultants encounter at least one instance during their on-call shifts where they have to report imaging performed for suspected CES or cord compression. The two pathologies have distinct presentations and management strategies, and cases are pass/fail when presented in the table viva or as long cases for FRCR 2B. For discussion purposes, cord compression is taken as metastatic spinal cord compression (MSCC), which mostly has acute presentation or rapid deteriorating symptoms. Chronic cord compression either due to long-standing disc–osteophyte complexes or spinal tumours are discussed in Chapter 2.3.

SUSPECTED CAUDA EQUINA SYNDROME (?CES)

CES is a clinical diagnosis confirmed by the presence of a combination of symptoms and clinical signs. MRI alone cannot diagnose CES; no single symptom or clinical sign is pathognomonic.

- Commonest causes: A large lumbar disc prolapse

- Uncommon causes: Trauma, epidural haematoma (following anaesthesia), epidural abscess (from spondylodiscitis or septic facet arthritis), tumour in the spinal canal

- Mimickers: Pelvic tumour or lymphadenopathy, presacral space irritation (recent ovarian cyst rupture), sacral insufficiency fractures (**Tip:** *Scrutinise localiser images of the MRI, assess the last/far sagittal or axial images carefully to rule out the mimickers, check STIR images when available for marrow oedema or replacement*)

Warning Signs

Sudden-onset bilateral radicular leg pain *or* unilateral radicular leg pain progressing to bilateral leg pain.

- Symptoms: Leg/back pain + recent onset (<14 days) or worsening of **any one** of the following:

  - Difficult initiation of micturition/Impaired urinary flow sensation

  - S2-S5 dermatome (perineal, perianal, or genital) sensation

  - Loss of sensation of rectal fullness

  - Sexual dysfunction

  - Progressive neurological deficit/major lower limb motor weakness (e.g. foot drop)

MRI is the best and most crucial imaging investigation (**Tip:** *Recent GIRFT guidance suggests the MRI certainly needs to be performed* **within 4 hours** *of the initial request to radiology*).

Critical Governance and Medicolegal Guidance Pertaining to MRI Requests for ?CES

- Most referrals come from the ED

- Discussion with on-call spinal services is **NOT** required before the MRI request

- An emergent ?CES MRI takes precedence over any routine or elective MRI

- MRI request should be discussed with ST4 equivalent or senior before referral

- If MRI is contraindicated, a CT scan or CT myelogram (at a neurosurgical centre) needs to be performed

- On-call surgical teams are happy to review the out-of-hours scans before a radiologist report

- Prevent image exchange portal delay

- Network-wide webPACS links should be available to surgical teams when imaging is acquired at different geographical sites

- See Table 1.6.1 for the common clinical team responses to common imaging outcomes

METASTATIC SPINAL CORD COMPRESSION (MSCC)

MSCC is an *oncological emergency*. It is defined as compression of the spinal cord and/or cauda equina by pathological vertebral collapse and/or direct tumour expansion. It presents as a past or current cancer diagnosis + presence of any one of the following:

- Bladder or bowel dysfunction

- Limb weakness

- Gait instability

- Radicular pain, numbness, paraesthesia, or sensory loss

- Neurological signs of spinal cord or cauda equina compression

Imaging Investigations of Spinal Metastases and/or Suspected MSCC

- To be overseen by a radiologist to ensure appropriate and complete imaging is (a) performed and (b) promptly reported

- MRI is the investigation of choice for suspected MSCC

- Offer an MRI to the patient with suspected MSCC *as soon as possible* (and always within 24 hours)

- Offer an MRI to the patient with clinical suspicion of spinal metastases but **NO** suspicion of impending MSCC *within 1 week* to guide treatment options

- Offer an overnight MRI only in clinical circumstances **where urgent diagnosis is needed to start the treatment urgently**

- In people with known spinal metastases, **DO NOT perform MRI** *solely for the detection of early cord compression* **when there are no clinical signs or symptoms of MSCC**

- If MRI is contraindicated, consider CT scan for suspected MSCC/spinal metastases

- Myelography should only be performed at a neuroscience or spinal surgical centre

- Do not perform a plain X-ray of the spine to diagnose or rule out spinal metastases or MSCC

- Multiplanar or 3-plane reconstruction of recent or new CT images to (a) assess spinal stability **and** (b) plan vertebroplasty, kyphoplasty or spinal surgery

Table 1.6.1 Imaging Findings and Clinical Team Actions

Imaging Outcomes	Action Required by Clinical Team
Confirmed cauda equina compression (no evidence of CSF around nerve roots/critical canal stenosis)	■ Urgent spinal surgical services referral ■ Keep the patient nil by mouth ■ If transfer required, cat 2 blue light ambulance transfer
Neural compression explaining the radicular symptoms but no confirmed cauda equina compression	■ Safety net against CES symptoms progression ■ Advice the patient that the pain is very much likely to improve ■ Referral to MSK triage services
No cause of CES found	■ Consider alterative diagnoses and referrals

Tip: All impending or confirmed MSCC patients need personalised care plans and involvement of acute oncology services. All NHS Trusts have MSCC referral and/or management policies. (*Make sure to convey the urgent need to communicate the report and document who was spoken to along with the time and date on the EPR/RIS. Trust-specified MSCC guidance if asked during the viva would be well-received by examiners.*)

ONWARDS SPINAL MANAGEMENT (PER NICE GUIDANCE)

When the person is diagnosed with confirmed MSCC, further management is usually directed to one of the following three pathways:

- Surgical intervention is suitable: Consider surgical decompression of the spinal cord + surgical stabilisation of the spine
- Surgical intervention is NOT suitable and no radiotherapy: Offer external spinal support such as halo vest or cervico-thoraco-lumbar orthosis in patient with suspected or confirmed mechanical instability AND the pain is not controlled by analgesics
- Radiotherapy is suitable but surgical decompression is NOT: Offer urgent radiotherapy (8 Gy single fraction) if the patient has paraplegia/tetraplegia for more than 2 weeks and pain is well controlled and overall prognosis is poor; if the patient develops spinal instability after treatment, consider halo vest or orthosis

SUGGESTED READING

- https://www.rcr.ac.uk/our-services/all-our-publications/clinical-radiology-publications/mri-provision-for-cauda-equina-syndrome/
- https://gettingitrightfirsttime.co.uk/wp-content/uploads/2023/10/National-Suspected-Cauda-Equina-Pathway-UPDATED-V2-October-2023.pdf
- https://www.nice.org.uk/guidance/ng234/chapter/Recommendations#imaging-investigations
- https://spinesurgeons.ac.uk/resources/Documents/News/Cauda_Equina_Syndrome_Standards_SBNS_BASS%20-%20Dec%202018.pdf

Chapter 1.7
Scoliosis

Tsz Shing Joshua Wong, Siddharth Thaker, and Harun Gupta

LEARNING OBJECTIVES

- To understand the significance of reporting nomenclature when interpreting radiological studies of scoliosis

- To explore the various causes of scoliosis and crucial factors influencing treatment strategies

- To gain insight into the different treatment approaches available for different types of scoliosis

- To evaluate the role of follow-up imaging in both treatment planning and monitoring disease progression

---

Scoliosis is defined by an exaggerated lateral curvature of the spine, diagnosed radiologically when the Cobb angle exceeds 10°. A Cobb angle of 10° or less is termed spinal asymmetry.

Idiopathic scoliosis is disease without an apparent cause. If it occurs before age 10, it is labelled early-onset or juvenile idiopathic scoliosis and adolescent idiopathic scoliosis if it develops after age 10. Idiopathic scoliosis predominantly affects the cervicothoracic spine, and it is progressive. **Neuromuscular scoliosis** occurs in cerebral palsy or muscular dystrophy, **congenital or infantile scoliosis** is present at birth, and **adult-onset degenerative scoliosis** occurs as a part of normal spinal degeneration. Sometimes vertebral fracture and infection can cause premature degeneration. Systemic causes include neurofibromatosis type 1, Marfan's syndrome, enzyme storage disorders, and genetic disorders.

IMAGING MODALITIES AND REPORTING NOMENCLATURE

Whole-spine radiographs (anteroposterior and lateral) serve as the primary modality for scoliosis imaging (to be requested by managing spinal surgeon). Radiographs may repeated during subsequent visits depending upon initial findings (see Section 1.7.4 on guidelines). Serial radiographs are compared for complete assessments of progression at each visit.

CT and MRI are utilised when structural abnormalities like neuropathic conditions (e.g. spinal cord tumours) are suspected. Cross-sectional studies also aid in surgical planning and assessing postoperative complications. Precise documentation of spinal curve characteristics is essential. Depending on institutional protocols, Cobb angle measurement may be part of standard reporting. Table 1.7.1 lists key descriptors for scoliosis evaluation.

TREATMENT

Scoliosis treatment is determined by the curvature's severity and rate of progression. Younger patients with skeletal immaturity are at greater risk of progression; once skeletal maturity is achieved, ongoing monitoring is only necessary for cases with a Cobb angle of 30° or greater.

CONSERVATIVE TREATMENT

- Treatment approaches encompass observation, bracing, physical therapy, and surgical intervention. Since the risk of progression reduces with age, serial clinical review may be preferred especially in milder cases, particularly in those close to skeletal maturity.

- In moderate cases (Cobb angle 20°–45°), bracing can be employed to stop or slow progression during skeletal growth, reducing the likelihood of surgery by slowing progression during skeletal growth. Please review the standards for imaging in bracing in the suggested reading. Bracing is not indicated for idiopathic scoliosis in skeletally mature individuals. Physical therapy exercises are designed to enhance postural alignment, optimise muscular symmetry, and improve spinal flexibility, thereby reducing the need for bracing or surgery.

DOI: 10.1201/9781003500247-8

Table 1.7.1 Imaging Abnormalities in Scoliosis

Nomenclature	Comments
Curve direction	A simpler way to characterise curvature is by describing the direction in which the **convexity** points
Cobb angle and end vertebrae	Used to measure the extent of spinal deformities The two most-tilted vertebrae (uppermost and lowermost) are identified; lines are drawn along their endplates Cobb angle is measured between the two lines of intersection Scoliosis is defined by a Cobb angle >10°. Cobb angle measurements should be interpreted with awareness of inter-observer discrepancies, variations in imaging projections, and shifts in patient positioning from prior studies, particularly when monitoring scoliosis progression
Apex/apical vertebrae	The vertebrae or disc spaces showing the greatest deviation from the expected central alignment of the spine
Neutral vertebrae	Usually found on either side of the apex and showing no axial plane rotation; can be the same as the end vertebrae, but are generally located several segments beyond the apex
Stable vertebra	The first vertebra situated below the lowest spinal curve, positioned close to the center of the central sacral vertical line
Sagittal and coronal balance	Erect whole-spine radiographs for evaluating sagittal and coronal alignment by drawing a vertical line from the C7 midpoint to the sacrum, with a deviation of more than 2 cm from the midline suggesting abnormal balance
Underlying bony abnormalities	Possible contributing factors to scoliosis can be identified through clues such as acute vertebral body fractures, infections, segmentation defects, congenital structural deformities, and sinister bony lesions

BRITISH SCOLIOSIS SOCIETY AND NICE GUIDANCE ON SURGICAL TREATMENT FOR SCOLIOSIS BEFORE SKELETAL MATURITY

Treatment of idiopathic scoliosis depends on age, severity and location of the spinal curve, and pattern/progression.

■ Mild scoliosis: Close monitoring (6- to 9-month clinical and X-ray follow-up by spinal surgeon) and physical therapy

■ Moderate to severe scoliosis: Casting and bracing

Vertebral body tethering is a non-fusion spinal treatment for idiopathic scoliosis that involves installing vertebral screws and rods through the convex side, restricting growth whilst allowing concave side free growth correcting the spinal deformity (Hueter–Volkmann Law). NICE recommendations for vertebral body tethering are that it is indicated (a) for patients with progressive scoliosis who still have significant growth potential, (b) when conservative treatments including bracing have failed, (c) when it does not preclude a subsequent posterior spinal surgery, and (d) when more than one device is available.

SURGICAL TREATMENT FOR SCOLIOSIS AFTER SKELETAL MATURITY AND ADULT-ONSET DEGENERATIVE SCOLIOSIS

■ Posterior instrumented correction and fusion

■ Adult degenerative scoliosis: Decompression alone, posterolateral fusion with decompression, posterior instrumented scoliosis correction with vertebral cages and osteotomies, and anterior and posterior instrumented scoliosis correction

■ Kyphosis: Posterior instrumented correction and fusion

■ Spondylolisthesis: Injections around the nerve roots or joints, posterolateral fusion with rods and screws and sometimes interbody cages (struts)

SUGGESTED READING

■ https://www.nice.org.uk/guidance/ipg728

■ https://britscoliosis.org.uk/Standards-of-Care (search for bracing in adolescent idiopathic scoliosis)

SECTION 2

IMAGING ASSESSMENT AND FEATURES OF MUSCULOSKELETAL PATHOLOGIES

Chapter 2.1
Acute and Chronic Spine Trauma

Rahoz Aziz and James Baren

LEARNING OBJECTIVES

- Appreciate the importance of understanding the anatomy and mechanism of injury when reporting traumatic imaging of the spine

- Understand the different imaging modalities used and when they are indicated

- Recognise the common and important injuries of the spine and how to determine spinal stability

- How to differentiate acute from chronic spinal injuries

Spinal trauma reporting is a core requirement of the RCR curriculum because all consultants and registrars face at least one polytrauma case during each on-call shift. This chapter is essential to those who are involved in A&E and on-call reporting. Chapters in Section 2 end with single best answer (SBA) questions and answers to review content.

INTRODUCTION

Spinal injury is a significant cause of morbidity and mortality globally with significant socio-economic implications. Injuries can be acute or chronic, and imaging has a central role in determining the chronicity when the clinical history is not available. Imaging confirms the location of the injury and allows for describing the injury pattern and assessing spinal stability. In order to effectively evaluate the traumatic spine, it is essential to understand the anatomy and recognise the mechanism of injury, which is often unknown. This will assist in providing a clinically relevant report and help determine the likelihood of associated ligamentous and neurological injury. There are various classifications systems used for spinal trauma, including the Denis three-column concept and the more recent AO system (much favoured by spinal surgeons). Most classifications are based on the imaging findings and the associated mechanism of injury, and the classification system used depends on local preferences.

ANATOMY

Bones

The spine is composed of 33 vertebrae: 7 cervical, 12 thoracic, 5 lumbar, 5 sacral, and 4 coccygeal segments. Each vertebra has a body, pedicles, laminae, and spinous and transverse processes. Intervertebral discs separate adjacent vertebrae and provide flexibility.

Ligaments

The spinal ligaments and paraspinal muscles provide stability to the spine. The anterior longitudinal ligament (ALL) runs along the anterior margin of the vertebral bodies. Superiorly, at the level of the body of the axis (C1), it continues as the anterior atlantoaxial membrane and then as the anterior atlantooccipital membrane. The posterior longitudinal ligament (PLL) extends from the posterior aspect of the vertebral bodies to the tectorial membrane, which in turn blends with the dura mater along the clivus. The ligamentum flavum connects the laminae of adjacent vertebrae from C2 to S1. The spinous processes are connected by the interspinous ligaments. The supraspinous ligament extends between the tips of the adjacent spinous processes from C7 to S1. The posterior ligamentous complex comprises the facet joint capsule, ligamentum flavum, and the interspinous and supraspinous ligaments and is frequently used in reports and classification systems. The posterior tension band also includes the osseous posterior vertebral elements. The anterior tension band refers to the ALL and disc. Figure 2.1.1 demonstrates the normal anatomy of the spinal ligaments. The craniocervical junction is complex and consists of multiple stabilising ligaments that are beyond the scope of this text.

DOI: 10.1201/9781003500247-10

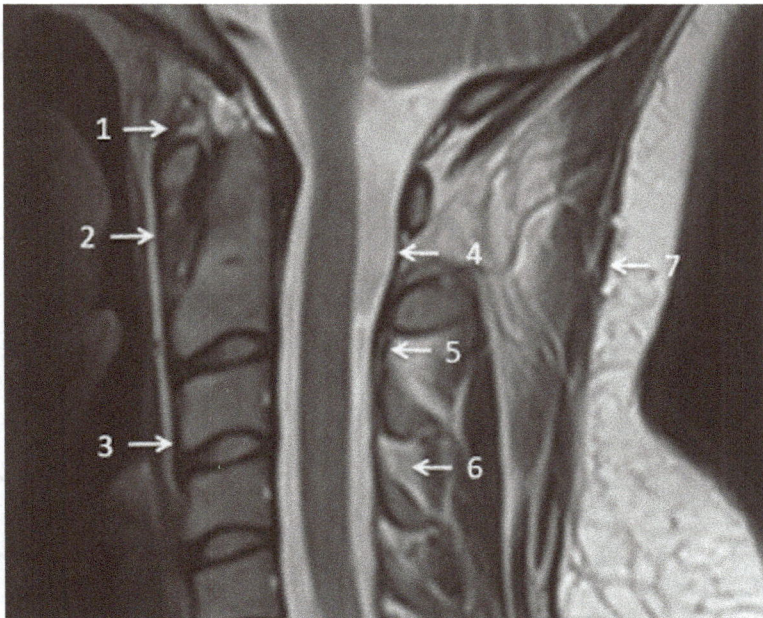

Figure 2.1.1 Normal anatomy of the cervical spine: 1, T2W sagittal MRI showing the apical ligament; 2, anterior atlantoaxial membrane; 3, anterior longitudinal ligament; 4, posterior atlantoaxial membrane; 5, flaval ligament; 6, interspinous ligament; 7, nuchal ligament.

Cord

The spinal cord extends caudally from the medulla oblongata below the foramen magnum. It descends through the spinal canal and terminates as the conus medullaris, typically at around the T12/L1 level in adults. The nerve roots that extend caudally from the conus are collectively called the cauda equina.

Nerves

There are 8 cervical, 12 thoracic, 5 lumbar, 5 sacral, and 1 coccygeal paired nerve roots (Table 2.1.1). The cervical exiting nerve roots exit through the neural (or intervertebral) foramen corresponding to the more caudal segment at the intervertebral disc level. For example, the C5 nerve root exits through the C4-C5 neural foramen. An exception is the C8 nerve roots, which exit through the C7-T1 neural foramen. The thoracic, lumbar, and S1 to S4 nerve roots all exit through the neural foramina corresponding to the more cranial segment at the intervertebral disc level. Thus, the L1 spinal exiting nerve lies below the L1 vertebra, in the L1–L2 intervertebral foramen, the L2 spinal nerve lies below the L2 vertebra, in the L2–L3 foramen, and so on. Lastly, the S5 and coccygeal nerve roots exit through the sacral hiatus.

TRANSITIONAL LUMBOSACRAL VERTEBRA

Lumbosacral transitional vertebrae (LSTV) are a frequent anatomical variant, observed in approximately 25% of the general population. It is defined as either sacralisation of the lowest lumbar segment or lumbarisation of the most superior sacral segment of the spine, with sacralisation of L5 being most common (Figure 2.1.2).

The degree of transition can range from partial to complete fusion. It is essential to accurately identify spinal levels and describe LSTV in the radiology report, as failure to recognise this variant or provide an accurate description of spinal levels can result in procedures being performed at incorrect levels.

Table 2.1.1 Spinal Nerve Roots and Their Corresponding Exit Levels

Spinal Region	Nerve Roots	Exit Level (Neural Foramen)
Cervical	8 pairs	Above corresponding vertebrae (C1–C8)
Thoracic	12 pairs	Below corresponding vertebrae (T1–T12)
Lumbar	5 pairs	Below corresponding vertebrae (L1–L5)
Sacral	5 pairs	Below corresponding vertebrae (S1–S5)
Coccygeal	1 pair	Sacral hiatus

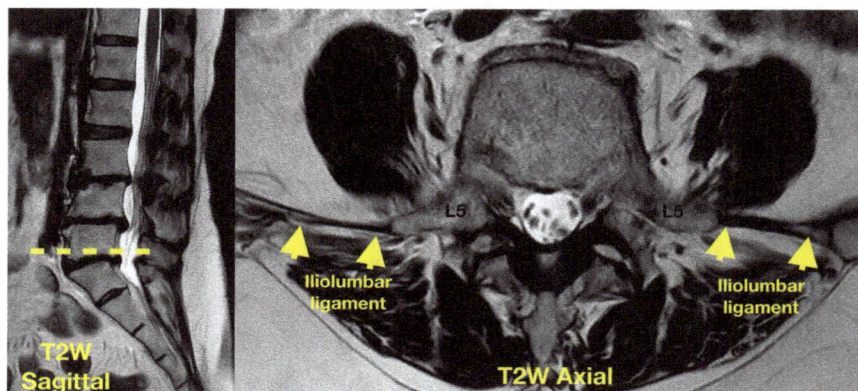

Figure 2.1.2 Lumbosacral transitional level.

HOW TO IDENTIFY LSTV AND CORRECTLY LABEL THE SPINE

- **Accurate enumeration:** The most precise method involves counting inferiorly from C2 if the whole spine has been imaged or using the whole-spine localiser sequences if available.

- **Iliolumbar ligaments:** They almost always arise from the L5 transverse processes and are therefore present at L5–S1.

IMAGING MODALITIES

In the acute traumatic setting with a high suspicion of significant injury, the initial modality of choice is CT (typically in the form of a polytrauma scan). Depending on the CT findings and/or the neurologic status of the patient, MRI is used to further assess ligamentous and neurological injuries. Plain radiographs have a role in chronic injuries and in paediatric patients but have little role in adult polytrauma patients (Table 2.1.2).

CT

CT is the imaging modality of choice for assessing the bones for fractures and alignment and is ideal for multiply injured patients as it is quick and can assess for injuries beyond the spine. A typical polytrauma protocol consists of volumetric imaging of the whole spine with sagittal, coronal, and axial reformats.

MRI

MRI provides excellent assessment of the spinal cord, ligaments, and surrounding soft tissues and is indicated if there is suspicion of injury to these structures either on the initial CT or clinically. MRI can also accurately identify epidural haematoma, the presence of which may influence surgical management. A typical imaging protocol includes axial and sagittal T2-weighted sequences as well as sagittal T1 and STIR sequences, but protocols will vary between institutions (Table 2.1.3). In traumatic setting, whole-spine MRI is recommended to detect potential multilevel spinal injuries.

Table 2.1.2 Primary Imaging Modalities in Spinal Trauma

	Plain Radiograph	CT	MRI
Benefits	• Quick and readily available • Lower radiation dose than with CT, particularly important in the paediatric population	• High sensitivity for detection of bony injuries • Quick and readily available	• Excellent soft tissue resolution; can accurately assess for ligamentous and neurological injuries • Can detect bone marrow contusions and fractures that may be occult on CT • No radiation
Limitations	• Low sensitivity and specificity for the detection of injuries • Assessment can be impaired by radiographic factors, the degenerative spine, and body habitus	• Cannot assess soft tissue structures, e.g. ligaments, nerves, spinal cord • High radiation dose	• Not as accurate as CT for assessing fractures • Availability is limited • Long acquisition time

MRI Protocol

Table 2.1.3 Different MRI Sequences and Their Uses

Sequence	Orientation	Benefits
T1W	Sagittal	• Mainly used for depiction of anatomy and fractures
T2W	Sagittal and axial	• Used to assess the cord, nerves, and spinal canal • Good at detecting bony and soft tissue oedema
STIR	Sagittal	• Very sensitive for detection of oedema, diagnosing soft tissue and ligamentous injuries, particularly of the interspinous or supraspinous ligaments

IMAGING ASSESSMENT

Assessing the Bones

CT is the imaging modality of choice for identifying fractures and traumatic dislocation. Each vertebral level should be assessed in all planes, paying close attention to any subtle vertebral body or facet malignment that could signify ligamentous injury. The spine should be scrutinised for prevertebral soft tissue swelling, which can be a sign of significant spinal trauma warranting further investigation. Cervical prevertebral oedema is common following intubation, so extra care is warranted in the assessment of ventilated patients. Comparison with any prior imaging can help in determining whether changes are acute or chronic.

Assessing the Cord

MRI provides excellent assessment of the spinal cord, particularly T2W sequences. The most common finding in spinal trauma is cord oedema, indicated by T2 hyperintensity and focal enlargement of the cord (Figure 2.1.3). The length of oedema within the cord correlates both with the neurological presentation and clinical functional outcome. Cord contusion and haemorrhage are the most important imaging prognostic factors in spinal cord trauma and are associated with poor prognosis. Contusions are demonstrated by a thin high T2 signal rim around a smaller, central low T1 signal. Cord haemorrhage appears similar but has a thick T2 signal rim rather than the thin rim seen in contusions. Cord transection is the most severe cord injury, demonstrated by a complete disruption of the cord with fluid signal seen between the portions of the severed cord on T2-weighted images.

Assessing the Ligaments

Ligaments normally are displayed as low signal intensity bands on all MR sequences. The notable exception is the interspinous ligament, which may have a striated appearance with low signal intensity areas interspersed with hyperintense foci related to fat on T1-weighted imaging. Ligamentous injuries can be partial or complete. Partial tears are hyperintense signal regions on STIR and T2-weighted sequences, relating to oedema or haemorrhage, with varying degrees of fiber disruption (Figure 2.1.3). With complete tears, there is a complete lack of intact fibers, with additional oedema and haemorrhage. Stripping of the ligaments can occur; in ALL, it can present as a focal area of discontinuity, with laxity/wavy appearance of the ligament that has stripped away from the bone.

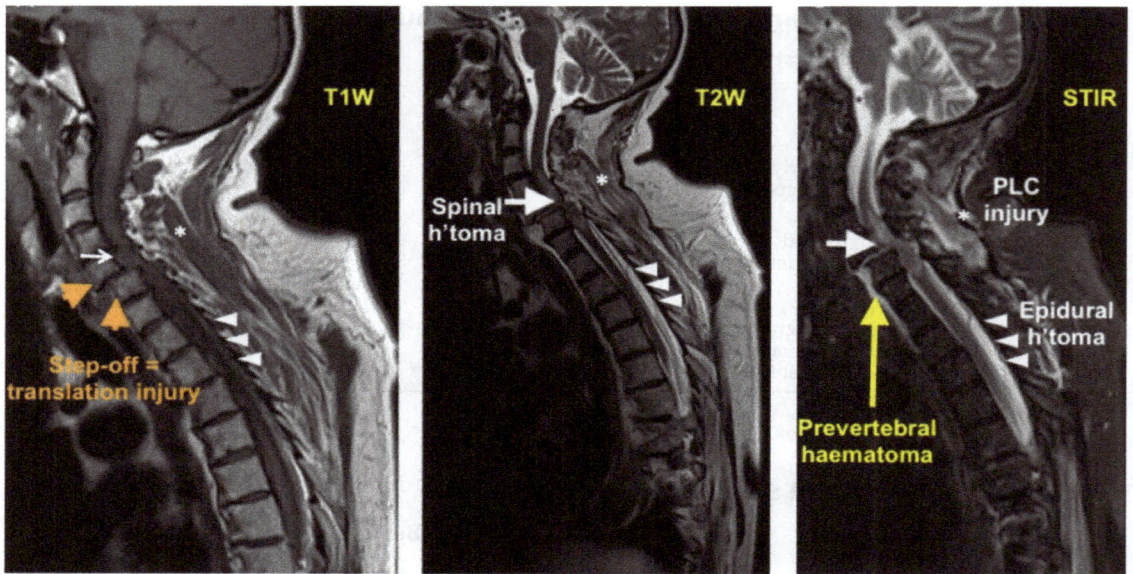

Figure 2.1.3 Spinal translational injury with cord damage and epidural haematoma.

Assessing for Haematoma

Epidural haematoma is a frequent finding in spinal trauma and is most common in the cervicothoracic region (Figure 2.1.3). The signal intensity of haematoma varies with age but is iso- or hyperintense to the cord on T1 imaging and heterogeneously hyperintense on fluid-sensitive sequences. It is important to describe any associated cord compression as well as the degree of cerebrospinal fluid effacement. The presence of epidural haematoma is also important information for the spinal surgical team, as posterior decompression may be required in addition to fixation.

CERVICAL SPINE

Cervical spine injuries are frequently encountered, with approximately 30% of injuries occurring at C2 and 50% at C6/C7. Cervical injuries can occur due to direct trauma, axial loading, rotation, hyper-flexion, or hyper-extension, with hyper-flexion injuries being most common.

Upper Cervical Fractures (C0–C3)

Occipital Condyle (C0)

C0 fractures are rare injuries that result from high-energy blunt trauma. As they may be associated with craniocervical instability, these fractures are important to identify and are best seen on coronal and sagittal CT reformats. Enlarged assymmetrical joint spaces can indicate injury; the occipitoatlantal joint should be <2 mm, and the atlantoaxial joint should be <3 mm (Figure 2.1.4).

Atlas (C1)

Atlas injuries are typically burst fractures of the ring of C1 with fractures in two or more places, commonly with lateral displacement of both articular masses (Figure 2.1.5). These fractures are the result of axial loading, with the forces driving the occipital condyles into the lateral masses of C1. The vertebral arteries are at high risk of injury (dissection and/or thrombosis) or spasm due to local inflammation that can result in neurologic deficit, and CT angiogram should be considered.

Odontoid Peg (C2)

Odontoid peg is the most common traumatic lesion of the C2, accounting for 10% to 15% of all cervical fractures and is rarely associated with spinal cord injury. The mechanism of injury can vary, occurring during either flexion or extension and with or without compression. When the fracture extends through the junction between the peg and the body of C2, which is the most common morphology of these fractures, these are classified as unstable injuries and have a high risk of non-union (Figure 2.1.6). The Anderson and D'Alonzo classification system is most used to describe odontoid fractures.

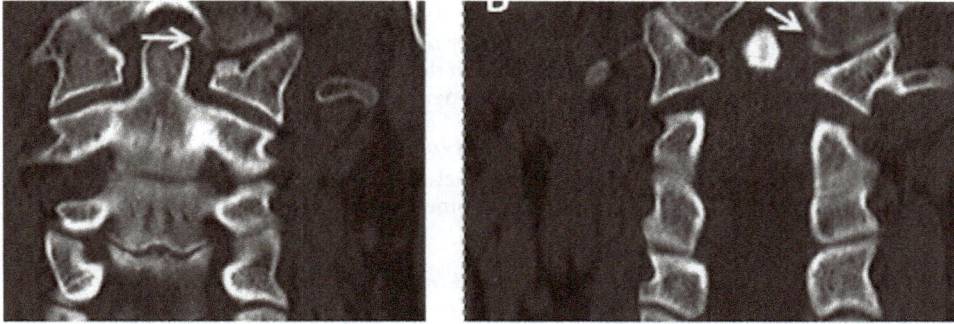

Figure 2.1.4 Occipital condyle fracture.

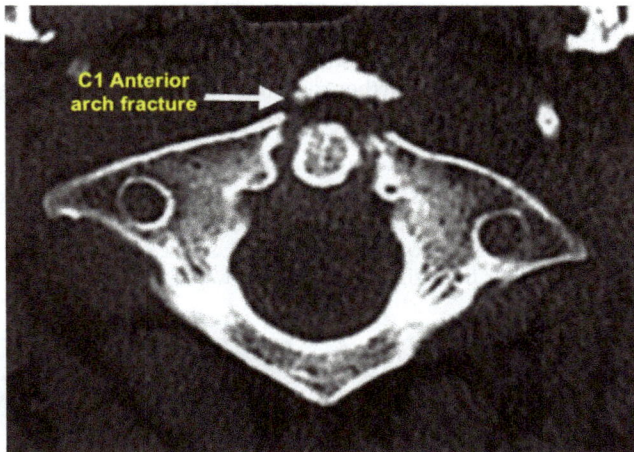

Figure 2.1.5 C1 fracture.

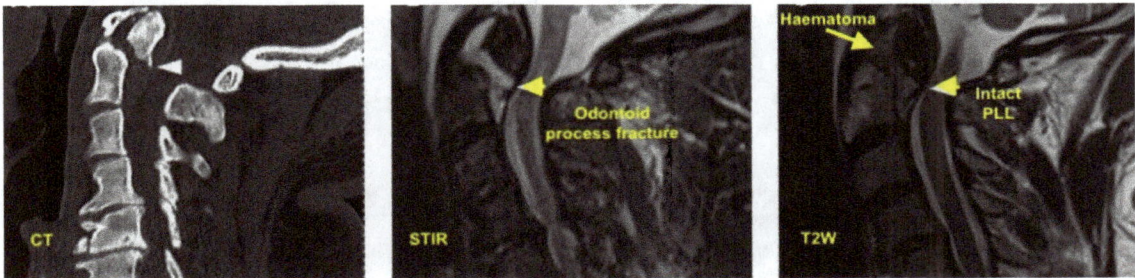

Figure 2.1.6 Odontoid fracture.

Hangman's Fracture (C2)

The hangman's fracture is a bilateral fracture that traverses the pars interarticularis of C2 with an associated anterolisthesis of C2 over C3. It is the most common cervical spine fracture and is usually the result of sudden hyperextension and distraction. CT angiogram of the vertebral arteries should be considered, as there is association with vascular injury.

Lower Cervical Region Injuries (C3–C7)

The lower cervical spine is vulnerable to traumatic injury due to its mobility, and the highest rate of injury is between C5 and C7. The injury morphology is crucial in determining injury severity, along with the integrity of the disco-ligamentous complex and the patient's neurological status.

Compression Injuries

Axial loading injuries result in vertical compression fractures ranging from simple endplate depression to split and burst fractures as seen in the thoracolumbar spine. Compression fractures are NOT usually associated with ligamentous injury.

Tension Band Injuries

These injuries involve disruption of either the posterior (bony or ligamentous) or anterior tension band and are potentially unstable. Tension band injuries are characterised by distraction, where there is separation of two vertebrae in the vertical axis.

Flexion–Distraction Injuries

In a flexion–distraction injury, the supraspinous ligaments first rupture posteriorly, followed by the interspinous then flaval ligaments and the facet capsule. Finally, in severe injuries, there is disc injury with widening of the posterior disc space. There can be widening of the interspinous distance on CT as well as facet joint injury, and any subtle findings warrant further investigation with MRI. MRI is the modality of choice for confirming posterior ligamentous injury in distraction injuries.

Extension–Distraction Injuries

In extension–distraction injuries, there is first rupture of the ALL and anterior disc space that progresses to injury of the posterior structures. Spinous process fractures are common due to posterior compression. Findings on CT can be subtle, and widening of the anterior disc space often with prevertebral swelling is an important finding, warranting further investigation (Figure 2.1.7).

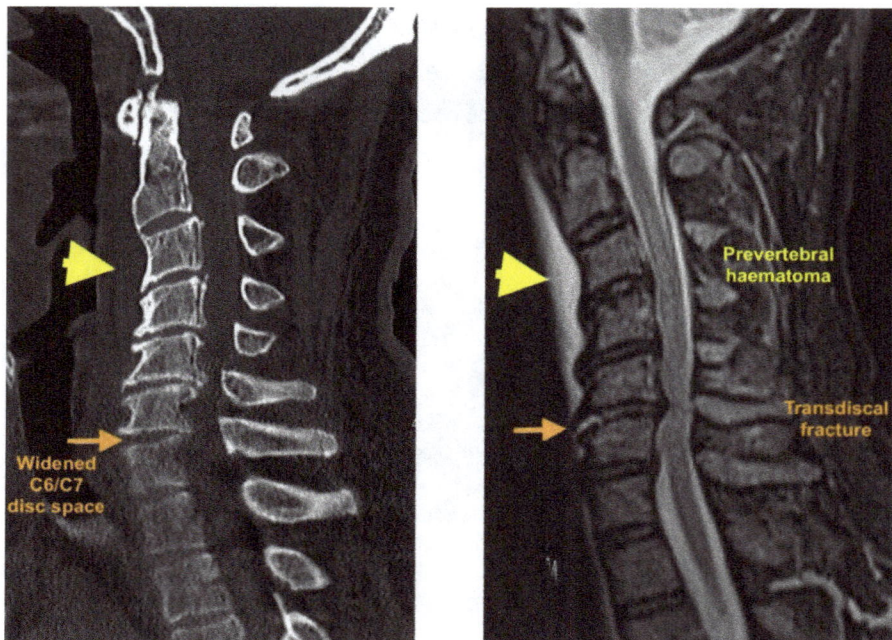

Figure 2.1.7 Extension–distraction injury.

Flexion Teardrop Fractures

These fractures are the result of cervical hyperflexion combined with axial loading and are associated with distraction and injury to the posterior tension band. A triangular anterior fragment is separated from the vertebral body, readily seen on CT (Figure 2.1.8). Forces can also cause the remaining posterior vertebral body fragment to displace posteriorly, leading to spinal cord injury. The ALL and disc are usually intact, but injury to the posterior ligamentous complex should be evaluated with MRI.

Extension Teardrop Fractures

Like flexion teardrop injuries, extension teardrop fractures present with a displaced anteroinferior bony fragment and disruption of the anterior tension band (Figure 2.1.9). Anterior disc widening can be seen on CT, as well as compression fractures of the spinous processes. C2 is the most common level in older patients due to ankylosis of lower levels, and the fracture fragment is usually smaller than in flexion teardrop fractures.

Translation Injuries

These are the most severe and most unstable cervical injuries, and they involve both the anterior and posterior ligamentous structures. On CT, there is displacement or translation of one vertebral body relative to another in any plane. The incidence of associated cord injury and epidural haematoma is highest after these injuries, warranting MRI for further assessment preoperatively.

Facet Injury

Facet injuries are usually the result of both flexion and rotation, and these dislocations can be unilateral (stable) or bilateral (unstable) (Figure 2.1.10). They occur to varying degrees and take on many appearances including subluxed, perched, and locked facets. When describing facet injury, it is useful to describe the size of the fracture fragment, with larger fragments (>1 cm) more likely to be unstable injuries.

Clay Shoveler Fractures

These are isolated spinous process fractures of a lower cervical vertebra, affecting mostly C7 (Figure 2.1.11). Several mechanisms can produce this injury, such as a direct blow to the posterior aspect of the neck and cervical hyperextension and hyperflexion injuries. These are relatively common and stable fractures.

Thoracolumbar Spine

Thoracolumbar fractures are common, and understanding the underlying mechanism is essential for determining injury severity and stability. Several classification systems have been described, but injuries can be broadly categorised as compression, distraction, or translational.

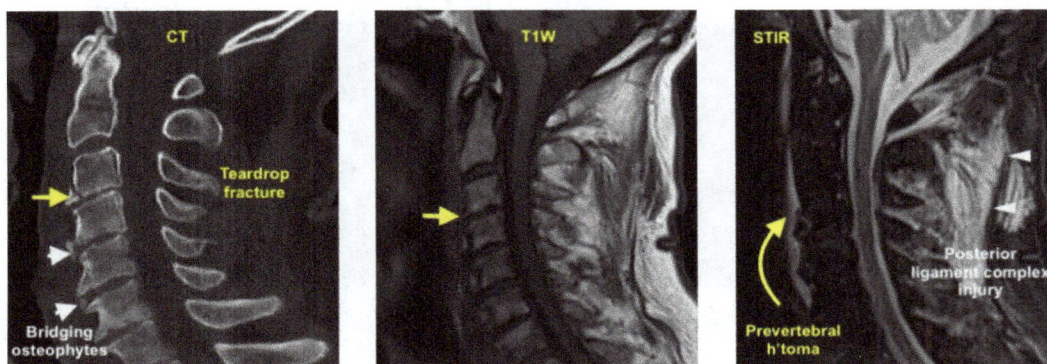

Figure 2.1.8 Cervical flexion teardrop fracture.

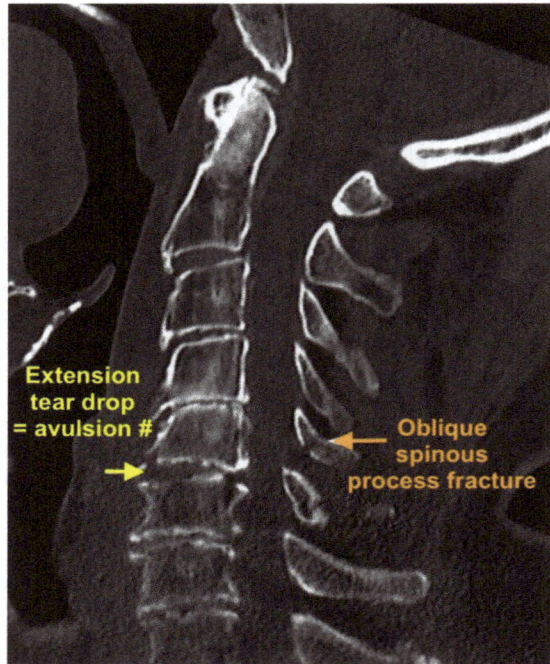

Figure 2.1.9 Extension teardrop fracture.

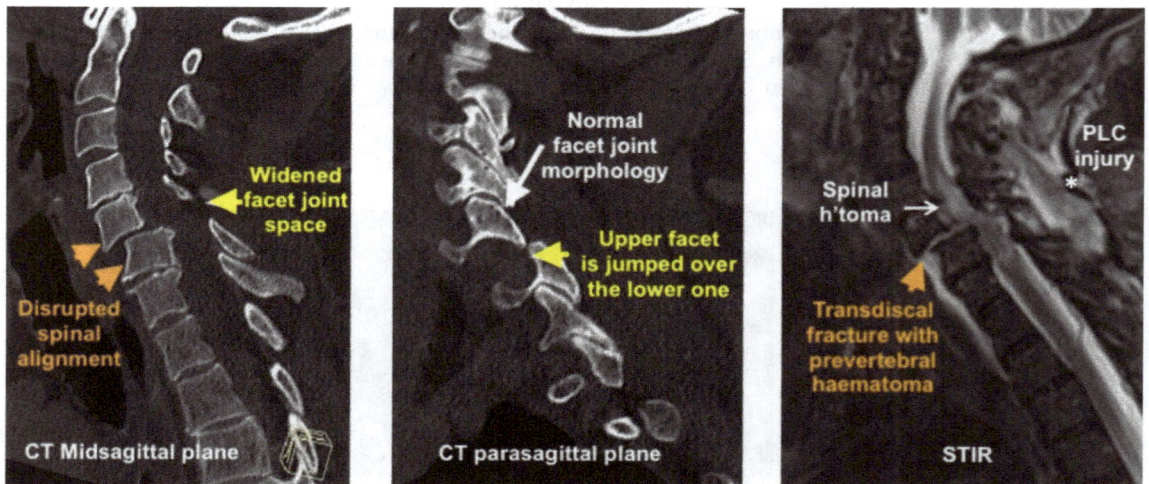

Figure 2.1.10 Facet joint injury.

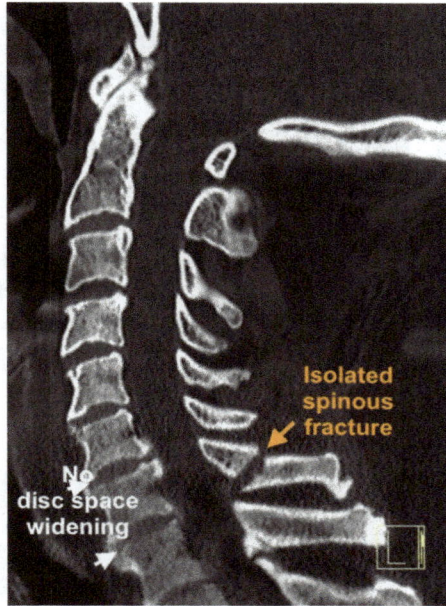

Isolated
spinous
fracture

No
disc space
widening

Figure 2.1.11 Clay Shoveler fracture.

Compression Fractures

Axial compression fractures are the most common injuries in the thoracolumbar spine and involve the vertebral body only.

Wedge Compression

Wedge fractures involve either loss of height of the anterior part of the vertebral body or the disruption of the vertebral endplate (Figure 2.1.12). The posterior cortex of the vertebral body is not involved, and the interspinous distance should be preserved. A horizontal dense band with cortical disruption may be seen on CT with an associated hypointense linear fracture line on MRI. The dense band can be confused with the sclerosis seen in chronic fractures, but this is a sign of trabecular impaction in an acute fracture.

Split Fractures

Split fractures are a variant of compression fractures. They are either sagitally or coronally oriented vertebral body fractures that involve the endplates of the superior and inferior vertebral body, however they do not involve the anterior or posterior cortices (Figure 2.1.13).

Burst Fractures

Burst fractures are more severe variant compression fractures associated with higher risk of neurologic deficit. The posterior cortex of the vertebral body is involved with frequent retropulsion into the spinal canal (Figure 2.1.14). A burst fracture can be complete or incomplete depending on whether one or both endplates are involved. They can be associated with a vertical fracture through the lamina and are best appreciated on CT.

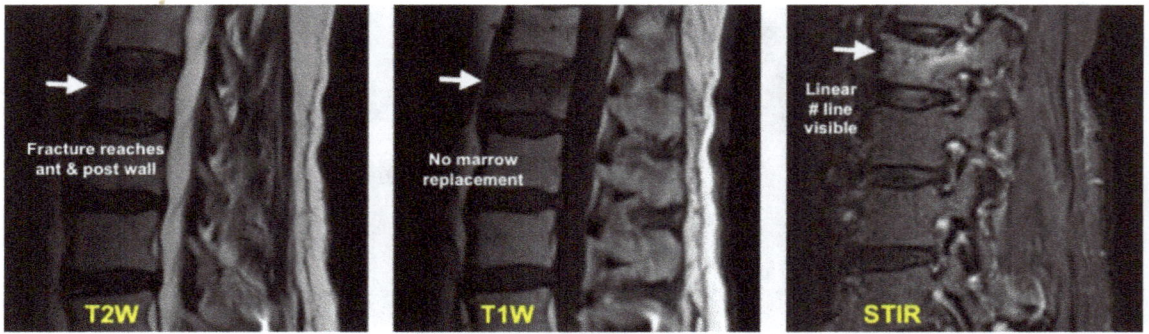

Figure 2.1.12 Acute compression fracture.

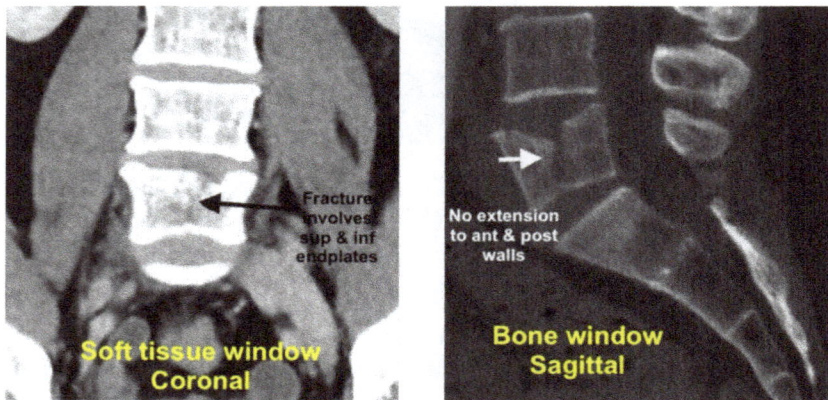

Figure 2.1.13 Split fracture.

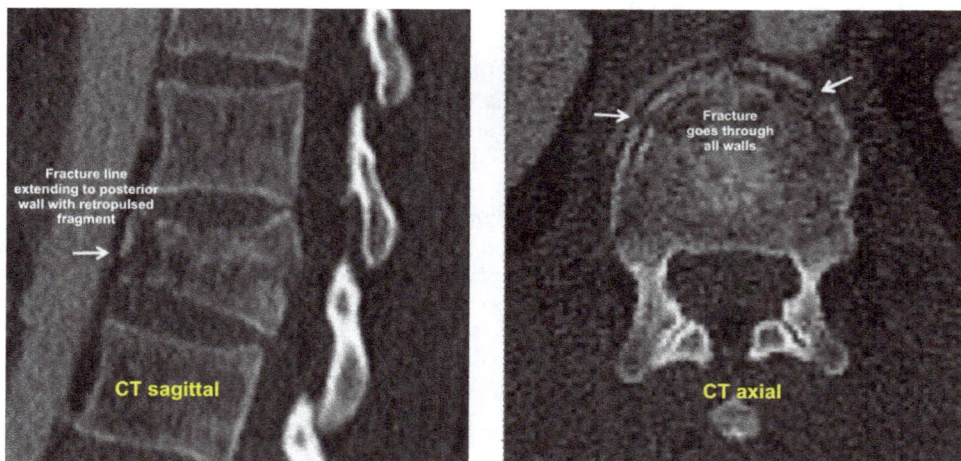

Figure 2.1.14 Complete burst fracture.

Distraction Injuries

Distraction injuries are potentially unstable injuries with dissociation in the vertical axis. Flexion–distraction injuries involve injury to the posterior tension band that can be osseous or ligamentous (Figure 2.1.15). Extension–distraction injuries involve disruption of the disc anteriorly. MRI is indicated for evaluation of the ligaments as well as associated haematoma or cord injury. Chance fractures are a type of flexion–distraction injury that involves the vertebral body and extends through to the posterior elements or involves distraction of the facet joints and spinous processes.

Translational Injuries

Translational injuries are uncommon but serious injuries due to shearing or torsional forces that result in disruption of the posterior ligamentous complex with displacement or rotation of one vertebra relative to another (Figure 2.1.16). The rate of neurological injury is high, and MRI is indicated for all patients.

Fused Spine

When the spine is fused, such as in patients with ankylosing spondylitis or diffuse idiopathic skeletal hyperostosis, the fused column acts as a lever and places greater than normal stress on the spine. Fractures can therefore occur following minor trauma and frequently extend through the vertebral body and posterior elements, leading to what is called a "chalk stick" fracture (Figure 2.1.17). In patients with a fused spine, it is important to assess for a subtle cortical defect on CT, which can indicate a significant fracture, as well as marrow oedema on MRI, which is also often very subtle.

Chronic Spinal Fractures

It can be difficult to assess whether a spinal injury is acute or chronic in the absence of a reliable history, but certain imaging findings can help determine the chronicity. Generally, acute injuries are denoted by sharp ill-defined cortical irregularities seen best on CT, as well as marked osseous marrow and soft tissue oedema best appreciated on MRI, whereas acute fractures are frequently associated with paravertebral or epidural haematomas.

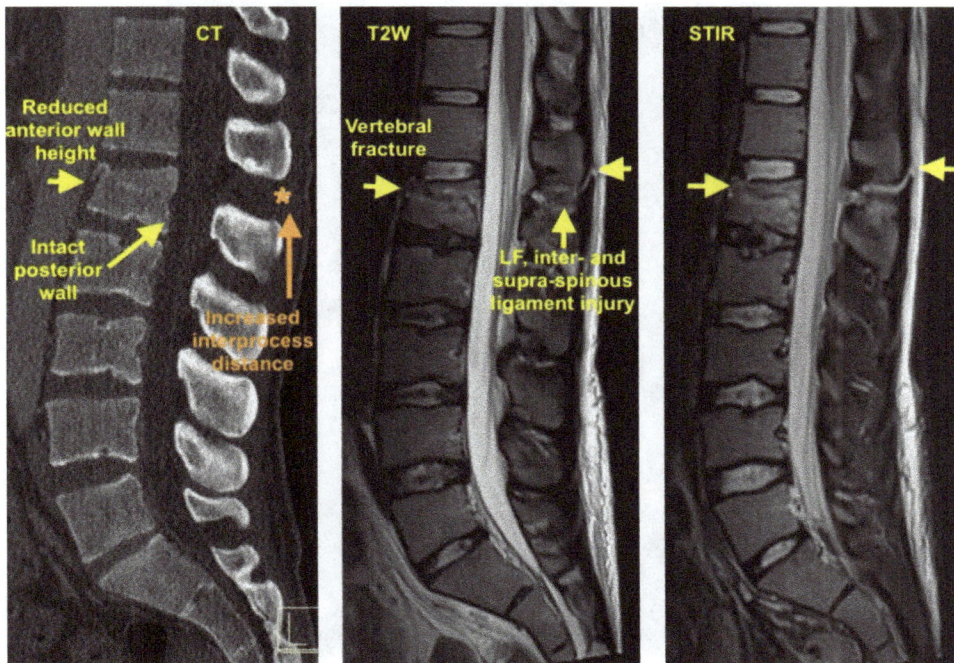

Figure 2.1.15 Flexion–distraction injury.

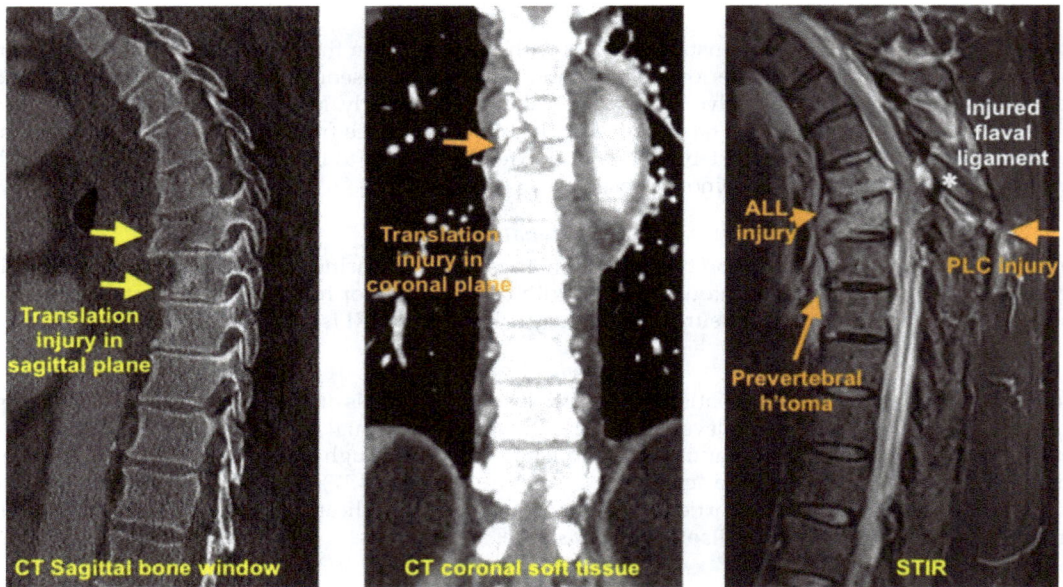

Figure 2.1.16 Translational injury.

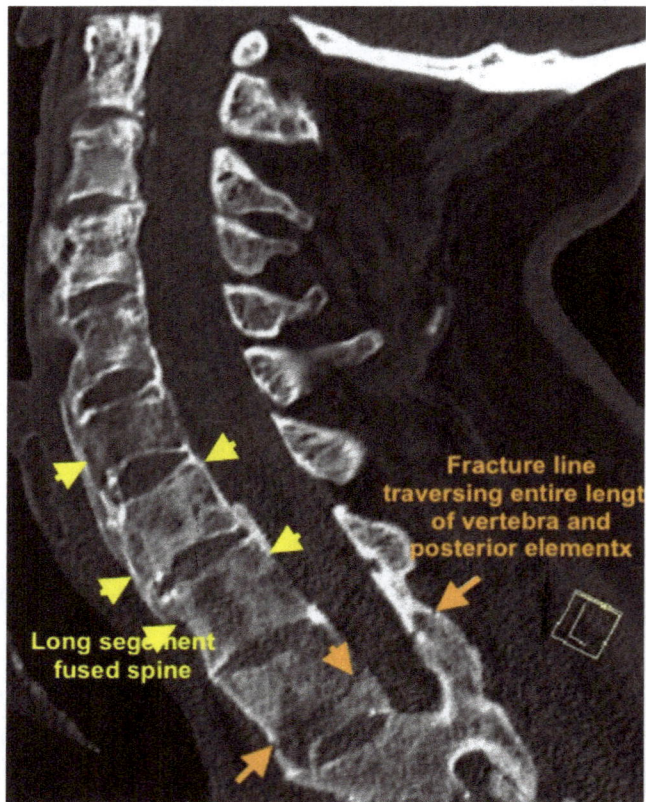

Figure 2.1.17 Fracture through the ankylosed/fused spine.

Chronic injuries can demonstrate bony sclerosis on CT (denoting healing), well-corticated fracture fragments, and less conspicuous or resolved marrow and soft tissue oedema (Figure 2.1.18). Marrow oedema can persist for months to years, signifying active healing, and is highly dependent on the severity of injury and the patient's physiology. Between definite acute and chronic injury is an indeterminate area which can be navigated by combining the history, constellation of imaging findings, and available previous imaging.

Osteoporotic Compression Fractures

These fractures are common in elderly or osteopaenic patients as a result of minor trauma or normal forces onto a weakened spine. A fracture should be diagnosed when there is loss of height in the anterior, middle, or posterior portion of the vertebral body that exceeds 20%. Fractures are classified as wedge, biconcave, or crush depending on whether the anterior, middle, or posterior aspect of vertebral body is most diminished in height. Osteoporotic spine fractures can be graded based on vertebral height loss in Genant classification as (Grade II and III requires referral to the ortho-geriatric team):

- Mild (Grade I): Up to 20%–25%

- Moderate (Grade II): 25%–40%

- Severe (Grade III): >40%

Differentiating between osteoporotic and pathological fractures can be difficult, but there are imaging findings that help support a diagnosis of one over the other (Table 2.1.4).

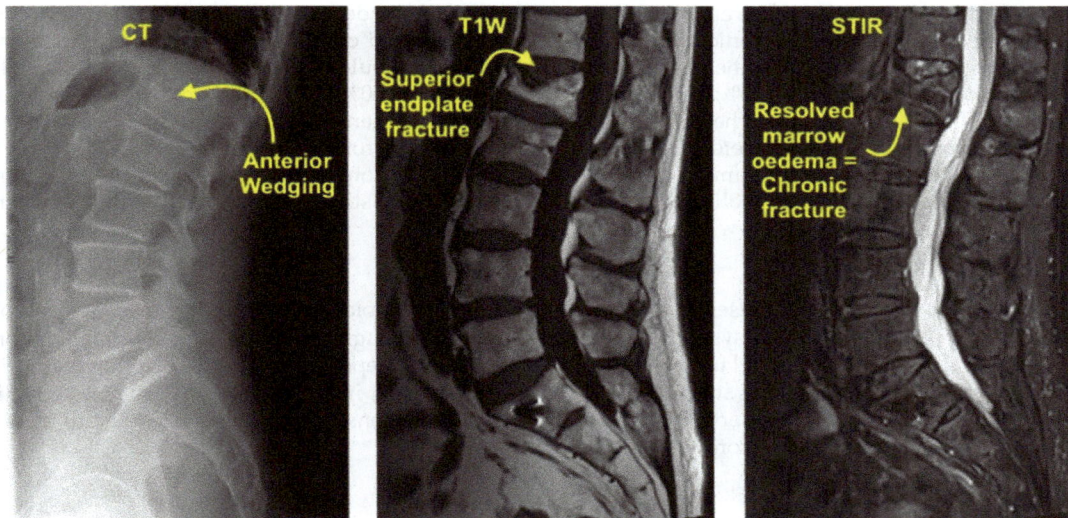

Figure 2.1.18 Chronic wedge compression fracture.

Table 2.1.4 Imaging Features Favouring a Pathological Fracture

Bony destruction
Loss of normal fat marrow signal on T1W images
Involvement of posterior elements
Convex bulging of the posterior vertebral cortex into the spinal canal
Associated soft tissue mass
History of malignancy

Pars Defects

Spondylolysis, commonly referred to as pars defect, is a fracture of the pars interarticularis that is most common in the lumbar spine and has a higher incidence in young adolescent athletes. It can be developmental or acquired and may lead to spondylolisthesis, a slip of one vertebral body relative to another. Acquired

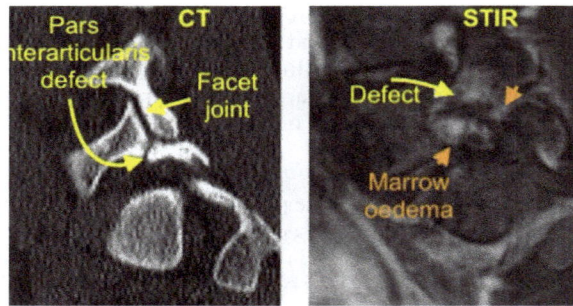

Figure 2.1.19 Chronic L5 pars defect.

causes include repetitive microtrauma (resulting in stress injuries from athletic activities or occupation), or they can be traumatic from hyper-extension of the spine. L5 pars defects account for 90% of all cases, with L4 accounting for the remaining ~10%. (Figure 2.1.19).

Radiographs and CT can reflect pars defects with or without spondylolisthesis; MRI has the added benefit of demonstrating marrow oedema relating to the pars interarticularis, denoting a stress injury that can eventually progress to a fracture. Chronic pars defects are well corticated on CT and are a common incidental finding on imaging. If spondylolisthesis is present, then the grade should be stated, with grade I reflected as anterior subluxation of less than 25%; grade II, 25% to 50%; grade III, 50% to 75%; and grade IV, 75% to 100%.

It can be difficult to determine whether the spondylolisthesis is degenerative or due to spondylolysis, and ancillary findings can be used to determine the aetiology. The neural foramina sign can be used; in patients with spondylolysis, the neural foramina often assume a horizontal configuration, whereas this sign is not present with degenerative spondylolisthesis. Degenerative spondylolisthesis is associated with spinal canal stenosis, which is not usually seen with lytic spondylolisthesis.

CONCLUSION

Traumatic injuries of the spine present a daunting challenge for radiologists due to the variety of pathologies and imaging appearances. A systematic approach, with a thorough understanding of spinal anatomy and injury mechanisms, is essential for providing a clinically useful report. Accurate description of injuries, along with an appreciation of the strengths and limitations of each imaging modality, ensures effective diagnosis and management. Further imaging with MRI should be considered, when necessary, to identify associated injuries such as spinal cord damage and haematoma.

SUGGESTED READING

- AO Spine Classification Systems. Available online.

SBA QUESTIONS

1) Which imaging feature suggests a pathological fracture rather than a simple fracture?

    A. Concave bulging of the posterior cortex

    B. Convex bulging of the posterior cortex

    C. Spondylolisthesis

    D. Retropulsion of fragments into the spinal canal

    E. High STIR signal

2) A patient who was involved in a road traffic collision has a CT C-spine as part of a trauma scan that demonstrates fractures of the C1 vertebral body extending through the transverse foramen. What should be the next step?

A. No further action

B. MRI C-spine with no contrast

C. MRI C-spine with contrast

D. CT angiogram of the cervical spine

E. Flexion and extension radiographic views

3) Patient has a traumatic spinal injury following a road traffic collision and has a subsequent CT (as part of a trauma scan). The scan demonstrates a fracture through the L4 vertebral body that is sagittally oriented and involves both the superior and inferior endplates but does not extend to the anterior or posterior cortices. Which pattern best describes the configuration of the fracture?

A. Flexion teardrop fracture

B. Burst fracture

C. Split fracture

D. Extension teardrop fracture

E. Osteoporotic compression fracture

Answers: (1) B, (2) D, (3) C

Chapter 2.2
Degenerative and Infective Spinal Disease

Saurabh Deore, Joshua Taylor, Lenetta Boyce, and Radhika Prasad

Infective Spinal Disease

LEARNING OBJECTIVES

- To identify imaging features of various types of spinal infection; prompt identification is critical to prevent severe and potentially irreversible complications

- To detect early imaging features of infective spinal disease on MRI given its high sensitivity to detect these changes and associated complications

- To understand normal spinal anatomy and appropriate MRI sequences and thereby distinguish between infective and non-infective aetiologies, which have different management pathways

---

INTRODUCTION

Infective spinal disease encompasses pyogenic spondylodiscitis, tuberculous spondylitis, epidural abscess, vertebral body osteomyelitis, and facet joint septic arthritis, which will all be discussed in this chapter.

Frequently Used Terms

Infective spondylitis is an umbrella term for infective spinal disease; infective discitis and spondylodiscitis are used interchangeably to describe intervertebral disc infection. Osteomyelitis refers to bony infection only. Technically, all infective spondylodiscitis (not facet arthritis) begins at the subchondral bone of the vertebral endplates where the blood flow is most sluggish, but for all these variations of spinal infection, imaging is invaluable. This chapter highlights the importance of understanding the common routes of infection, typical multimodality imaging findings and appropriate management strategies for each manifestation of spinal infection.

Background

- **Three common routes of spread:** (a) Secondary via haematogenous spread from a recent infection (most common), (b) direct implantation from recent surgical procedure, and (c) contiguous spread from sites close to the spinal canal.

- **Risk factors:** Immunocompromised status; transplant history; chronic disease such as diabetes mellitus or chronic renal and lung disease; concurrent infection such as infective endocarditis; history of intravenous drug use or presence of a long-term external vascular access device.

- **Origin of hospital requests:** Most clinical requests arise from EDs, medical and infectious disease wards, decision making units, ITUs, and transplants units.

- **Demographics:** Patients in 50s and 60s, Male: Female = 2:1.

- Pyogenic spondylodiscitis can also occur in the paediatric population, usually starting in the intervertebral disc (preserved direct blood supply) versus starting in the endplate in adults.

- Usually a bacterial infection, the commonest organisms being *Staphylococcus aureus*, *Streptococcus* and *Pneumococcus* with fungal, viral, and parasitic causes (uncommon). *Mycobacterium tuberculosis* is also possible, as will be covered later.

- The lumbar spine is the most commonly affected part.

DOI: 10.1201/9781003500247-11

Presenting Complaints

- Severe back pain in the presence of fever is the typical presentation for infective spinal disease, but fever is frequently absent.

- Constitutional symptoms include fatigue, night sweats, and weight loss, especially in the setting of tuberculous infection or more chronic infections.

- Focal sensory/motor deficits, bowel/bladder dysfunction or paralysis (due to inflammatory phlegmon, epidural abscess, or collapsed vertebra causing neural compression).

HOW TO REVIEW SPINAL MRI IN THE CONTEXT OF INFECTION

MRI Sequences

Always consider whole-spine MRI for suspected spinal infection; multilevel spondylodiscitis is a common occurrence (Figure 2.2.1). Sequence combinations include the following:

- T1W, T2W, fat-suppressed T2W imaging, or short-tau inversion recovery (STIR) sequences: Sagittal through whole spine

- T1W and T2W axials: Through involved levels (preferably a block)

- Pre- and post-contrast T1W sequences (with or without fat suppression); use of gadolinium for suspected spinal infection differs by hospital in the NHS

- Diffusion-weighted imaging (DWI): Very infrequently used for epidural abscess

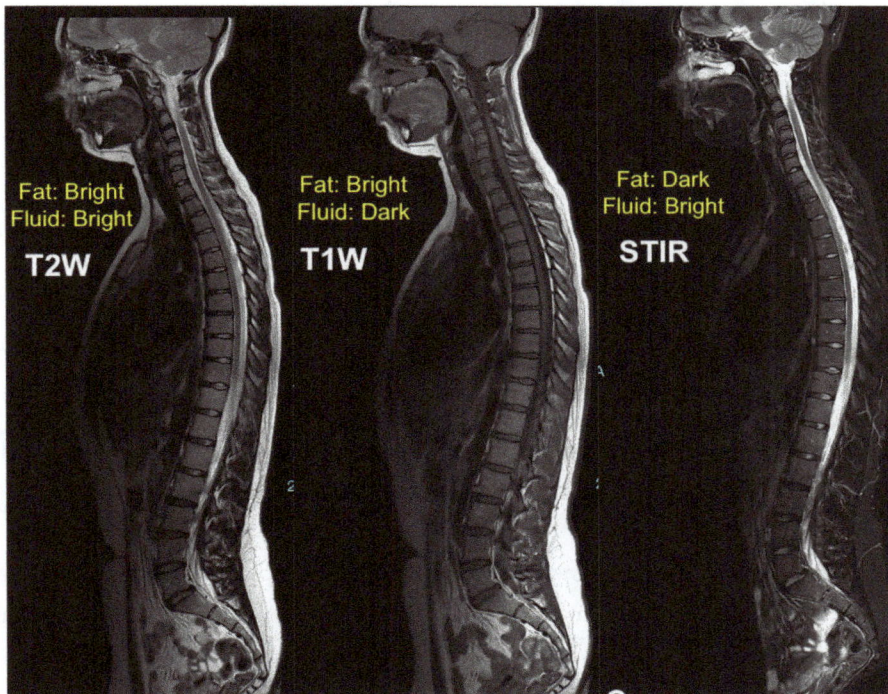

Figure 2.2.1 Standard MRI sequences of the whole spine: Sagittal T2, T1, and STIR. As mentioned, axial T2 and T1 pre- and post-sequences can be selected if there is an area of concern on the sagittal imaging.

INTERPRETATION

- **Step 1:** Review the clinical information, patient demographics, and previous imaging if available. Review associated imaging if available, e.g. chest X-rays in the setting of suspected tuberculous spondylitis. Raised CRP and white cell counts help narrow down the differentials but non-specific.
- **Step 2:** Scout images; check to ensure that other body areas included do not demonstrate relevant incidental findings.
- **Step 3:** Label the vertebrae from C1 caudally to ensure that the vertebral segmentation and vertebral body numbers are conventional and save a key image of the vertebral body count to ensure consistency with surgical colleagues.
- **Step 4:** Assess the MRI sequences for:
  - Signal abnormalities in the vertebrae, endplates, or disc or paraspinal tissues (psoas muscles, pre- and paraspinal spaces, and posterior paraspinal muscles).
  - Oedema is indicated by high STIR and T2W signal, which corresponds with low T1W signal.
  - Post-contrast enhancement of the bones or disc suggests hypervascularity as would be seen in infective spinal disease and can highlight associated abscess (walled-off collection) or phlegmon (no walls to the collection).
  - Structural abnormalities such as vertebral body/endplate destruction or erosion, loss of intervertebral disc height, obvious spinal canal stenosis, cord and cauda equina compression.

IMAGING FEATURES OF INFECTIVE SPINAL DISEASE

Pyogenic Spondylodiscitis and Epidural Abscess
Radiographs

- Often normal in the early stages of spondylodiscitis.

- In advanced stages, radiographs show reduced intervertebral disc space height at the affected vertebral level with irregularity, destruction, and sclerosis of the affected vertebral endplates and vertebral body collapse (Figure 2.2.2).

- Endplate sclerosis with intervertebral disc height reduction is common in Modic degenerative disease.

- Vertebral body collapse is common in the setting of osteoporosis.

CT

- CT is more sensitive than X-rays.

- Endplate erosive changes and vertebral body collapse are easier to identify, and paraspinal abscesses can usually be seen clearly on contrast enhanced CT (Figures 2.2.3 and 2.2.4). This feature is helpful in identifying spinal infection as a potential cause of unidentified sepsis in a patient being investigated in the wards.

- Disc enhancement is less appreciable on CT and marrow oedema cannot be assessed.

MRI

- MRI is the most sensitive and specific modality to assess infective spondylodiscitis.

- In adults, subchondral marrow oedema affecting at least half the vertebral body height and contrast enhancement are early signs of infective spondylodiscitis.

- High STIR and T2 signal, low T1 signal, high post-contrast T1 signal.

- It can spread to the adjacent disc, appearing as endplate oedema and enhancement with erosion/irregularity/collapse and disc oedema and enhancement with disc height loss (Figures 2.2.5 and 2.2.6) in a few days. *Therefore, follow-up MRI in the same protocol after 10–14 days is a safer approach.* This is particularly recommended in cases of clinical suspicion with first MRI showing equivocal changes.

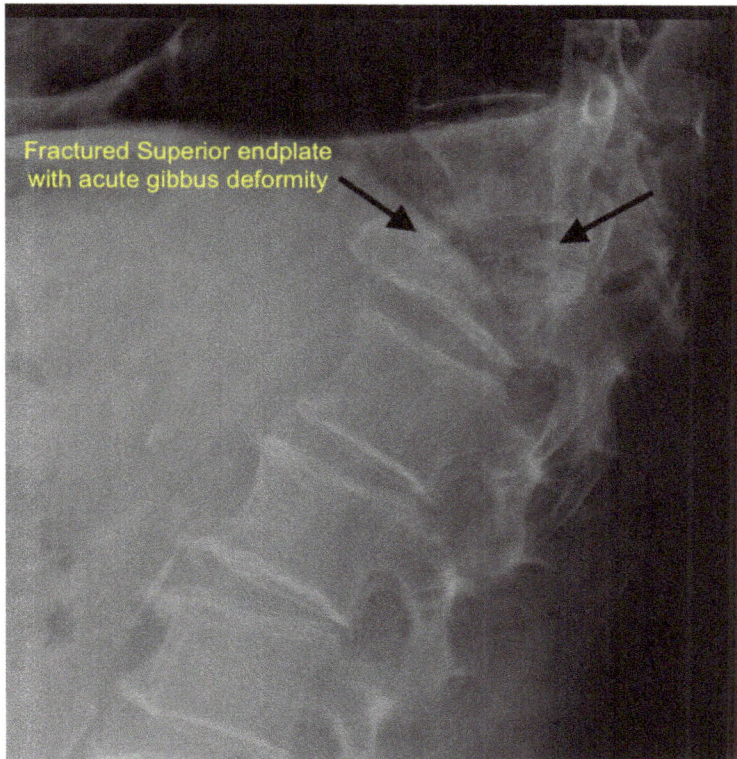

Figure 2.2.2 X-ray features of chronic T11/12 infective spondylodiscitis with complete collapse of the T11 vertebra body and mild collapse of the T12 superior endplate.

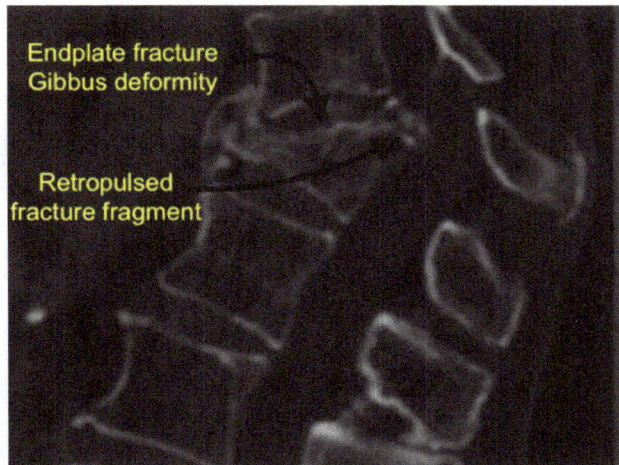

Figure 2.2.3 CT features of chronic T11/T12 discitis with vertebral body collapse and kyphosis, and the endplates are sclerosed.

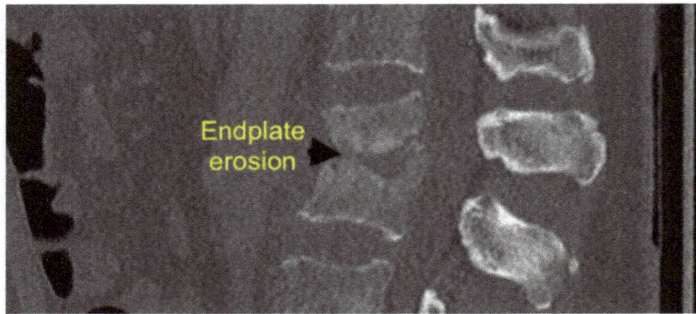

Figure 2.2.4 CT features of acute spondylodiscitis with irregular ill-defined endplates and vertebral body height loss.

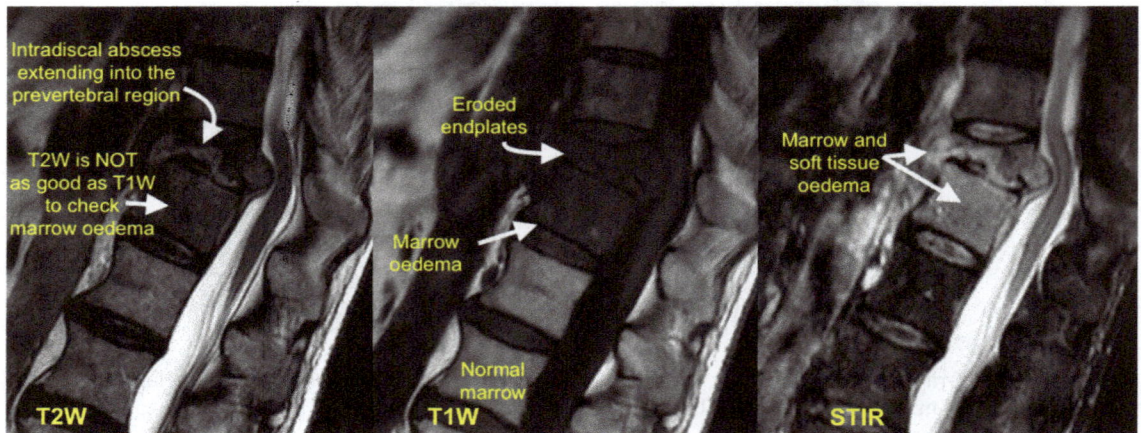

Figure 2.2.5 T11/T12 infective spondylodiscitis with fluid signal (high T2, low T1, and high STIR) in the T11/T12 IV disc and marrow oedema in the adjacent T12 and T11 vertebral body, which is collapsed and retropulsed, causing moderate-severe spinal stenosis.

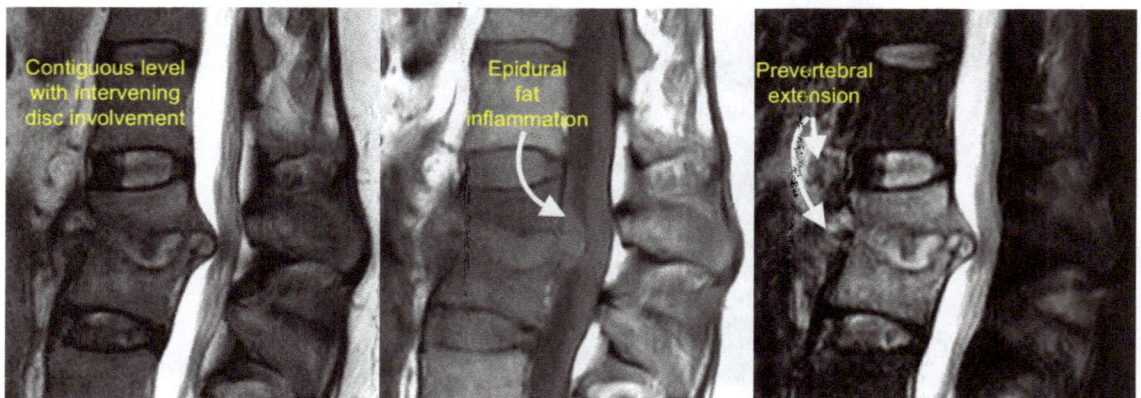

Figure 2.2.6 Acute pyogenic spondylodiscitis with fluid signal in the IV disc and adjacent vertebral body oedema and collapse. There is an epidural abscess/phlegmon which is contained by the PLL but is causing moderate spinal stenosis.

- Epidural abscess is a known complication, usually contained by the posterior longitudinal ligament (PLL) (Figure 2.2.7). Epidural abscesses can extend far distant to the level of infection. Therefore, it is essential to review all images to see entire extension of the epidural abscess.

- Paraspinal soft tissue spread can occur as phlegmon, which is demonstrated by uniform enhancement or walled-off abscess, which is demonstrated by peripheral enhancement (Figures 2.2.8 and 2.2.9).

- Epidural abscess usually occurs secondary to spondylodiscitis but may be primary indicated by irregularly enhancing mass in the epidural space +/– dural enhancement without the endplate and disc features of spondylodiscitis (Figure 2.2.10), uncommonly.

- Abscess can also occur within the vertebral body and disc.

- Mass effect on the cord and caudal equina can be best assessed on the axial sequences and sagittal sequences.

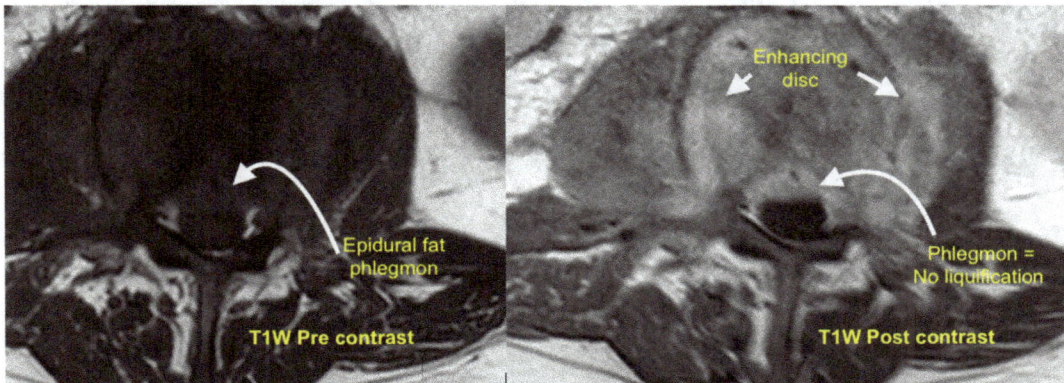

Figure 2.2.7 Pre- and post-contrast T1 images showing enhancing material in the epidural space in a patient with other radiological features of IV spondylodiscitis, in keeping with epidural abscess.

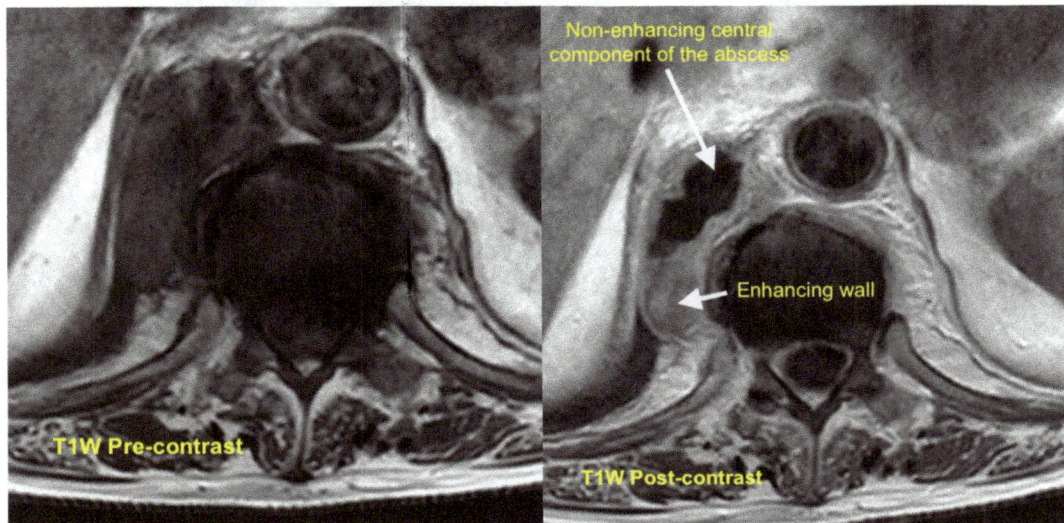

Figure 2.2.8 Paraspinal abscess: Peripheral enhancement sparing the centre is typical.

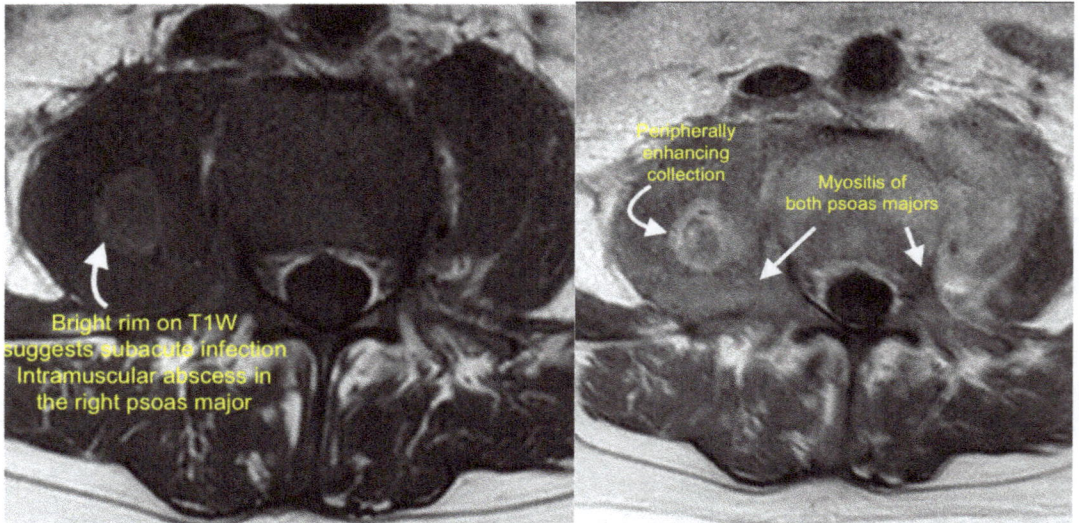

Figure 2.2.9 Paraspinal abscess and phlegmon: Abscess with peripheral enhancement is only seen in the right psoas muscle. In the left psoas muscle, there is uniform enhancement in keeping with phlegmon.

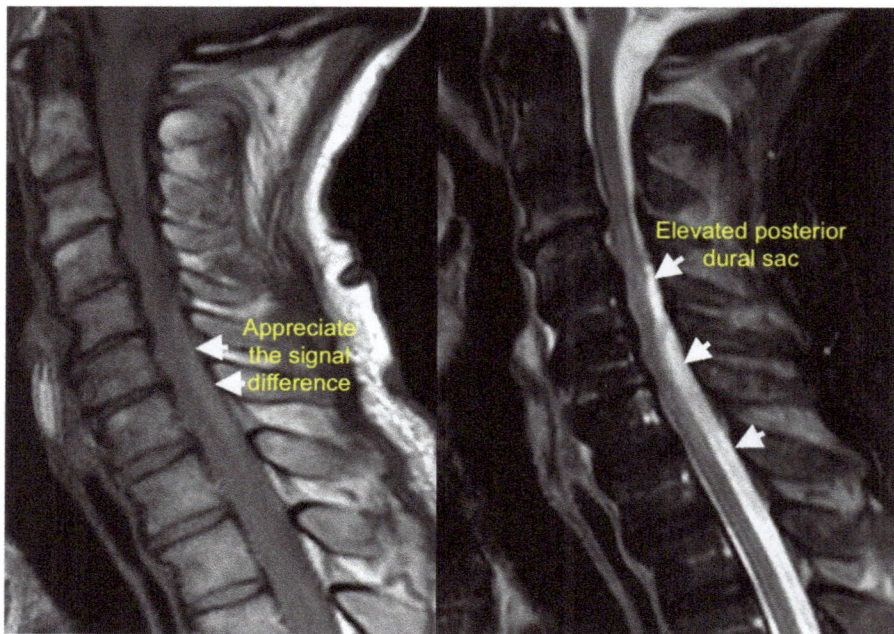

Figure 2.2.10 Cervical epidural abscess in an immunocompromised patient. No radiological evidence of concurrent osteomyelitis or spondylodiscitis.

Tuberculous Spondylodiscitis (Pott Disease)

- Tuberculous (TB) spondylitis accounts for less than 1% of all cases of TB.
- Most common spread is haematogenous from lung or GI tract TB.

- The thoracolumbar and lumbar spine are most commonly affected, in the anterior subchondral vertebral body, with subligamentous spread to adjacent discs and vertebral bodies leading to contiguous extension along several vertebral segments.

- Non-contiguous "skip" infected lesions can also occur.

- The intervertebral disc is relatively spared in comparison to the vertebral body and endplate bony erosion.

- Large paraspinal and epidural abscesses are common, e.g. retropharyngeal space, mediastinum, and psoas muscles.

- Associated arachnoiditis, meningitis, and spinal cord infection are also possible.

Radiography and CT findings

- TB spondylitis shows similar findings with pyogenic spondylitis on X-ray and CT.

- Gibbus deformity is a short segment angular deformity causing significant thoracolumbar kyphosis secondary to significant vertebral body collapse and destruction.

MRI findings

- TB spondylitis will demonstrate similar vertebral body, endplate, disc, and paraspinal signal and structural abnormalities as pyogenic spondylitis, but if there are contiguous vertebral bodies affected with relative sparing or the discs with large paraspinal collections, TB should be suspected (Figure 2.2.11).

- TB collections demonstrate copious volume and tend to insinuate along the areas of least resistance far from the site of infection (Figure 2.2.12)

- Arachnoiditis is demonstrated by clumping of the caudal nerve roots, and meningeal and spinal cord infection is demonstrated by post-contrast enhancement.

Vertebral Body Osteomyelitis and Facet Joint Septic Arthritis

- Pyogenic vertebral osteomyelitis/abscess without involvement of the disc is rare, as is facet joint septic arthritis; the latter is usually unilateral. However, it can happen bilaterally.

- Clinically, in facet joint septic arthritis, the patient will present with unilateral back pain and muscle spasm, and this will usually occur in the lumbar spine.

MRI findings

- Vertebral body osteomyelitis is shown by ill-defined oedema in the vertebral body.

- Vertebral body abscess is shown by a well-defined encapsulated intermediate signal intensity lesion with variable surrounding signal intensity due to central fluid with surrounding sclerosis (T1W hyperintense rim is the most specific finding).

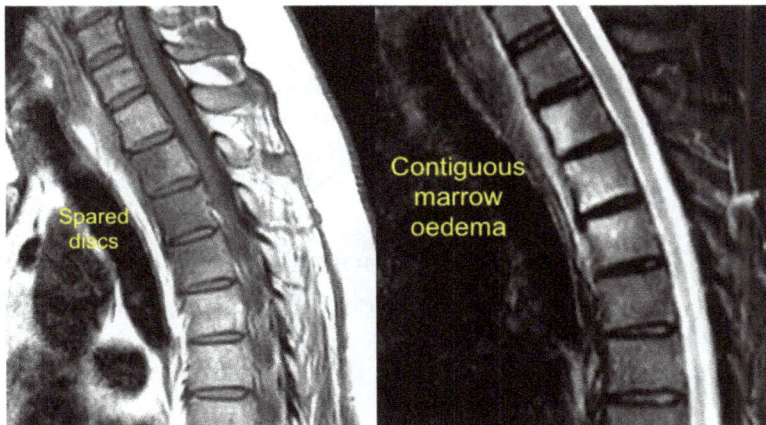

Figure 2.2.11 TB spondylitis: Contiguous marrow oedema in thoracic vertebrae with relative sparing of the IV discs and prevertebral extension and large associated paraspinal abscess (not shown).

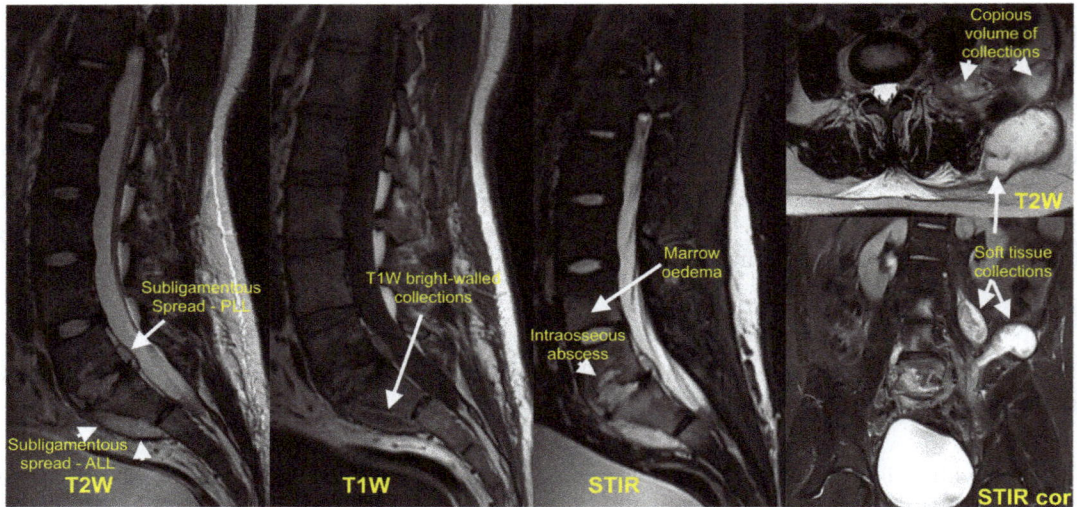

Figure 2.2.12 Classic TB spondylodiscitis: Sizable collections from L5/S1 spondylodiscitis extending beneath the anterior and posterior longitudinal ligaments, retroperitoneum, and posterior paraspinal soft tissue.

- Facet joint septic arthritis is demonstrated by facet joint widening and erosion with joint effusion as demonstrated by high T2/STIR signal material in the joint. Posterior epidural abscess is a frequent complication.

Radiological Follow-up in a Diagnosed Case of Spinal Infection

- Usually, a diagnosed case of infective spondylodiscitis does not require further imaging unless there are new symptoms such as progression of neurological deficit or no or suboptimal treatment response.

- Radiological appearances of improvement lag clinical improvement. Follow-up MRIs should not be used to prove or assess for improvement.

- Post-interventional procedures such as surgical drainage in complex cases might require follow-up to guide direct intervention or other medical/surgical management if required.

Mimickers of Infective Spinal Disease (Top Tips for Differential Diagnoses)

INFECTIVE DISEASE MORE LIKELY IF

- Fluid in disc or endplate erosion, destruction or enhancement with epidural, and/or paraspinal abscess/phlegmon

Alternative differentials are more likely if there is an absence of the symptoms of infective disease with the following more specific features

DEGENERATE TYPE 1 MODIC CHANGES ARE MORE LIKELY IF

- Presence of "vacuum sign" (air in the disc space) can be due to a degenerate disc

- Features remain stable over time

SCHMORL'S NODE IS MORE LIKELY IF

- Focal smooth irregularity of only one endplate

TRAUMATIC FRACTURES MORE LIKELY IF

- Appropriate clinical history of trauma
- Low T1 and high T2/STIR line indicating fracture in a common fracture pattern, e.g. wedge compression fracture

VERTEBRAL NEOPLASM MORE LIKELY IF

- Marrow replacement, i.e. low T1 and T2 signal in the vertebral bodies

INFLAMMATORY SPONDYLOARTHRITIS MORE LIKELY IF

- Typical inflammatory vertebral body lesions such as Andersson and Romanus lesions in the presence of sacroiliitis (described in detail in Chapter 2.13)

Degenerative Spinal Disease

LEARNING OBJECTIVES

- Identifying potential causes of low back pain on MRI, which provides detailed images of the intervertebral discs, vertebrae, and surrounding soft tissues.
- To appreciate biomechanical changes in response to age-related degeneration or trauma led to a cascade of changes in the intervertebral discs, vertebral body endplates, bone marrow, facet joints, and the spinal canal, which are reflected in various modalities.
- To identify sites of neural compression and localised inflammatory changes can cause symptoms within the spinal canal, the lateral recess, or the neural foramen.
- *Speak the same language as your local spinal surgeons.* To guide management, it is necessary to adopt the commonly accepted terminology in relation to spinal degenerative changes (spondylosis vs spondylolysis vs spondylolisthesis) and be consistent with the accepted terminologies at local levels.
- In general, non-operative management is opted as first line treatment for degenerative disc disease (DDD). Surgical management is reserved for patients with neurological symptoms and varies with the pattern of degenerative change seen within the spine.

Introduction

- DDD is one of the most common causes of back pain.
- MRI is the imaging modality of choice for assessing DDD due to its ability to provide detailed images of intervertebral discs, vertebral bodies, and adjacent soft tissues.
- Spondylosis is an umbrella term for degeneration affecting the spinal discs, vertebrae, and facets. It is further categorised by its location into cervical, thoracic, and lumbar spondylosis.

This chapter provides a focused approach to reading a spinal MRI for the evaluation of degenerative disc disease.

Aetiopathogenesis of the DDD

- Trauma or age-related degeneration can lead to spondylosis, with the earliest sign being intervertebral disc desiccation.
- This process begins with the dehydration of the nucleus pulposus, the central core of the disc, which reduces disc height.
- As degeneration progresses, the posterior portion of the annulus fibrosus, the outer layer of the disc, develops small fissures. These tiny tears cause loss of the normal radial tension in the disc's architecture and can eventually allow the disc to herniate.

- In response to progressive degeneration, the vertebrae above and below undergo bony osteophytosis.

- Eventually, progression of these spinal column changes involves distant structures such as ligamentum flavum hypertrophy or facet joint arthrosis in the posterior column, with severe disease leading to spinal canal stenosis, degenerative fusion, and ultimately spinal nerve compression.

Frequently Used Terms and Their Associated Findings

- **Spondylosis** refers to degenerative changes within the spine. On plain radiographs, spondylosis is characterised by disc space narrowing, endplate sclerosis, and osteophyte formation. MRI can provide a more detailed view, showing disc desiccation, loss of disc height, and signal changes in the vertebral endplates (Modic changes).

  - Spondylolysis is characterised by a defect or fracture in the pars interarticularis, typically seen in the lumbar spine. It is often visualised as a break in the "neck" of the "Scotty dog" on oblique radiographs and more commonly seen in adolescent athletes. CT is the gold standard for assessing this bony defect. A high proportion of patients with spondylolysis progress to spondylolisthesis.

- **Spondylolisthesis** occurs when one vertebra slips forward over the one beneath it. (*Tip: Spondylolisthesis is always described in reference to the superior vertebra over the inferior one. For instance, anterolisthesis of L4 over L5 vertebra, NOT retrolisthesis of L5 over L4 vertebra*) Radiologically, it is best seen on lateral X-rays where the degree of slippage is assessed using the Meyerding classification (grade I: 0%–25%, grade II: 26%–50%, grade III: 51%–75%, grade IV: 76%–100%, and grade V: >100%).

  - Spondylolisthesis suggests underlying spinal instability. Spinal surgeons are usually interested in the cause for anterolisthesis, being degenerative (facet arthritis), lytic (pars interarticularis defects), dysplastic (congenital deformity of the posterior elements), neoplastic (due to tumoral destruction), and iatrogenic (failed surgery). Surgeons usually begin with flexion and extension lateral views of the spine to detect positional aggravation of spondylolisthesis. Once confirmed, they request MRI and CT scans to see structural abnormalities like facet joint degeneration, foraminal narrowing, or pars defects.

IMAGING FEATURES OF DEGENERATIVE SPINAL DISEASE

What to Look for in MRI Sequences

Axial and sagittal planes are useful in evaluating degree of DDD including disc dehydration, annular fissures, disc herniation, osteophyte formation, or in severe cases facet joint arthrosis, ligamentum flavum hypertrophy, and spinal stenosis.

Endplate Changes

Modic endplate changes refer to MRI signal alterations in the vertebral endplates and adjacent bone marrow, commonly associated with degenerative disc disease. They are classified into three types based on their MRI appearance. See Table 2.2.2.

Table 2.2.1 Different MRI Structures to Assess on Specific Sequences

Sequence	What to Assess?
T1-Weighted	Excellent for evaluating the anatomy of the vertebral bodies and for detecting bone marrow changes
T2-Weighted	Useful for assessing disc hydration, the spinal canal, and nerve roots
STIR	Highly sensitive for detecting subtle changes in bone marrow and soft tissues, such as oedema or inflammation

Table 2.2.2 Modic Changes and Their MRI Appearances

Modic Type	Description	T2W Signal	T1W Signal
Type 1	Acute degenerative changes with inflammation and marrow oedema	High	Low
Type 2	Fatty degeneration	Iso to High	High
Type 3	Reactive fibrosis or sclerosis	Low	Low

Remember that type 1 Modic changes (acute degenerative endplate changes with inflammation and marrow oedema) can simulate infective spondylodiscitis. In such cases, it is worth checking bloods on electronic patient record for elevated CRP and white cell counts. Normal counts are reassuring for type 1 Modic changes. When posed with indeterminate CRP or white cell counts, it is worth repeating MRI after 10–14 days. No progression favours Modic type 1 changes (indolent infections are less common in the spine), whereas progressive destruction of endplates suggests infective spondylodiscitis (Figures 2.2.13 and 2.2.14).

Disc Herniations

The presence of disc tissue beyond the limits of intervertebral disc space can be due to a diffuse disc bulge or due to focal disc herniation. Focal disc herniation can be classified into four zones: central, paracentral or subarticular, foraminal, and extraforaminal (Figure 2.2.15).

On the axial plane, the disc can herniate through the anterior or posterior margins. Based on the morphology of the imaging findings, this can be divided into the three subtypes described in Table 2.2.4. Note that normal disc anatomy is presented in Figure 2.2.16a.

Disc sequestration is more prone to causing severe spinal symptoms. Figures 2.2.16 through 2.2.18 present a series of sagittal images of herniated discs.

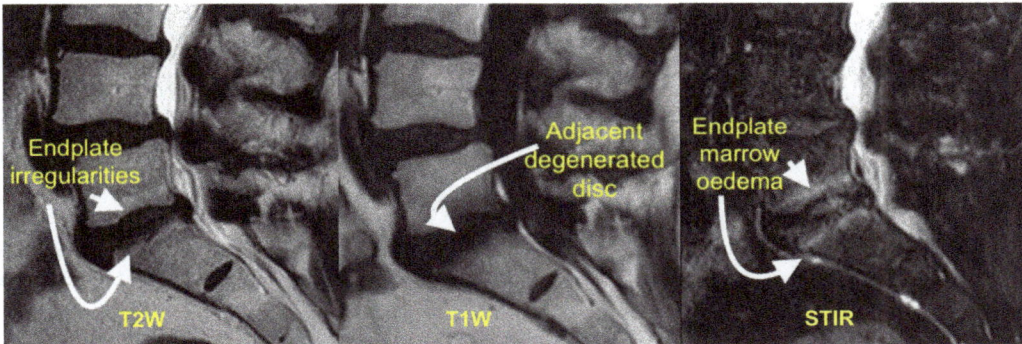

Figure 2.2.13   Modic type I endplate change at L5/S1 with low T1 and high T2 and STIR signal intensity.

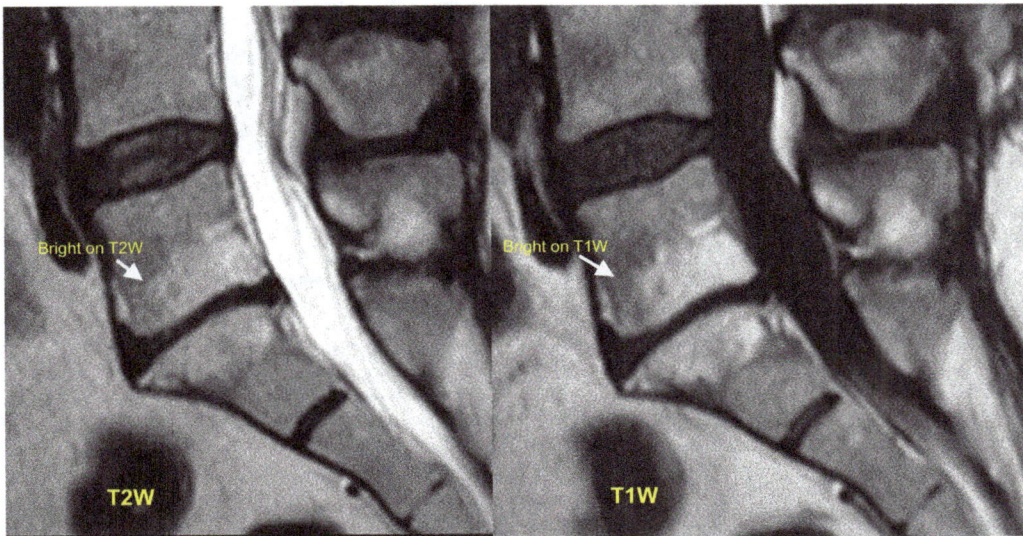

Figure 2.2.14   Modic type II endplate change at L5/S1 with bright T1 and T2 signal intensity.

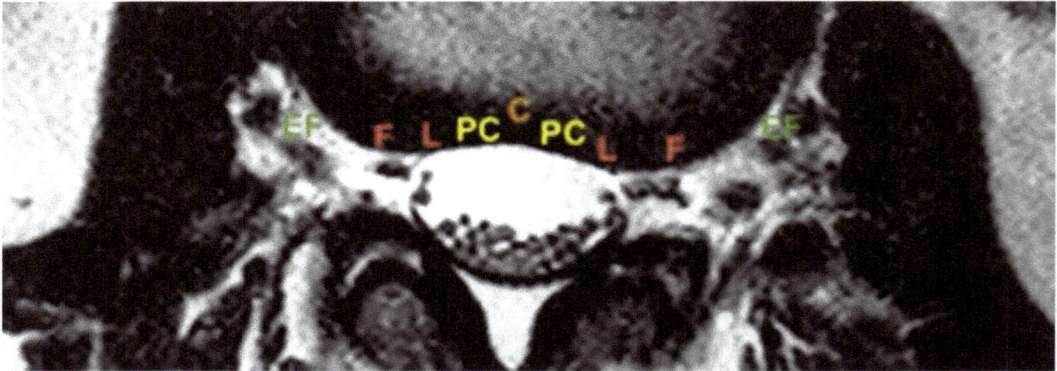

Figure 2.2.15 Locations of disc herniation: central zone (C), paracentral zone (PC), lateral recess (L), foraminal zone (F), and extraforaminal (EF).

Table 2.2.3 Disc Herniations According to Their Locations

Zone	Appearance
Central	The disc herniates left or right of the central canal zone due to the presence of a thick posterior longitudinal ligament in this location.
Paracentral	This is the commonest zone for a disc herniation.
Foraminal	5%–10% of disc herniation occur in this zone and can cause symptoms due to irritation of the dorsal root ganglion in this region.
Extraforaminal	Relatively uncommon to get disc herniation in this zone.
	• (*An extraforaminal disc is a commonly missed pathology in the spine, and this is an important review area. See Chapter 2.3.*)

Table 2.2.4 Disc Herniations According to Their Morphology

Terminology	Appearances
Disc protrusion	When disc herniation (involving more than 25% of the circumference of the disc) base is wider than its outward extension (Figure 2.2.16b)
Disc extrusion	When the outward extension of the herniated disc is larger than its base (Figure 2.2.16c)
Disc sequestration	When a fragment of the intervertebral disc (typically the nucleus pulposus) breaks off as a free fragment and is not in continuity with the parent disc

Central Canal Stenosis Assessment

- Can happen at one level or multiple levels.

- Usually due to ligamentum flavum hypertrophy or facet osteophytes posteriorly and disc herniations anteriorly.

- Do not measure the anteroposterior diameter of canal. Use the shape of the canal and the thecal sac instead.

- No agreed-on definition of mild, moderate, or severe canal stenosis. Following is the rough guide of the central canal stenosis: *Mild*: Majority of CSF around intrathecal nerve roots or cord is preserved. *Moderate*: Paucity of CSF with crowding of intrathecal nerve roots or flattening of cord. *Severe*: Complete loss of CSF around intrathecal nerve roots or complete flattening or kinking of the cord without or with cord signal abnormalities.

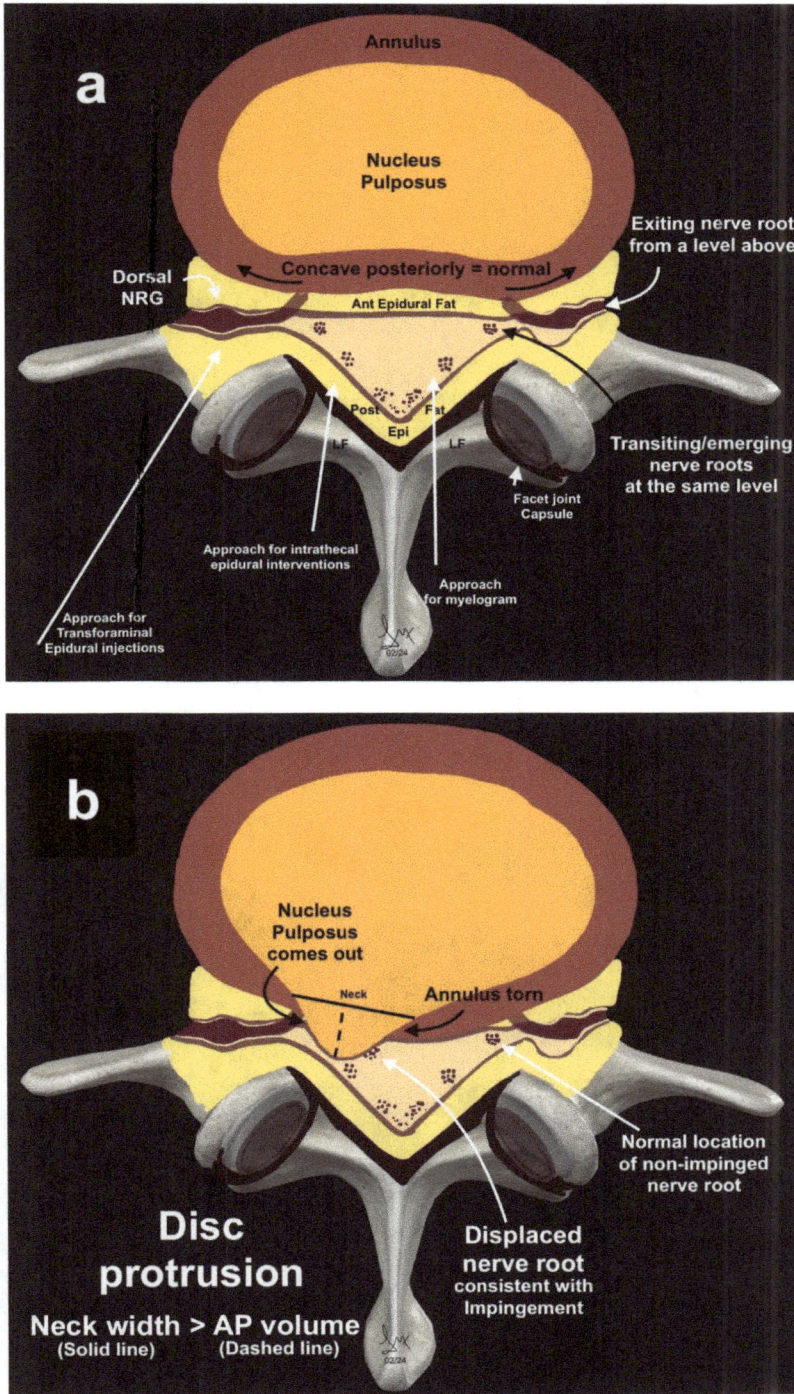

Figure 2.2.16 Graphic figures illustrating (a) normal disc anatomy and features and differences of (b) disc protrusion, and (c) disc extrusion. (Courtesy of Dr Siddharth Thaker, Leicester, UK.)

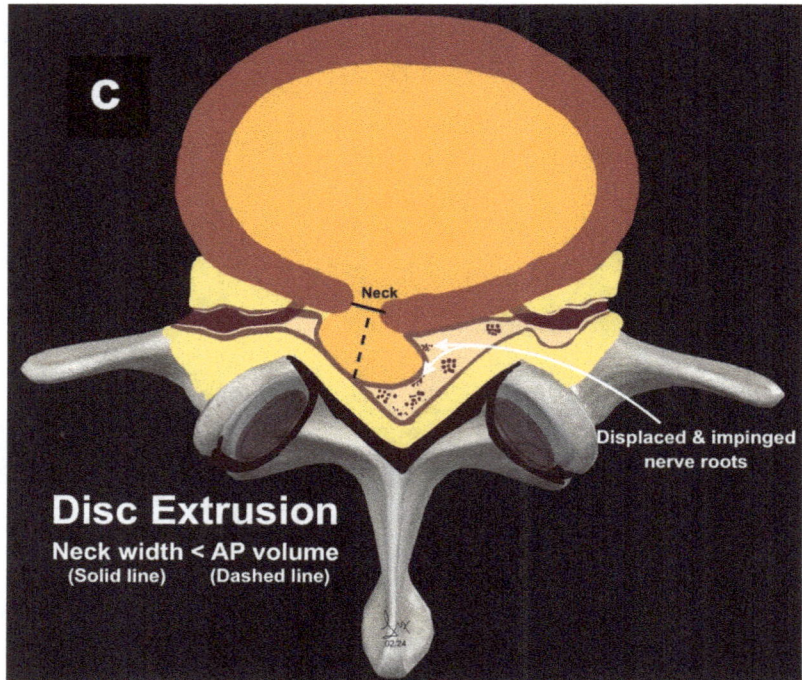

Figure 2.2.16 (Continued)

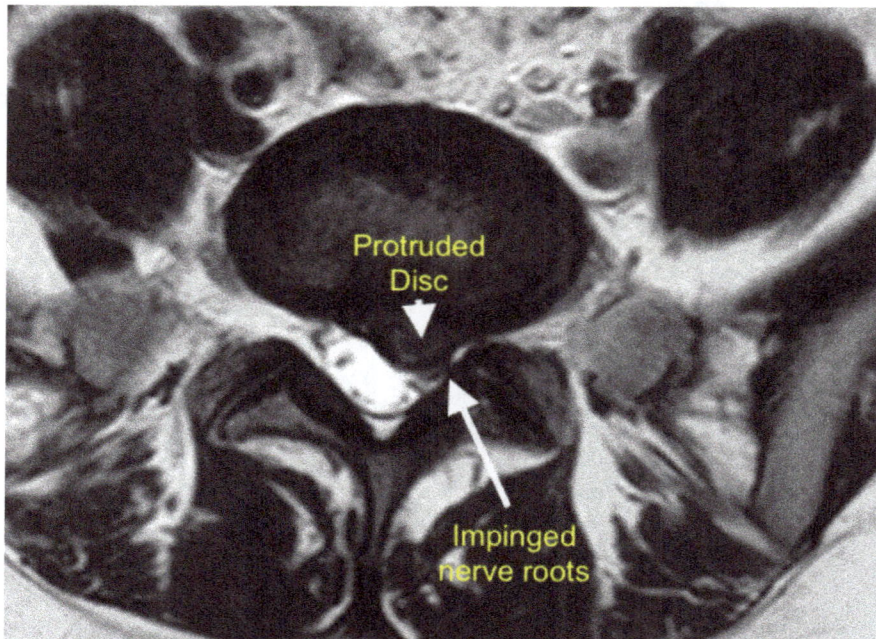

Figure 2.2.17 Left paracentral disc protrusion causing stenosis of the left subarticular recess and impingement of the traversing left L5 nerve root.

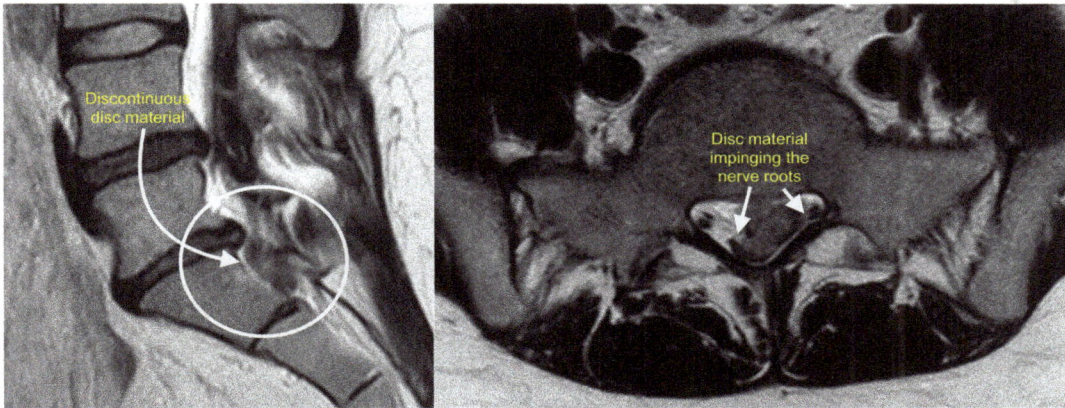

Figure 2.2.18 Sagittal T2 sequence of the lumbar spine demonstrating disc protrusions as L4/5 and also L5/S1. There is a sequestered disc fragment lying posterior to the S1 vertebral body on the axial T2.

Facet Joint Degeneration

- Facet osteophytes, joint irregularities, and effusion are commonest features.

- Prominent osteophytes cause neural impingement in the foraminal region.

- Sometimes, a synovial cyst develops from the degenerated synovial joint, which can extend dorsally in the paraspinal region or within the central canal, compressing the intrathecal nerve roots.

HOW TO LOOK AT A SPINAL MRI IN CONTEXT OF DDD

Step 1. Assess Disc Hydration

A healthy intervertebral disc should appear T2 hyperintense due to the high water content. Disc desiccation is one of the earliest signs of DDD; it is indicated by a loss of this hyperintense T2 signal, resulting in a darker disc. Compare the height of the affected disc with the adjacent levels; disc height loss is a sign of advanced degeneration. The presence of gas within the disc space (vacuum phenomenon) is also a sign of advanced disc degeneration and is best appreciated on CT. On MRI, it is seen as an intensely hypointense signal on T2-weighted images (Figure 2.2.19), the presence of gas within the disc space, seen as a hypointense signal on T2-weighted images, is a sign of advanced disc degeneration.

Step 2. Evaluate Disc Contour and Integrity

Hyperintense T2 signal at the margins of the annular fibrosis can be a sign of annular fissures, which are associated with back pain. Assess the contour of the disc on the axial plane (disc bulge vs disc herniation). Evaluate the extent and impact on the spinal canal and nerve roots.

Schmorl's nodes are vertical herniations of the intervertebral disc material (nucleus pulposus) into the adjacent vertebral body endplates and can be incidental findings associated with DDD.

- T1-weighted images: Low signal intensity within the vertebral body

- T2-weighted images: Variable signal intensity

Step 3. Examine the Adjacent Structures

- Assess for Modic type vertebral endplate changes, best seen on the T1- and T2-weighted sagittal planes.

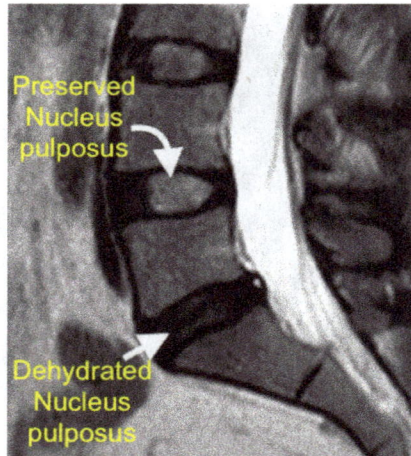

Figure 2.2.19 T2 sagittal image of the lumbar spine demonstrating disc desiccation and reduced intervertebral disc height at L5/S1 with a small posterior annular fissure.

- Assess for osteophytes, which appear as bony outgrowths at the edges of the vertebral bodies, visible on both T1- and T2-weighted images.

- Assess for signs of facet joint osteoarthritis, such as joint space narrowing, subchondral sclerosis, and osteophyte formation. A synovial cyst and ligamentum flavum hypertrophy are further findings that can be associated with facet arthropathy (Figure 2.2.20). Osteophytes and facet joint arthrosis can contribute to spinal canal stenosis.

Step 4. Evaluate the Spinal Canal, Lateral Recess, and Neural Foramina

- Central canal stenosis: Assess the anteroposterior diameter of the spinal canal on the axial plane T2-weighted images (Figure 2.2.21). Signs of stenosis include effacement of the thecal sac to compression of the spinal cord (if prolonged, this can lead to myelopathic change seen as abnormal T2 signal intensity within the cord itself). Various classifications have been proposed for cervical, thoracic, and lumbar spinal stenosis that generally grade the degree of stenosis as normal, mild, moderate, or severe.

- Lateral recess stenosis: Assess the traversing nerve roots in the lateral recess on the axial plane T2-weighted images. The degree of stenosis can be classified as normal, abutting the nerves, or compressing the nerves (Figure 2.2.22).

- Neural foraminal stenosis: Assess the foramina on the T1-weighted sagittal planes for signs of nerve root impingement. The degree of stenosis can be classified as mild, moderate, or severe based on the extent of effacement of the epidural fat surrounding the exiting nerve in the neural foramina (Figure 2.2.23).

Step 5. Spondylolisthesis

Assess for any anterior or posterior slippage of one vertebral body over another. The Meyerding classification, discussed earlier, is used to grade spondylolisthesis. It is most often seen in the lumbar spine and can lead to spinal instability and cauda equina syndrome.

Step 6. Review Areas

Do not forget to assess conus, pre- and paravertebral and pre-sacral regions, and scout or localiser images for actionable findings.

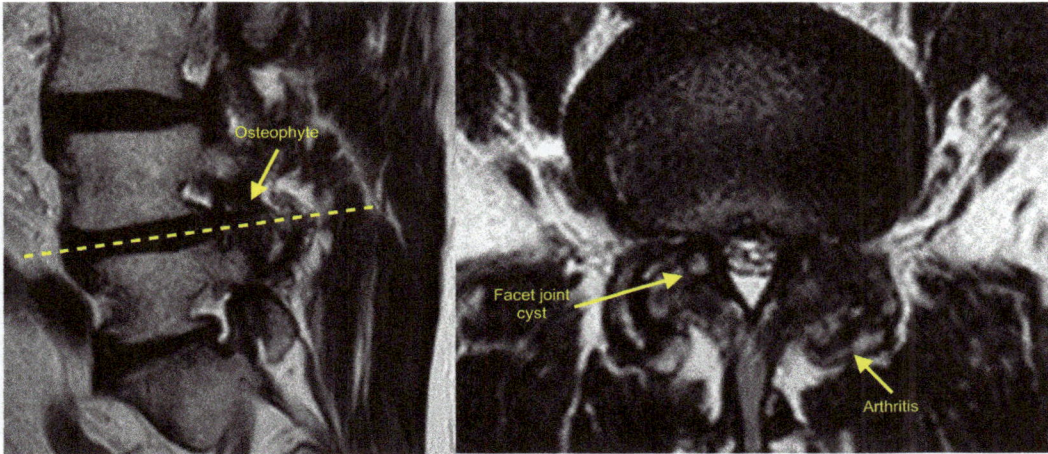

Figure 2.2.20 Sagittal and axial T2 sequences demonstrating severe bilateral facet joint arthritis and hypertrophy of the ligamentum flavum.

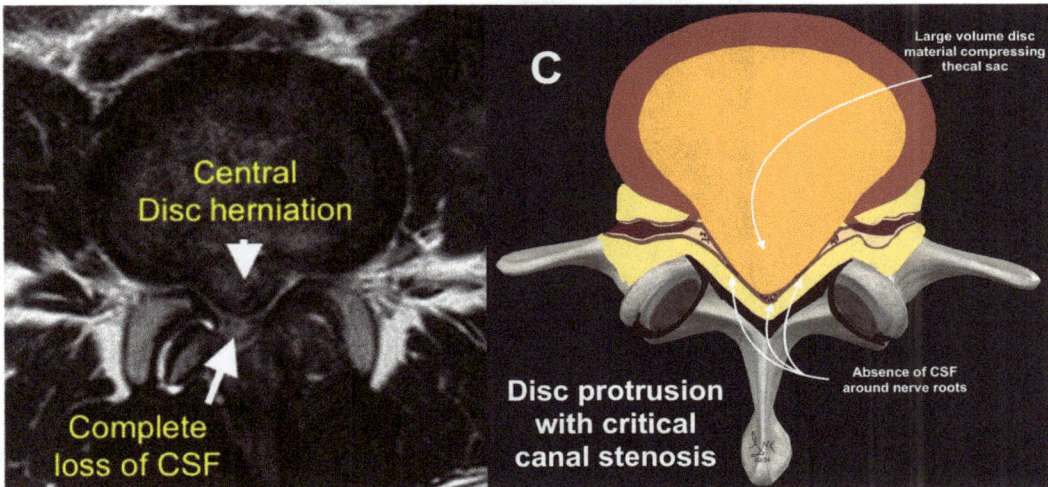

Figure 2.2.21 Axial T2 and corresponding graphic image demonstrating a large central disc protrusion causing severe central canal stenosis and compression of the cauda equina. The cauda equina roots are packed tightly together with no interfacing bright CSF signal. The posterior epidural fat pad is also compressed.

TREATMENT

- Non-operative treatment is the first choice for most patients with degenerative spine disease unless there are acute neurological concerns. If medical therapy is ineffective, imaging and spinal surgery are the next steps.

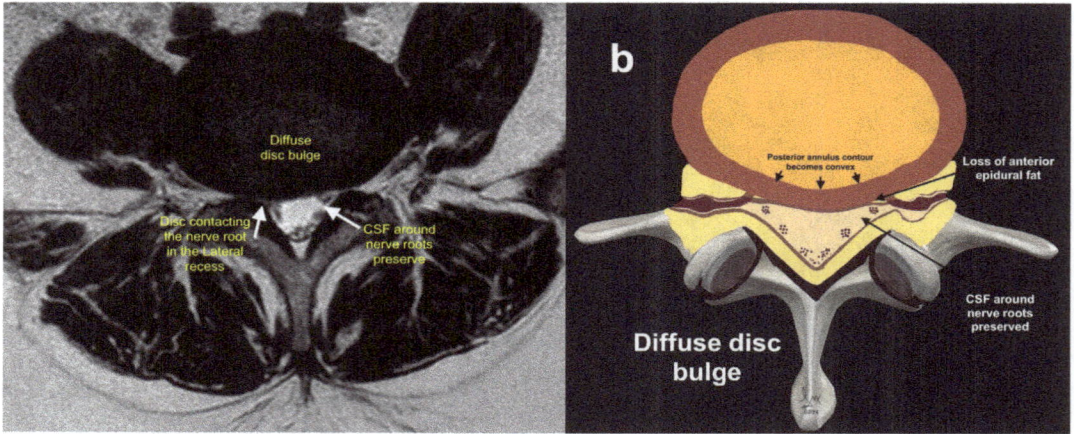

Figure 2.2.22 Axial T2 and corresponding graphic image demonstrating a generalised posterior disc bulge along with ligamentum hypertrophy causing stenosis of the right subarticular recess and abutment of the traversing right L5 nerve root.

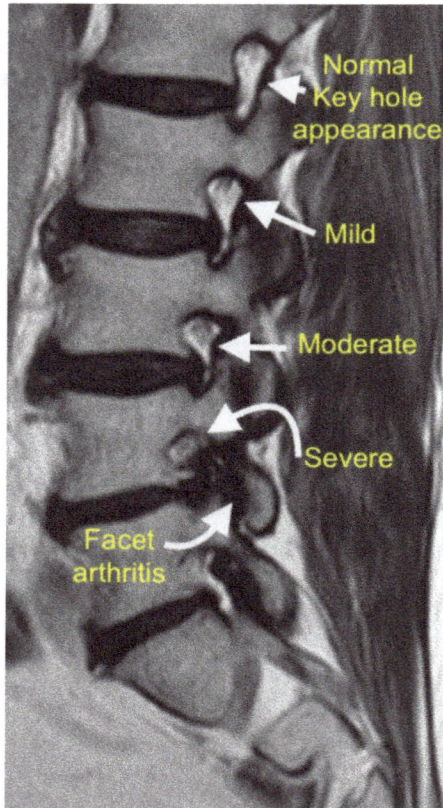

Figure 2.2.23 Sagittal T1 image through the lumbar spine with variable degree of foraminal narrowing at multiple levels.

- Surgical options vary based on the degenerative pattern. Microdiscectomy can help with symptomatic disc herniations, while surgical fusion may be necessary if the degeneration causes spinal instability. Interbody fusion implants are used to restore disc height and support the spine.

- Spondylosis typically does not require surgery.

CONDITIONS MIMICKING DEGENERATIVE SPINAL DISEASE

Several conditions can mimic DDD due to overlapping radiological features. Differentiating these conditions from DDD requires careful consideration of the specific imaging characteristics and clinical context for each case:

- **Intervertebral disc space:** Conditions like infection, trauma, and ankylosing spondylitis can lead to disc space narrowing. Crystal deposition, for example in calcium pyrophosphate deposition disease, can lead to calcific deposits in the intervertebral discs. Similar changes with disc space narrowing or calcifications are sometimes seen in advanced degenerative disc disease.

- **Vertebral body endplate:** Vertebral endplate changes, including fractures, erosions (crystal arthropathies), and inflammation (infection and ankylosing spondylitis), can resemble the Modic type changes in DDD.

- **Bone marrow oedema:** Bone marrow oedema is a non-specific and common finding in infections, trauma, and inflammatory conditions, but you would expect the other features in those conditions to distinguish it from DDD.

- **Osteophyte-like formations:** The formation of syndesmophytes in ankylosing spondylitis, bony outgrowths at the edges of the intervertebral discs, can appear similar to osteophytes seen in DDD. However, syndesmophytes are finer in appearance and are more vertically oriented than the more horizontally inclined vertebral osteophytes.

SUGGESTED READING

- Helms CA, Major NM, Anderson MW, Kaplan P, Dussault R. *Musculoskeletal MRI e-book*. Elsevier Health Sciences; 2008 Dec 9.

- Baert AL. *Spinal Imaging: Diagnostic Imaging of the Spine and Spinal Cord*. Springer Science & Business Media; 2007 Dec 27.

SBA QUESTIONS

1) A 67-year-old man undergoes an MRI of his lumbar spine following an episode of acute or chronic lower back pain. The MRI shows vertebral body endplate signal abnormality at L5/S1 with low T1 and high T2 signal intensity. What is the most likely diagnosis?

    A. Modic type I change

    B. Modic type II change

    C. Modic type III change

2) A 56-year-old woman with a recent history of infective endocarditis presents with thoracolumbar back pain and low grade fevers. There are features of infective spondylodiscitis at T12/L1. Which feature would suggest the formation of an associated paraspinal abscess rather than phlegmon?

    A. Uniformly enhancing lobulated paraspinal soft tissue adjacent to the level of infective spondylodiscitis.

    B. Uniformly enhancing area in the epidural space.

    C. Peripherally enhancing and centrally non-enhancing lobulated paraspinal soft tissue adjacent to the level of infective spondylodiscitis.

3) Which of these features are more commonly seen in TB spondylitis rather than pyogenic spondylitis?

A. Small paraspinal abscess/phlegmon formation.

B. Non-contiguous vertebral body involvement.

C. Contiguous vertebral body involvement with relative sparing of the IV disc with large paraspinal abscess/phlegmon formation.

Answers: (1) A, (2) C, (3) C

Chapter 2.3
Spinal Cord and Cauda Equina Compression

Siddharth Thaker and Harun Gupta

LEARNING OBJECTIVES

- Understanding MRI sequences, normal appearances of various tissues on different pulse sequences, abnormal appearances, and variant anatomy

- Cauda equina compression: Various causes and imaging appearances, the clinical importance of such findings and how to convey them, and differential diagnoses when the CES MRI is negative

- Spinal cord compression: Extrinsic causes of the cord compression (spinal cord tumours are described separately in the oncology volume), cord compression scoring and SINS, benign vs malignant vertebral fractures, imaging appearances of metastases, lymphoma, and myeloma

---

INTRODUCTION

Please refer to Chapter 1.6 to understand the importance of various imaging appearances. The RCR/NICE dictates a particular set and order of MRI sequences to be performed as soon as possible, certainly within 4 hours of the clinical request.

MRI SEQUENCES FOR CAUDA EQUINA SYNDROME (CES)

First, perform sagittal T2W 2D fast spin echo (FSE) or turbo spin echo (TSE) through the lumbar spine. Then, if lumbar T2W sagittal is positive for compression, additional (2) T1W sagittal and (3) T2W axial images are obtained at the level to aid potential surgical intervention.

OR

IF lumbar T2W sagittal is negative for compression, T2W sagittal images through the cervical and thoracic spine are obtained with additional axial images through the level of compression if present or the patient is sent to clinical review if no compression. Please see Table 2.3.1 to understand the normal and abnormal appearances of anatomical structures.

Causes, Mimics, and Imaging Appearances of Cauda Equina Compression

The most common cause on imaging for suspected CES is a large lumbar disc prolapse. Degenerated discs show different shapes and volumes. Numerous terms are used to define disc shape and neural irritation, and unfortunately, there is no consensus on standardisation across regions and practitioners. We described the normal disc and various types of disc shape change with degeneration in Chapter 2.2.

Degenerated Disc and Status of the Canal

Degenerated disc disease, alone or in combination with degenerated and hypertrophied flaval ligaments and facet joints, is the most common cause of low back pain and may be associated with cauda equina-type symptoms.

Surgical Reasoning Behind the MRI Scan

- Severe central canal stenosis by disc and posterior elements degeneration requires posterior decompression.

- If only disc herniation is causing severe canal stenosis with normal posterior elements, a variety of disc removal procedures can be tried, with laminotomy and microdiskectomy being the most common.

- If any spinal instability is causing the patient's symptoms, recurring discs, scoliosis, or spondylolisthesis, choose lumbar interbody fusion with posterior stabilisation with rods and screws.

Anatomical Divisions of the Posterior Annulus

The extraforaminal location is also known as the far lateral region. Extraforaminal disc herniation impinges completely exited nerve roots, causing radiculopathy. (**Tip:** *It is common to miss extraforaminal disc herniation*

DOI: 10.1201/9781003500247-12

Table 2.3.1 Normal and Abnormal Appearances of Various Spinal Structures on Different MRI Sequences

Sequence	Assessed Structures	Normal Appearances	Abnormal Appearances
T2W sagittal	Thecal sac containing the conus and the intrathecal nerve roots Spinal alignment and vertebral heights Intervertebral disc heights and degenerative changes	Preserved CSF around the conus and cauda equina nerve roots Preserved disc heights and differentiation between annulus fibrosus and nucleus pulposus Clear prevertebral and presacral spaces for retroperitoneal and presacral fat, respectively	Loss of CSF around the conus and cauda equina nerve roots due to external tissue involvement, whether from disc, tumour, or soft tissue extension from the adjacent vertebra Retroperitoneal and presacral lymphadenopathy or masses
T1W sagittal	Vertebral marrow Endplate and disc changes	Normal vertebral marrow Brighter compared to the intervertebral discs (normal) and paraspinal muscles Endplates: Regular with no discontinuity or erosion	Marrow replacement (most important) Loss of normal bright signal with dark signal on T1W images (Figure 2.3.6) Focal area of fat signal near the posterior vertebral wall surrounding the basivertebral vein is a normal finding (Figure 2.3.1) Typical vertebral haemangioma appears bright (hyperintense on T1) and dark (hypointense on STIR) images
T2W axial	Thecal sac containing the conus and the intrathecal nerve roots Degree of neural compression Facet joint assessment and synovial cysts	Plenty of CSF around the intrathecal nerve roots Uncompressed nerve roots sag down on supine MRI (tip: floating nerve roots indicate compression at the level above or below; check the T2W sagittal to confirm)	Degenerative disc disease at various stages (Figure 2.3.1; for better understanding of disc shape changes, see Figure 2.2.16) Complete loss of CSF around nerve roots = critical canal stenosis

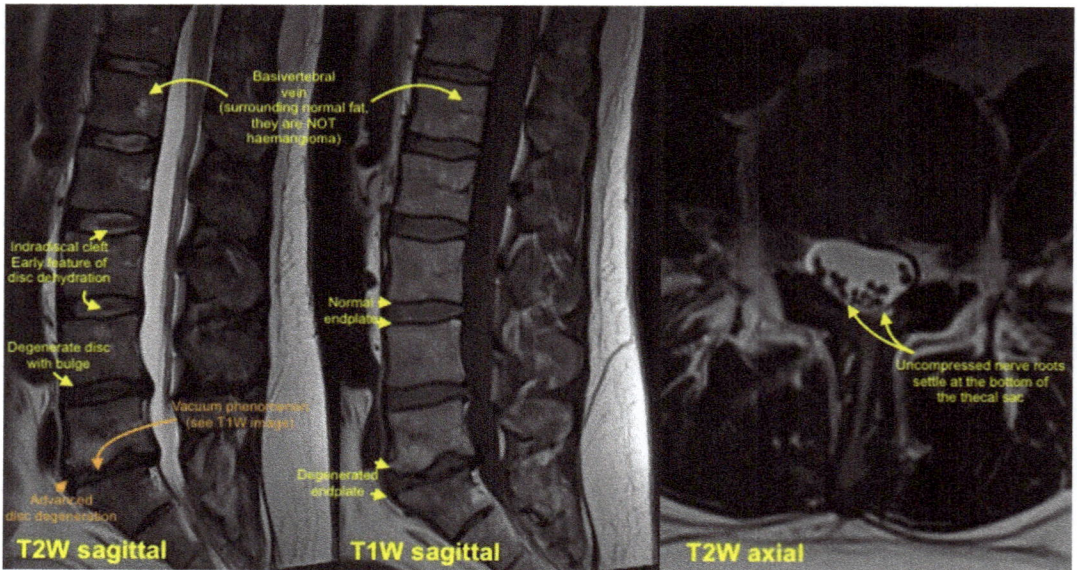

Figure 2.3.1 Routine sequences for cauda equina compression.

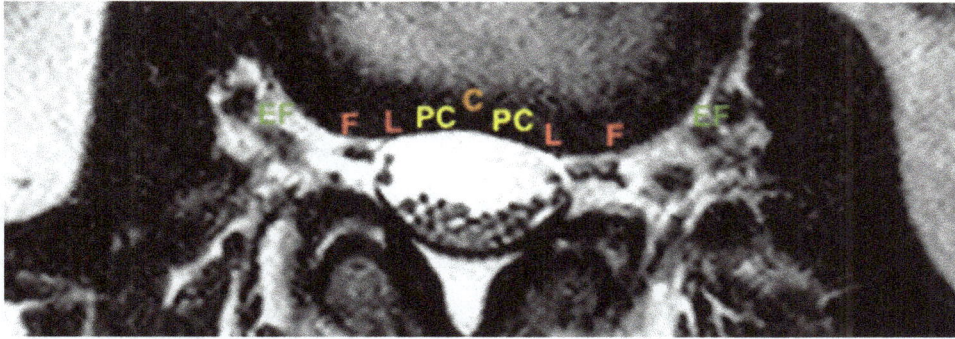

Figure 2.3.2 Locations of disc herniation in relation to the central canal and neural foramina. C = central, PC = paracentral, L = lateral recess, F = foraminal, EF = extraforaminal.

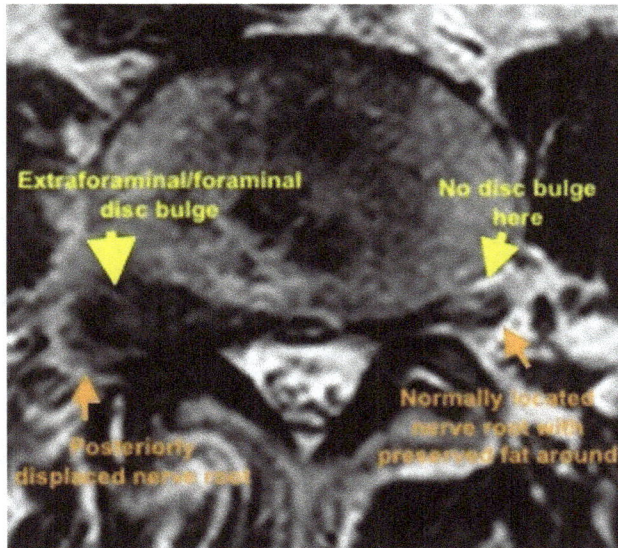

Figure 2.3.3 Right-sided extraforaminal/foraminal disc herniation with neural impingement.

during busy on-call shifts. Carefully assess the first and last sagittal images to diagnose it. It can be confirmed on corresponding axial images as an asymmetrical disc bulge with loss of the fat plane and angulation or posterior displacement of exited nerve roots when compared to the opposite side; Figure 2.3.3). Disc herniations can occur in different locations at a single level. Therefore, mentioning specific details, as in Figure 2.3.2, would provide the reading clinician a better understanding of the herniation.

Importance of Contrast in Certain Cases

Uncommonly, post-contrast spinal imaging is performed when attempting to differentiate a herniated disc from a neurogenic tumour. The herniated disc will show peripheral enhancement (Figure 2.3.4), whereas the neurogenic tumour will show solid, intense enhancement (not shown here).

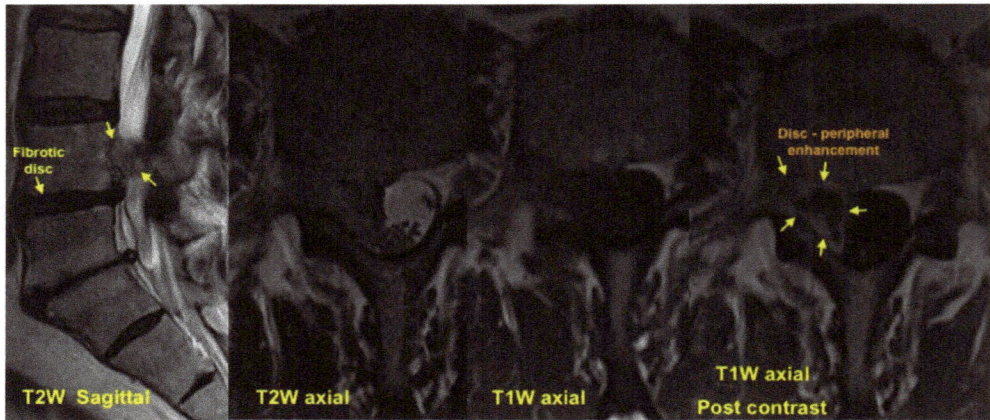

Figure 2.3.4   Post-contrast imaging for differentiating disc herniation from neurogenic tumours.

Important Differentiating Features

Patients with Recurrent CES Symptoms with Recent Spinal Surgery for Similar Symptoms

Spinal surgeons who request repeat MRIs in the early postoperative period are looking for treatable causes that might have developed after spinal surgery, such as the following:

- Epidural haematoma or abscess (discussed in Chapters 2.1 and 2.2 in detail)

- Residual or recurrent disc (at the operated level; Figure 2.3.5)

- New disc herniation (at the level above or below the operated level)

Early postoperative MRI findings might be normal. Make sure NOT to overcall them:

- Postoperative seroma in the posterior paraspinal tissues/surgical bed can persist up to 6 months after the surgery. The diagnosis of infected seroma is clinical based on assessing the wound for pus discharge and serial CRP measurement. Fluid aspiration is rarely required.

- Some endplate irregularity and oedema at the operated level are normal. If the clinical suspicion persists for postoperative spondylodiscitis, a follow-up MRI at 10–14 days interval with serial CRP measurement is required. Progressive endplate destruction, epidural or paravertebral abscess, or new soft tissue oedema beyond the surgical field on STIR images indicate postoperative spinal injection.

- Dural tear/CSF fistula does not present with recurrent CES symptoms. Headache with postural changes is the most common symptom. It requires a fluid-sensitive 3D CISS sequence for further assessment.

Table 2.3.2 Herniated Disc versus Neurogenic Tumour on MRI

Herniated Disc	Neurogenic Tumour
• Usually shows connection in T1W or T2W images with the native degenerated disc	• Separate from the adjacent discs and surrounded by CSF, nodular, can be multiple
• Teardrop shaped, acute disc if T2W increased signal (more painful and high inflammatory component)	• Round to ovular, usually dark (hypointense on T1W and T2W images)
• Peripheral enhancement on post-contrast T1W images	• Continuous intense enhancement on post-contrast T1W images

Spinal Tumours

Spinal cord and primary vertebral column tumours can present as CES. The oncoradiology volume describes them in detail.

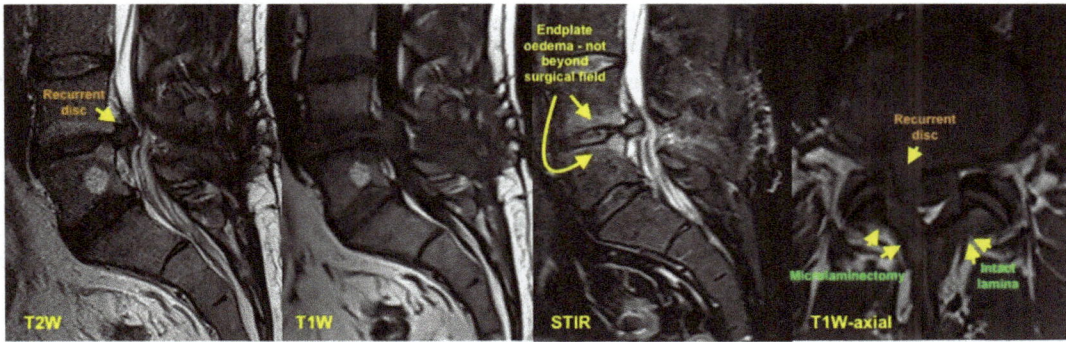

Figure 2.3.5 Recurrent disc herniation presenting with right lower limb radiculopathy and an episode of urinary incontinence.

SPINAL MIMICKERS OF ?CES

Pelvic Tumour or Lymphadenopathy Compressing the Lumbosacral Plexus

Important review areas on the lumbosacral spine MRI:

- Presacral and retroperitoneal space (for pelvic mass, lymph nodes, fluid/blood irritating the lumbosacral nerve roots; common following haemorrhagic adnexal cyst rupture), and aortic aneurysm.

- Edge of kidneys on axial images (for renal masses).

- Compare marrow fat for visible portions of the pelvis; any marrow replacement (Figure 2.3.6) raises suspicion of bony metastases or less likely primary bone lesion.

- On localiser images, look for very large and obvious (do NOT overcall; when in doubt, ask for help!) intraabdominal and pelvic masses, aneurysmal aorta, hip osteonecrosis, and lung masses.

Sacral Insufficiency Fractures

Imaging features and onward referral conditions are as follows:

- Usually involves both sacral alae and the mid-sacrum, usually at S2 or S3 level.

- Linear, wavy lines on T1W images around or involving neural foramina (Figure 2.3.7) and variable degree of oedema on STIR images. The presence of marrow oedema suggests acute or subacute fractures, and movement at fracture sites.

- When seen in elderly and with trivial/no trauma, these T1W or STIR image findings suggest insufficiency fractures requiring further workup for osteoporosis, and rheumatology/ortho-geriatric team referral depending upon the local guidelines.

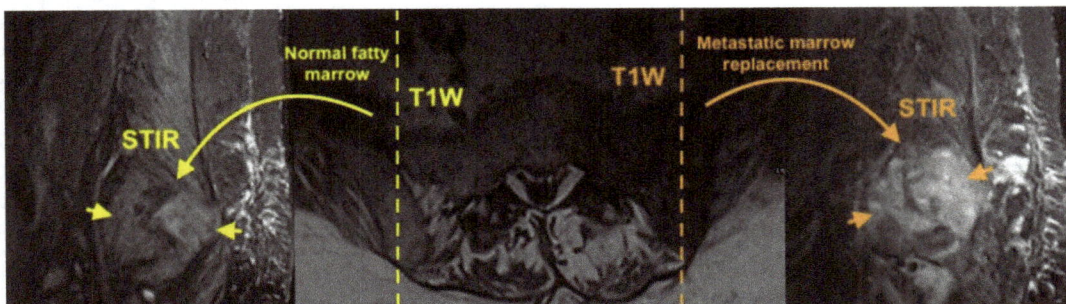

Figure 2.3.6 Axial T1W image showing normal marrow on the right side (yellow annotations) with corresponding sagittal STIR image with normal appearing right sacroiliac joint, compared with marrow replacement of the left hemisacrum (amber annotations) with diffuse bone metastases around the left sacroiliac joint.

- DEXA and serum vitamin D, calcium, phosphate, ALP, and sometimes additional renal functions are carried out for osteoporosis assessment.

- If there is pelvic instability on clinical assessment, CT pelvis can confirm or rule out superior and inferior pubic rami.

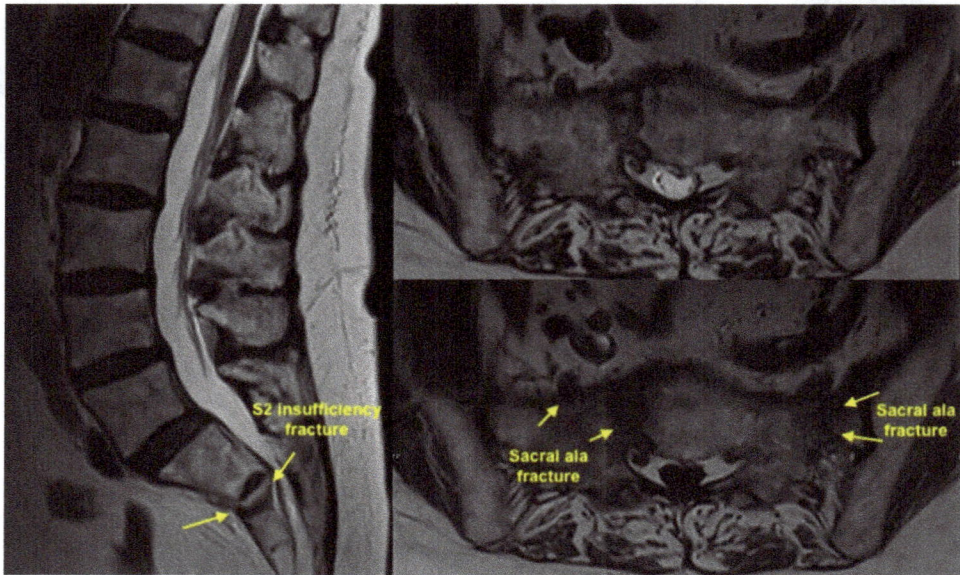

Figure 2.3.7 Classic sacral insufficiency fractures in elderly presented as possible CES.

METASTATIC SPINAL CORD COMPRESSION

- MRI sequences: T1W, T2W, and STIR sagittal images through the whole spine, followed by T2W axial "block" through the area of interest (where the cord compression is suspected to see the CSF around the cord).

- No compression: At the level of spinal metastases, CSF around the cord and cauda equina is maintained circumferentially, and there is no pathological fracture of the vertebra or retropulsion. Such cases can be safety netted and discharged by the clinical team.

- Confirmed cord compression: There is complete and circumferential loss of the CSF; cord is displaced, angulated, and/or oedematous; or severe pathological fracture with retropulsed component in the central canal obscuring the CSF around the cord. This is an oncological emergency. The patient should be immediately flagged to the ED/referring team as it requires urgent acute oncology and spinal team inputs. It is good practice to convey the critical findings to the referrer via telephone (in addition to electronic alerts if available) and document them on report or EPR.

  - Impending cord compression is the most challenging both radiologically and clinically. Key imaging appearances are a new pathological fracture with oedema, which suggests that it can progress; mild cord deformity but CSF and epidural are still present around the cord; and no cord oedema.

Benign (Osteoporotic) vs Malignant (Pathological) Fractures

Sspinal instability neoplastic scoring is less important from the examination point of view. Spinal surgeons might ask for the score during MDT discussions to formulate a surgical plan.

MSCC CAUSES, IMAGING FEATURES, AND MANAGEMENT
Vertebral Metastases
Imaging Features

- Focal or multiple, nodular or diffuse, homogenous or heterogenous involvement

- Osteolytic metastases: T1W—dark and T2W/STIR—bright (variable degree)

- Osteoblastic metastases: Dark on all pulse sequences

- Variable degree of marrow oedema

- Bone islands, Paget's disease, and atypical haemangioma can mimic metastases (focal CT or DIXON imaging in cases of atypical haemangioma are helpful)

- MRI can dictate the treatment response following local or systemic therapy

Table 2.3.3 **MRI Appearances of Benign versus Malignant Vertebral Fractures**

Benign Fractures	Malignant Fractures
• Abnormal signal (T1W—dark, STIR—bright) limited to the body	• Abnormal signal (T1W—dark, STIR—bright) involves posterior wall and posterior elements of vertebra
• Involves adjacent vertebrae (domino pattern); usually thoracic and lumbar vertebrae are involved	• Shows skip levels; can involve any vertebra and sacrum
• Preserved fatty marrow signal	• Complete replacement of fatty marrow
• Concave posterior margin resembles crumbled empty box; fracture line often visible	• Convex posterior margin resembles crumbled box with spillage of internal content; no visible fracture line
• NO associated soft tissue mass	• Soft tissue mass present

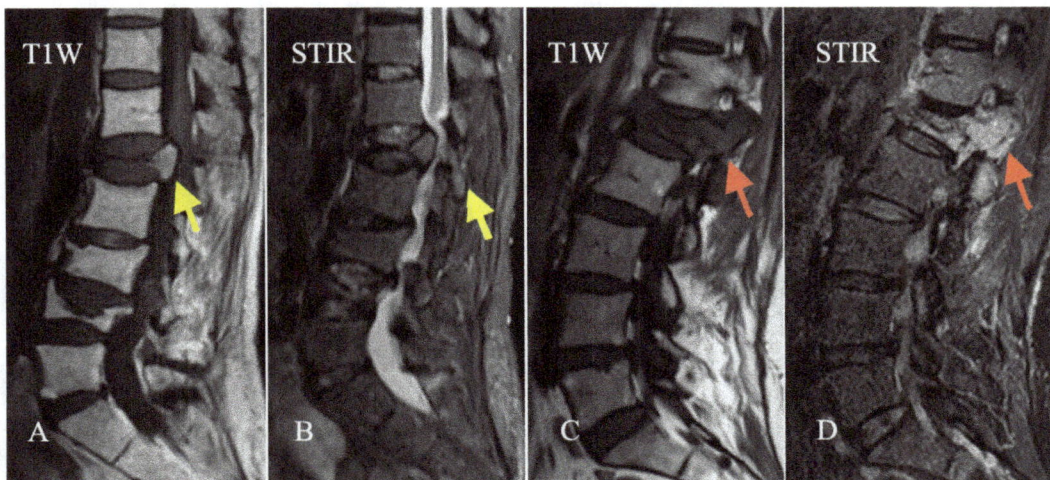

Figure 2.3.8 Vertebral compression fractures: (A) MRI lumbar spine: T1W and (B) STIR sagittal images demonstrate compression of L1 vertebral body with retropulsion of the posterior cortex and preserved normal fatty marrow signal (yellow arrows) suggesting benign or osteoporotic fracture. Conversely, (C) T1W and (D) STIR sagittal images demonstrates infiltrative lesion in L1 vertebral body replacing the normal fatty marrow and extending to the posterior elements (red arrows) suggesting malignant aetiology. (Courtesy: Dr Ankit Tandon, Tan Teck Song Hospital, Singapore.)

Imaging Recommendations If Newly Diagnosed

- Contrast-enhanced CT chest, abdomen, and pelvis identify the primary and relevant MDT referral.
- If no primary tumour identified on staging CT, MDT for unknown primary referral.

Lymphoma

- Approximately 95% of marrow involvement in lymphoma is secondary.
- Most common spread: Haematogenous, circulating lymphoma cells deposited in the marrow from an extra skeletal primary site.

Imaging Features

- Non-specific; may mimic metastases
- T1W, T2W, and STIR—mild dark
- Large soft tissue component, extensively infiltrating surrounding structures without displacing them
- Diffusion restriction on diffusion-weighted and ADC images
- Intense post-contrast enhancement

Imaging Recommendations If Newly Diagnosed

- Contrast-enhanced CT of the neck, chest, abdomen, and pelvis in 2-week wait protocol
- Lymphoma MDT referral
- PET-CT for the staging, treatment response, and restaging

Myeloproliferative Disease/Myeloma

- Plasmacytoma, multiple myeloma, Waldenström's macroglobulinemia (associated with osteonecrosis), and amyloidosis appear similar on MRI.
- Unchecked proliferation of plasma cells stimulates osteoclasts and inhibits osteoblasts, leading to trabecular destruction and diffuse osteopaenia.
- Myeloma screen, bone marrow aspiration, and biopsy are definitive.

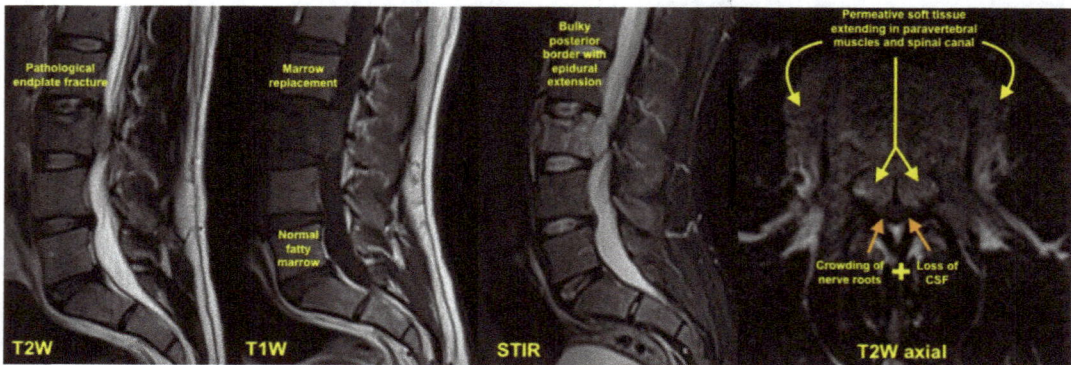

Figure 2.3.9 Biopsy-proven lymphoma showing all features of malignant fracture and cord compression from a large infiltrative soft tissue component.

Imaging Features

- MRI patterns of multiple myeloma change with change in the disease severity.

- Normal marrow appearances (low disease burden) –> focal lesions (mimics metastases, "mini brain" appearances) –> variegated involvement (heterogenous appearance, like cracked black pepper sprinkled on the marrow) –> diffuse skeletal involvement (homogenous involvement)

- Pre-treatment MRI appearances: T1W—iso to hypo (dark), T2W—hyper to hypo (bright to dark), and STIR (bright) to adjacent muscles or intervertebral disc, post-contrast—enhances.

- Post-treatment MRI appearances: Resolution of lesions and/or no/rim enhancement indicates complete response. Persistent lesions with enhancement indicates incomplete response.

- Whole-body MRI uses diffusion imaging to further characterise lesions and treatment response. No diffusion restriction following treatment in previously diffusion-restricted lesion indicating treatment response.

Imaging Recommendations If Newly Diagnosed

- Whole-body MRI is used for staging and response assessment.

- PET-CT could be negative (no osteoblastic response).

- Myeloma MDT referral.

CONCLUSION

Cauda equina and metastatic cord compression present unique challenges for reporting radiologists and registrars. To steer patient management in the right direction, they require a thorough understanding of diverse patient presentations, pathologies, mimickers, and appropriate imaging recommendations for each.

SUGGESTED READING

- Helms CA, Major NM, Anderson MW, Kaplan P, Dussault R. *Musculoskeletal MRI e-book*. Elsevier Health Sciences; 2008 Dec 9.

- Baert AL. *Spinal Imaging: Diagnostic Imaging of the Spine and Spinal Cord*. Springer Science & Business Media; 2007 Dec 27.

SBA QUESTIONS

1) A 29-year-old female athlete presents with increasing low back pain, bilateral radiculopathy, and equivocal clinical assessment for cauda equina syndrome. The A&E has requested an urgent MRI scan, which reveals no disc herniation or canal stenosis. However, there is some bilateral symmetrical marrow oedema affecting pedicles of L4 vertebra with linear dark signal within them on T1W images. What is the most likely diagnosis?

   A. Vertebral haemangiomata

   B. Bilateral pars interarticularis fractures

   C. Seronegative spondyloarthritis

   D. Early spondylodiscitis

2) A 69-year-old woman with a history of treated breast cancer presented to A&E with gradually increasing mid-thoracic back pain now causing band-like area altered sensation in the anterolateral and posterior chest wall. Whole-spine MRI was requested to assess for treatable cause by the A&E registrar. It revealed multilevel vertebral metastases with a large metastatic deposit at T8 level. There is marked loss of CSF around the cord, which shows some deformity anteriorly due to epidural soft tissue. However, a sliver of

CSF is still preserved posteriorly. There is no cord oedema by moderate loss of involved vertebral height. What is the most appropriate management for this case?

A. Provide reassurance and wait and watch as such findings are very common in metastatic cancer, and symptoms improve gradually with palliative management.

B. Alert the referrer about the potential need to involve acute oncological services for impending cord compression and document the discussion.

C. Repeat the whole-spine MRI with contrast, alert the referrer for the need for further MRI, and document it.

D. Refer the patient to a weekly breast cancer MDT and assign appropriate MDT code.

3) An MRI performed for suspected cauda equina syndrome can demonstrate which of these?

A. Disc herniation with canal stenosis

B. Normal discs

C. Marrow replacing lesions

D. All of the above

Answers: (1) B, (2) B, (3) D

Sandeep Singh and Amit Shah

LEARNING OBJECTIVE

- To highlight appendicular fractures encountered in clinical practice and a few common classification systems used to guide management

---

INTRODUCTION

FRCR candidates are not always asked for details about fractures, but they are regular occurrences in routine clinical practice. This chapter can be helpful to musculoskeletal radiologists who are involved in orthopaedic trauma MDTs.

- Fracture: A discontinuity in a bony cortex (described according to the location/alignment of the distal fracture fragment).

- Dislocation: A loss of anatomical congruency of bones at a joint level (described by the position of the distal bone comparted to the proximal one).

  - Subluxation: An incomplete dislocation with bones still touching each other.

  - Fractures according to orientation: Transverse, oblique, and spiral fractures.

  - Avulsion fracture: Due to pull from a ligament or a tendon attachment.

  - Overuse/fatigue fracture: Abnormal stress applied to a normal bone.

  - Insufficiency fracture: Normal stress applied to an abnormally weak bone.

  - Pathological fracture: Underlying bone lesions (benign or malignant) and comminuted, open, and intra-articular fractures require definitive (surgical) treatment.

UPPER LIMB AND CLAVICLE FRACTURES

Upper limb and clavicle fractures are frequently due to a fall onto the shoulder and infrequently due to direct trauma or fall onto an outstretched hand (FOOSH). The fractures are categorised according to its anatomical location (Figure 2.4.1). In children, they present as greenstick fractures (Figure 2.4.2). Patients present clinically with palpable or visible deformity due to the cranial pull of the sternocleidomastoid and/or shoulder drop from the inward and downward pull from the latissimus dorsi and pectoralis major.

Complications

- Clavicular fractures are commonly isolated. However, consider injury to the subclavian vessels and/or brachial plexus give its proximity.

- Closed fractures can be converted to open if there is fracture displacement or severe angulation (Figure 2.4.3). They are also at increased risk of skin necrosis and converting a closed fracture to an open fracture. These fractures are also at risk of mal-union, non-union, and neurovascular compromise from mechanical compression or from callus encasing them.

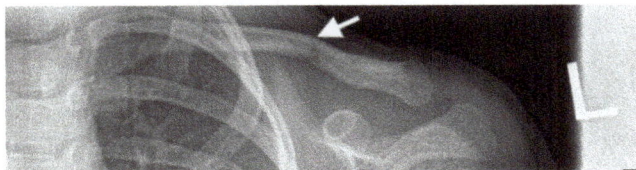

Figure 2.4.1　Middle third clavicle demonstrating a horizontal fracture at the thinnest segment.

DOI: 10.1201/9781003500247-13

- Medial clavicle fractures are difficult to identify, are associated with high-energy trauma, and can pose risk of mediastinal injuries.

Management

- Uncomplicated fractures are managed conservatively.

- Patients at risk of neurovascular compromise or severe skin tenting are managed with open reduction internal fixation (ORIF).

SCAPULA FRACTURES

Scapular fractures are relatively uncommon and are usually associated with high-energy trauma with 80%–90% associated with concomitant injuries. Blunt trauma in road traffic collisions and direct trauma are common injury mechanisms. Isolated glenoid inferior rim fractures following anterior shoulder dislocations (Figure 2.4.4), usually with an associated Hill–Sachs deformity. Management is heavily dependent on the complexity of injuries: Non-displaced scapular fractures tend to be managed conservatively; operative

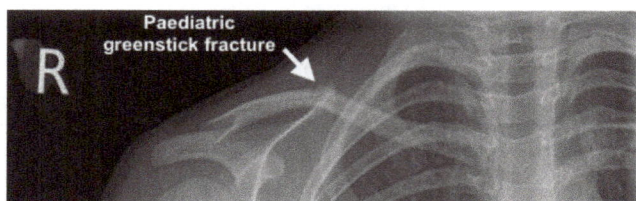

Figure 2.4.2   Greenstick clavicular fracture with angulation in a paediatric patient.

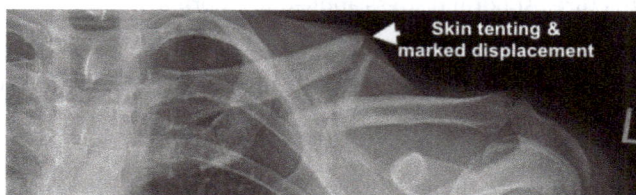

Figure 2.4.3   Markedly displaced clavicle fracture causing skin tenting, with a potential to be open fracture.

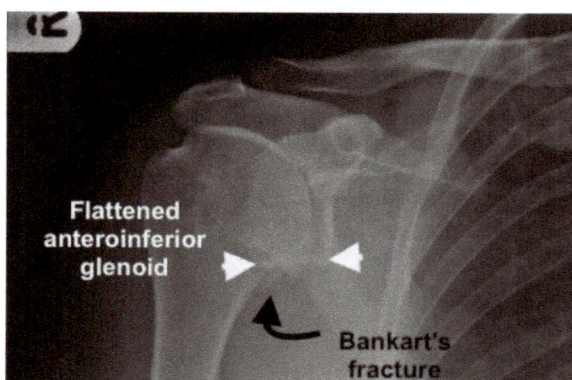

Figure 2.4.4   Inferior glenoid rim fracture in keeping with a Bankart's lesion with a small fracture fragment in the axillary pouch.

management needs to be considered in the contexts of limited shoulder movement, displacement, and concomitant fractures.

PROXIMAL HUMERUS FRACTURES

- Fractures are associated with low-energy impact in elderly patients with osteoporosis and high-energy trauma in young patients.

- Fractures are categorised according to their locations including the anatomical neck, surgical neck (weakest point), and greater and lesser tuberosities. They can require further CT scan depending upon the fracture patterns.

- CT usually aids in surgical decision-making about whether to treat fractures conservatively or surgically. If proximal humerus fractures are not treated sufficiently, osteonecrosis of the humeral head and premature osteoarthritis follow.

Neer Classification

Categorises fracture complexity into four broad groups based on the anatomical and surgical neck and the greater and lesser tuberosities. A fragment is considered separate/displaced if it is angulated >45° or separated by 1 cm:

- A one-part fracture with no displacement is treated conservatively.

- With two-part fractures with displacement of one segment, the patient needs to be followed up.

- Operative management is called for with three-part fractures (Figure 2.4.5) that include displacement of two segments including one tuberosity and the surgical neck.

- Four-part fractures with displacement of three segments are considered complex with possible vascular compromise to the humeral head, and operative management is also called for.

Complications

- Weakened deltoid function with loss of sensation at the inferior deltoid in keeping axillary nerve injury.

- Avascular necrosis of the humeral head is common in the elderly and complex fractures.

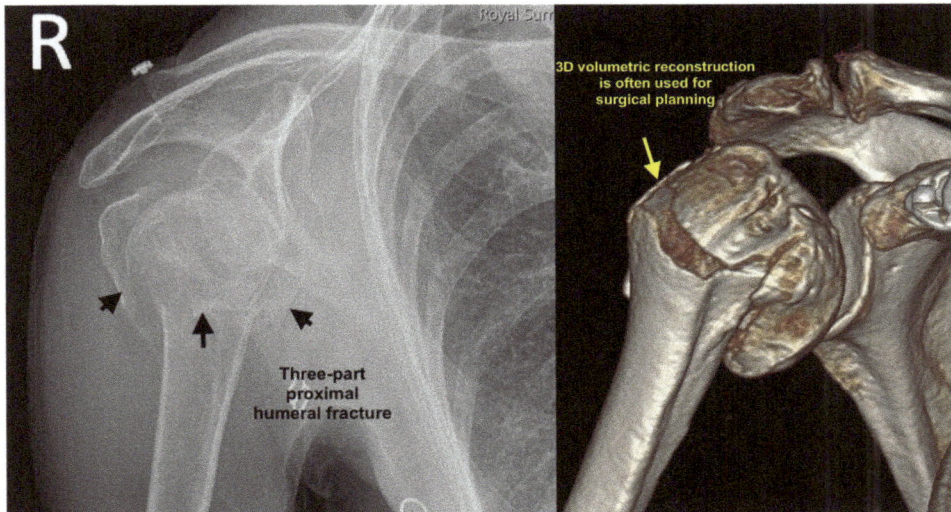

Figure 2.4.5 Comminuted fracture of the humeral head. Neer classification is a three-part fracture as there are >3 fracture fragments including the greater tuberosity. CT could be helpful in preoperative assessment.

Management

- Non-operative management is offered to patients with minimal displaced fractures.

- Surgical management includes ORIF, hemi-arthroplasty, and reverse shoulder arthroplasty and is determined by patient's bone quality, age group, and complexity and Neer classification.

SUPRACONDYLAR FRACTURES

The supracondylar bone is the distal segment of the humerus and is weak in children. FOOSH fractures occur in hyperextension. Non-displaced fractures can be occult with normal anterior humeral line and raised anterior and posterior fat suspicious for an acute fracture.

Complications

Displaced fractures need urgent reduction because of risk of injury to the brachial artery. The median, radial, and ulnar nerves are also at risk.

LATERAL HUMERAL CONDYLE FRACTURES

The second most common fracture in childhood is following FOOSH, considered Salter–Harris IV. High risk of complication if misdiagnosed. Articular displacement determines treatment options (Figure 2.4.6).

Management

Conservative management includes long arm casting for up to 6 weeks, in contrast with operative management involving ORIF with casting.

Complications

Delayed/missed diagnosis can cause stiffness, non- or mal-union, avascular necrosis, and growth arrest given involvement of the growth plate.

FOREARM FRACTURES

Radial Head Fractures

Common intra-articular fractures associated with elbow instability are frequently due to FOOSH and infrequently due to direct trauma. Radial head fracture (Figure 2.4.7) can occur in isolation or as part of complex elbow fracture dislocation. Isolated radial head fractures which are not comminuted can be treated

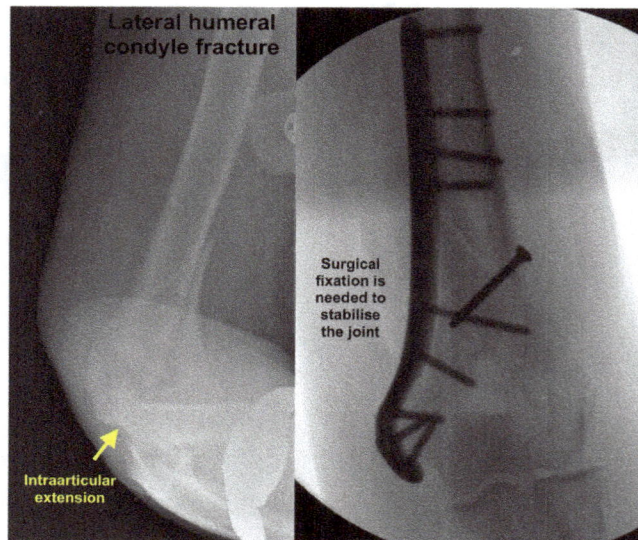

Figure 2.4.6 X-ray showing lateral humeral condyle fracture with intra-articular extension and its treatment (surgical fixation).

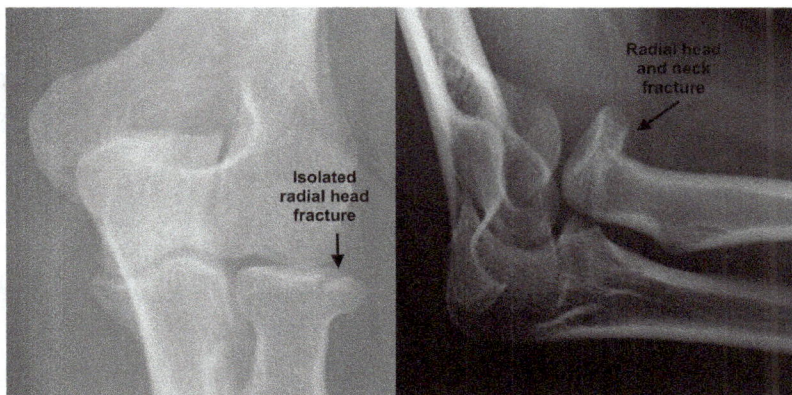

Figure 2.4.7   Isolated radial head and head–neck fractures.

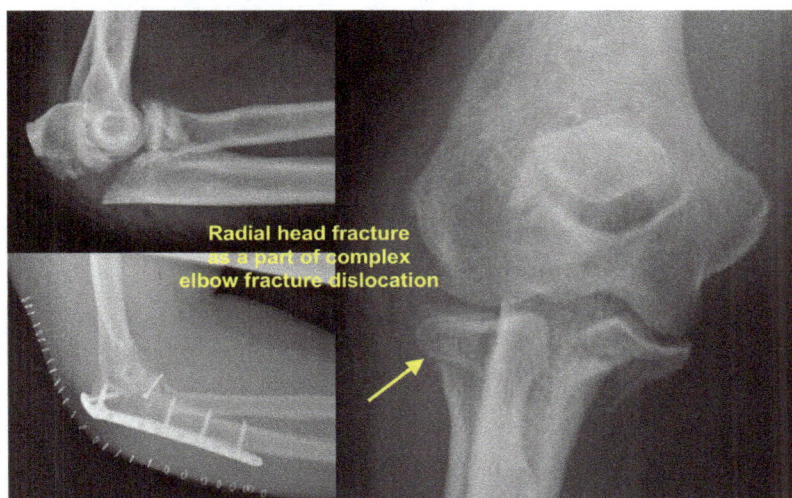

Figure 2.4.8   Radial head fracture as a part of complex elbow fracture–dislocation.

conservatively. Conversely, fractures which are multifragmented, displaced, and associated with more complex injuries require operative management (Figure 2.4.8).

Complications

Elbow instability, stiffness in the absence of early mobilisation, postoperative avascular necrosis, and post-trauma arthritis are common complications following radial head fracture.

ULNA AND RADIUS FRACTURES

Galeazzi, Monteggia, and Essex–Lopresti fractures commonly occur following FOOSH and occur less commonly due to direct trauma.

Galeazzi Fracture

- Distal 3rd radius fracture with an associated distal radioulnar joint (DRUJ) dislocation (Figure 2.4.9). Radial nerve is commonly injured.

- Conservative approach in children with immobilisation, closed reduction, and splitting; in adults, surgery avoids non-union.

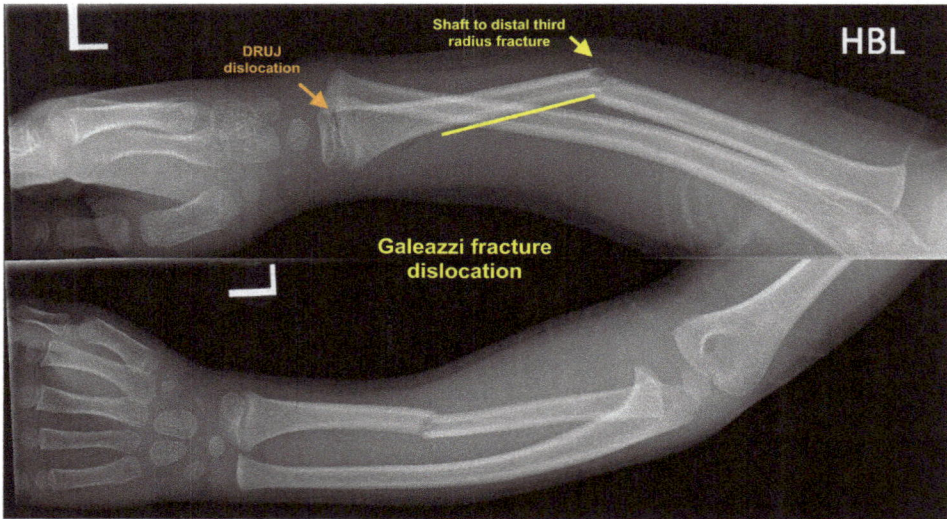

Figure 2.4.9 Galeazzi fracture pattern.

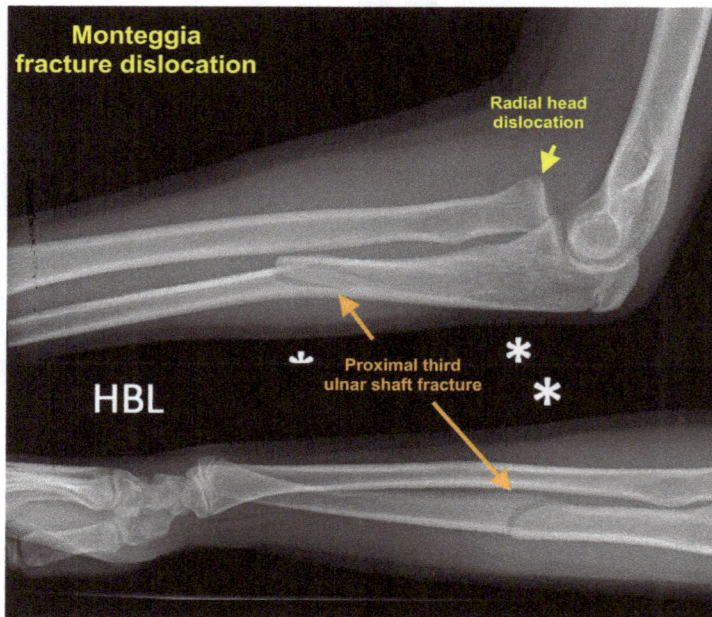

Figure 2.4.10 Monteggia fracture pattern.

Monteggia Fracture

- Proximal ulna fracture with an associated dislocation of the radial head (Figure 2.4.10).

- Radial and median nerve are commonly injured.

- Considered unstable and requires operative management. In paediatrics, plastic deformity, or greenstick fracture, non-operative management is considered.

Essex–Lopresti Fracture

- Radial head fracture, dislocation of the DRUJ, and disruption of the interosseous membrane
- Surgical approach

DISTAL RADIUS FRACTURES

Caused by FOOSH in elderly osteoporotic bones or high-energy impact in young patients. Fractures can be managed operatively or non-operatively if certain criteria have been satisfied. Often associated with ulna styloid fractures (Figure 2.4.11).

Colles Fracture

- Extra-articular fracture with dorsal angulation
- "Dinner fork" deformity

Smith Fracture

- Extra-articular fracture with volar angulation
- "Garden spade" deformity

Barton Fracture

- Intra-articular fracture of the distal radius with dorsal tilt of the distal fragment

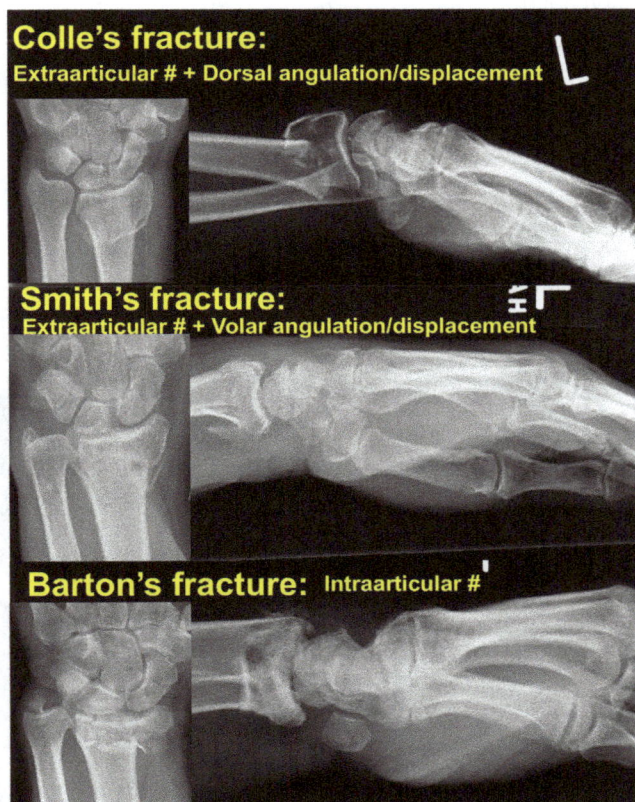

Figure 2.4.11   Distal radius fracture patterns.

HAND FRACTURES

Scaphoid Fracture

Most common and difficult to diagnose. Fractures may be initially occult on X-ray, consider further imaging; MRI most sensitive, but CT readily available. Commonly occurs following FOOSH and infrequently stress fractures in athletes. Retrograde blood flow from distal to proximal increases the risk of osteonecrosis in middle and proximal scaphoid fractures.

- Mayo Classification: Middle (waist), 70% (Figure 2.4.12); distal, 20%; proximal, 10%

- Scaphoid series (DP view, DP view with ulnar deviation, oblique view, and lateral view) are used to detect scaphoid fractures. Sometimes, scaphoid fracture is not visible on initial radiographs, and follow-up radiographs after 10–14 days are recommended. If the patient remains symptomatic after 2 weeks, clinical suspicion is still high, and no fracture is visible on follow-up X-rays, CT or screening MRI is used to detect or rule out potential fracture.

- Non-operative management in non-displaced fractures or <1mm displacement. Operative management improves morbidity, stiffness, healing and grip strength and reduces the immobilisation period.

- CT is commonly used to follow up treated fractures. It can readily detect complications including osteonecrosis, delayed union, scapholunate non-union advanced collapse, and scapholunate advanced collapse (SLAC) if there is associated scapholunate dissociation (see Figures 2.16.30 and 2.16.32).

CARPAL FRACTURES (FIGURE 2.4.13)

Triquetral Fractures

- The second most common fracture
- "Pooping duck sign" on lateral projection
- Typically managed conservatively

Hamate Fractures

- Uncommon
- Classified as type I (hook of hamate) or type II (body of hamate)
- Often associated with base of 4th and 5th fracture/dislocation
- Ulnar nerve and artery are commonly injured

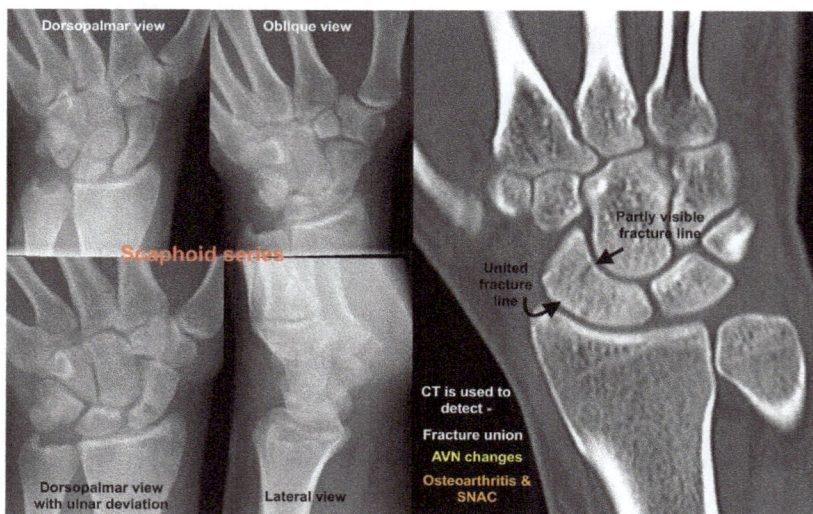

Figure 2.4.12 Radiographic series showing scaphoid fracture.

METACARPAL FRACTURES (FIGURE 2.4.13)

Rolando vs Bennett Fractures

- Both considered intra-articular fractures at the base of the 1st metacarpal

- Bennet fracture separates the palmar ulna aspect of the 1st metacarpal

- Roland fracture is a comminuted fracture forming Y- or T-shape fragments at the base of the 1st metacarpal

Boxer's Fracture

- Direct trauma transmitted from a closed fist

- Fracture at the neck of the 5th metatarsal with volar angulation of the head

- Minor angulation is treated conservatively with immbolisation and buddy splint

- Significant angulation needs to be managed operatively with K wires

PHALANX FRACTURES

Gamekeeper's Thumb (Figure 2.4.14)

- Avulsion fracture at the base of the proximal phalanx of the thumb

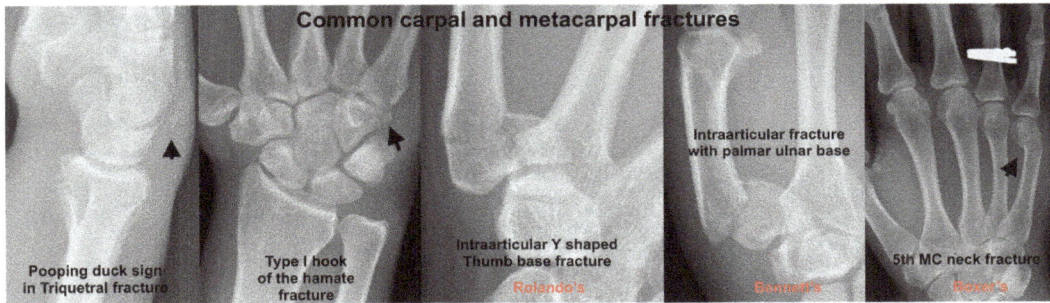

Figure 2.4.13 Common carpal and metacarpal fractures.

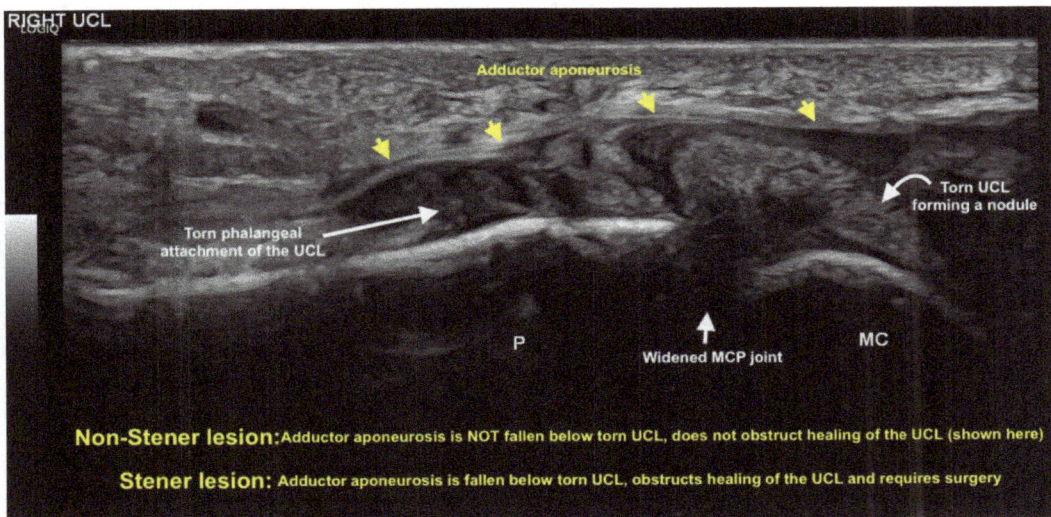

Figure 2.4.14 Ultrasound appearances of the injured UCL of the thumb.

- Interposition of the adductor pollicis aponeurosis between the UCL and MCP joint suggests a Stener lesion and calls for MRI/US evaluation. With a non-Stener lesion, adductor aponeurosis falls between the torn UCL and the MCP joint and can heal with conservative treatment.

Mallet Finger

- Hyperflexion injury causing an avulsion fracture at the fragment at the base of the distal phalanx at the attachment of the distal extensor tendon.

- Distal interphalangeal joint is held in flexed position.

- Conservative management with a splint held in hyperextension for 6 weeks is preferred.

- Complications include post-traumatic arthritis, extensor lag, and swan neck deformity.

Tuft Fractures

- Comminuted fracture of the distal phalanx, usually because of crush injury.

- If the nail bed is avulsed, it is considered as an open fracture and antibiotics cover is required.

- Commonly treated conservatively unless very comminuted, in which case K wire stabilisation is called for.

LOWER LIMB FRACTURES

Femur Fractures

- Neck of femur fractures are common following a fall/trauma in the elderly with osteoporotic bone or high-velocity injury in young patients.

- Often classified as an intracapsular or extracapsular.

- Intracapsular fractures are at risk of avascular necrosis (AVN); the medial femoral circumflex artery supplies the femoral head via retrograde blood flow from the femoral neck. Displaced fractures disrupt the blood flow and lead to femoral head AVN.

- Intracapsular fractures can also be described in relation to the neck of the femur as subcapital (most common), transcervical and basicervical (Figure 2.4.15).

- Extracapsular fractures are defined as subtrochanteric fracture when the femoral fracture is within 5cm of the lesser trochanter and intertrochanteric fracture when at the level of the greater and lesser trochanter (Figure 2.4.15).

- Extracapsular fractures are treated differently than intracapsular fractures (usually dynamic hip screw and, if the femoral head and neck are not salvageable, total hip replacement.

- It can be difficult to differentiate between baso-cervical and intertrochanteric fractures.

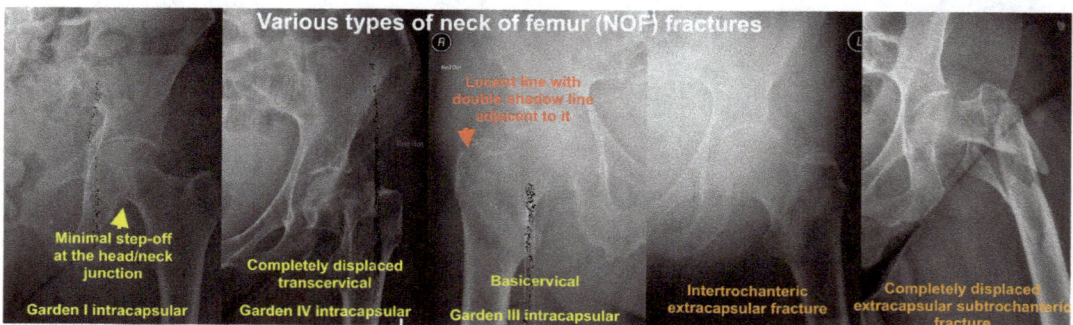

Figure 2.4.15 Intracapsular and extracapsular neck of femur fractures.

Management and Complications

- Non-operative management in patients who are non-ambulatory or postoperative shows high morbidity. Closed reduction with cannulated screw fixation in young, healthy individuals with Garden I & II fractures.

- Open reduction and internal fixation in young patients (<60). However, with fixation there is a high risk of mal-union and avascular necrosis.

- Hemi-arthroplasty in less active elderly patients with co-morbidities, and total hip replacement in active elderly patients. Risk of dislocation with arthroplasty.

KNEE FRACTURES

Tibial Plateau Fracture

- Commonly seen following high-energy trauma in young patients.

- Often associated with neurovascular and/or ligamentous and menisci injuries.

- Suspected individuals need to undergo a throughout ATLS assessment; patients are at high risk of compartment syndrome.

- CT is often used in preoperative planning.

Schatzker classification defines tibial plateau fractures according to fracture depression, displacement, and location (Figure 2.4.16):

- I   Split   Lateral plateau

- II Split depressed   Lateral plateau

- III Central depression   Lateral plateau

- IV Split   Medial plateau

- V Bicondylar fracture

- VI Bicondylar fracture with metaphysis and diaphysis dissociation

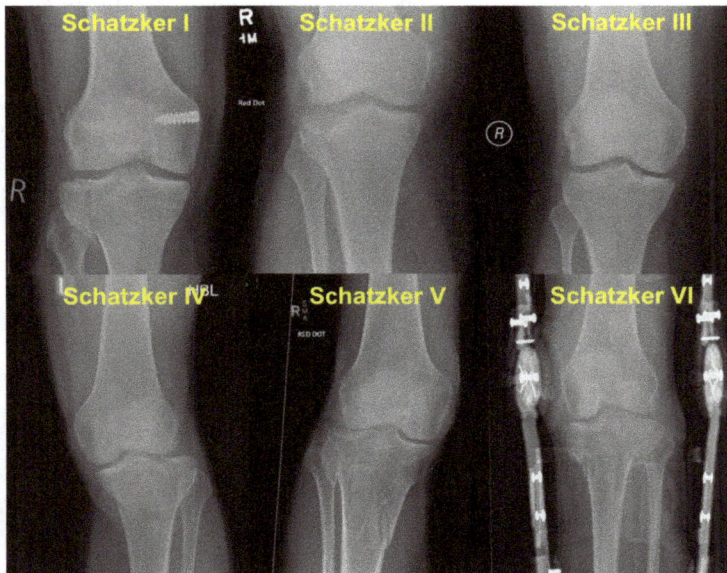

Figure 2.4.16   Tibial plateau fracture with Schatzker classification.

Management

- Non-operative management in minimally displaced fractures or non-ambulatory patients with non-weight-bearing or partially weight-bearing supported by a hinged knee brace.

- The purpose of operative management is to restore articular surface and joint stability. Open reduction internal fixation in fractures with significant displacement and depression.

- External fixation with limited fixation in patients in open fractures with marked contamination. Arthroplasty is considered in elderly osteoporotic patients.

Complications

- Chronic pain, postoperative arthritis, and gait abnormalities are common complications.

Patella Fracture (Figure 2.4.17)

- Largest sesamoid bone, often fractured by direct trauma or by indirect eccentric contraction during active contraction of the quadriceps and rapid knee flexion.

- Fractures can be displaced or non-displaced; the latter demonstrates an intact extensor mechanism.

- Bi-/tri-partite patella is often in superolateral position and can be mistaken for non-displaced fractures.

- Comminuted fracture of the patella with displacement. Lipohaemarthrosis is noted in the lateral projection.

- Bipartite patella in the superolateral position can be often mistaken for a fracture.

Management

- Non-operative management with knee immobilisation held in extension with full weight bearing in patients with an intact extensor mechanism non-displaced fracture.

- Operative management with open reduction and internal fixation with displaced fractures.

- Partial patellectomy in comminuted fractures involves removal of the bone fractures with patella or quadricep tendon advancement via suture tunnels or anchors.

- Common complications are high risk of osteonecrosis, symptomatic hardware and/or implant failure, infection in open fractures, non-union, and postoperative arthritis.

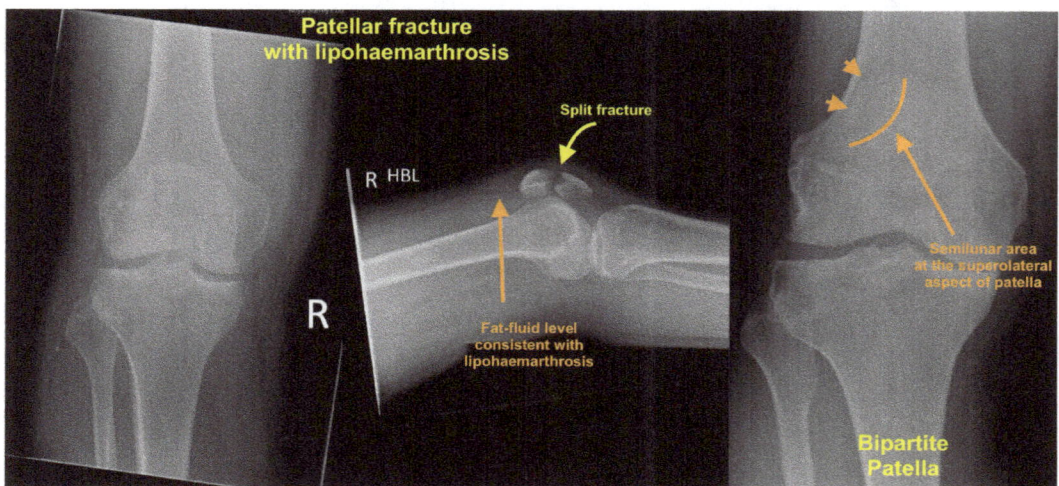

Figure 2.4.17   Patellar fracture and its mimic, bipartite patella.

Segond Fracture (Figure 2.4.18)

- Avulsion fracture at the proximal lateral tibia associated with anterior cruciate ligament injury

- Represents bony avulsion of the anterolateral ligament

- MRI to assess ACL and meniscus injury

Reverse Segond Fracture

- Avulsion fracture at the medial proximal tibia associated with the posterior cruciate ligament injury

- Bony avulsion of the menisco-tibial deep fibres of the medial collateral ligament

ANKLE FRACTURES

Ankle injuries are a common presentation in the emergency department following direct trauma, fall, or twisting. Fractures can be isolated to the distal fibula, and these can be defined as lateral malleolar fractures and/or involve the distal medial and/or posterior tibia, respectively, medial or posterior malleolar fractures (Table 2.4.1).

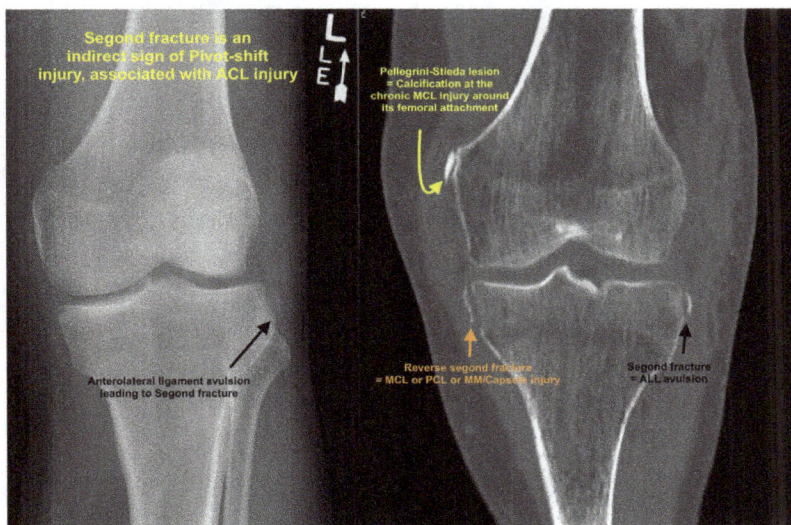

Figure 2.4.18 Segond and reverse Segond fractures and Pellegrini Stieda lesion.

Table 2.4.1 Types of Ankle Fracture–Dislocations by Traumatic Mechanisms

Weber A	Infrasyndesmotic injury (mostly transverse orientation)	• Tibiofibular syndesmosis intact • Conservative management
Weber B	Trans-syndesmotic injury (oblique orientation)	• Tibiofibular syndesmosis is usually intact. Stress views sometimes demonstrate widening of the syndesmosis • Lateral talar shift with increased medial space > 4 mm indicated deltoid ligament injury • May required ORIF if syndesmosis or deltoid ligament injury
Weber C	Suprasyndesmotic injury	• Tibiofibular syndesmosis is usually disrupted • Deltoid ligament injury +/– medial malleolus fracture • Usually treated with ORIF

Lateral Malleolar Fracture

The Weber classification corresponds to the level of lateral malleolar fracture in relation to the distal tibiofibular syndesmosis, which determines the management. Weber is a mechanism-based classification of ankle fractures (Figure 2.4.19). CT is frequently used to ascertain the level, intra-articular extension, and morphology of fractures and to assess the status of the syndesmosis. Delayed wound healing, postoperative arthritis, complex regional pain syndrome, and range limitation are common complications.

Isolated Medial Malleolar and Bi-/Trimalleolar Fractures

These are considered unstable; fractures involving the medial malleolar involve deltoid ligament injury, which can present as lateral talar shift with medial space >4 mm. Posterior malleolar involvement (AITFL avulsion) in addition to bimalleolar fractures make any ankle fracture dislocation trimalleolar in nature; these are severe injuries that require urgent surgical referral (Figure 2.4.20). ORIF is indicated in view of unstable injury, and thromboprophylaxis is indicated to avoid DVT until fully weight bearing.

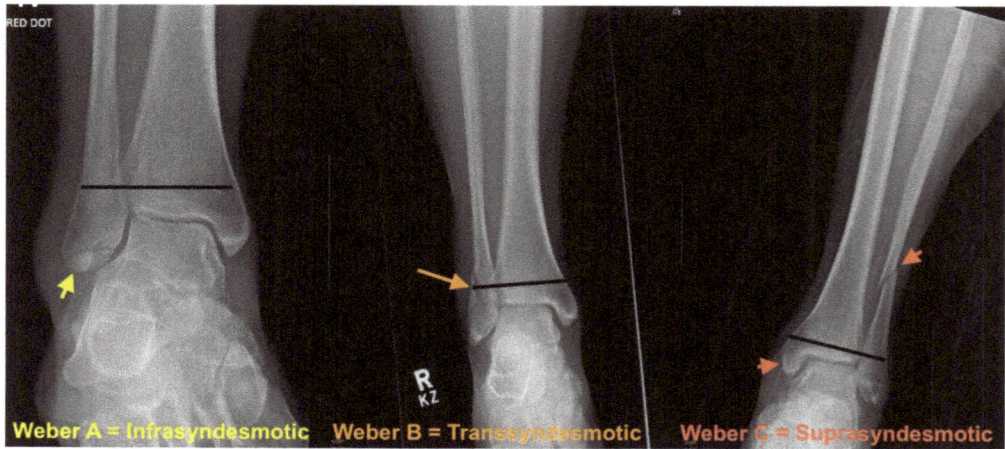

Figure 2.4.19   Ankle fracture dislocations at the syndesmosis.

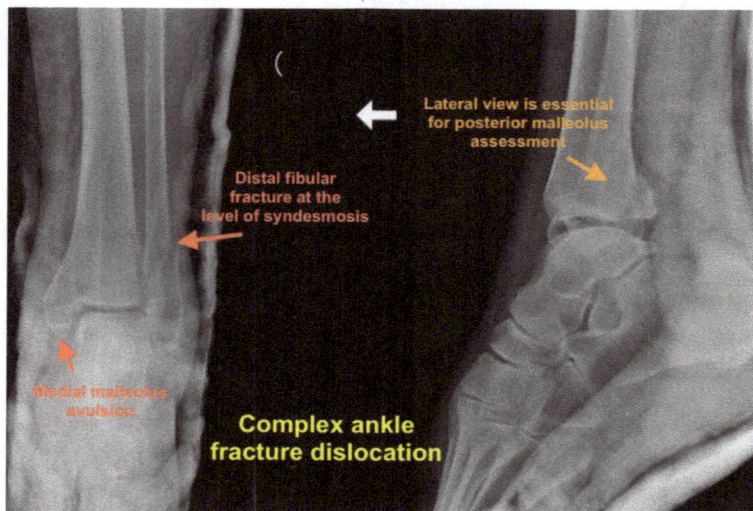

Figure 2.4.20   Using two orthogonal views to detect trimalleolar fracture of the ankle.

Tibial Plafond Fracture

- Intra-articular distal tibial fracture following axial loading, which drives the talus into the tibial plafond following fall from height or road traffic accidents.

- Fracture patterns can vary from minimal displacement to market comminution. Fractures often involve the fibula.

Calcaneal Fractures

- Intra-articular burst fractures of the calcaneus often occur following axial loading in young patients. Fractures can be subtle, and Bohler's angle can be used to demonstrate depression of the calcaneus (Figure 2.4.21).

- Extra-articular fractures often occur at the tuberosity following Achilles tendon avulsion.

- Calcaneal fractures described here represent acute traumatic fractures. The calcaneus is also a common site for stress fractures in runners and athletes (see Chapter 2.16).

Lisfranc Injury

- Tarsometatarsal fracture dislocation involving the second metatarsal base and medial cuneiform disrupts the Lisfranc ligament. The ligament is responsible for the stability of the 1st and 2nd tarsometatarsal joints and transverse midfoot arch. It is classified as a homolateral or divergent injury (Figure 2.4.22).

- Fractures are often subtle; if clinical suspicious remains, orthopedic opinion with further imaging (mostly CT) is advised.

Proximal 5th Metatarsal Fractures

Figure 2.4.23 demonstrates common injury patterns around the base of the 5th metatarsal. Note oblique/ vertical orientation of the unfused apophysis. Peroneus brevis avulsion fracture is usually located within 1 cm of the most posterior edge of the metatarsal base and has transverse orientation (due to pull of the peroneus brevis tendon), whereas the Jones fracture is usually more than 1 cm from the joint line.

The rest of the metatarsal, predominantly metatarsal neck regions, are susceptible to insufficiency fractures in patients with osteopaenia or osteoporosis and stress fractures in athletes (see Chapter 2.16).

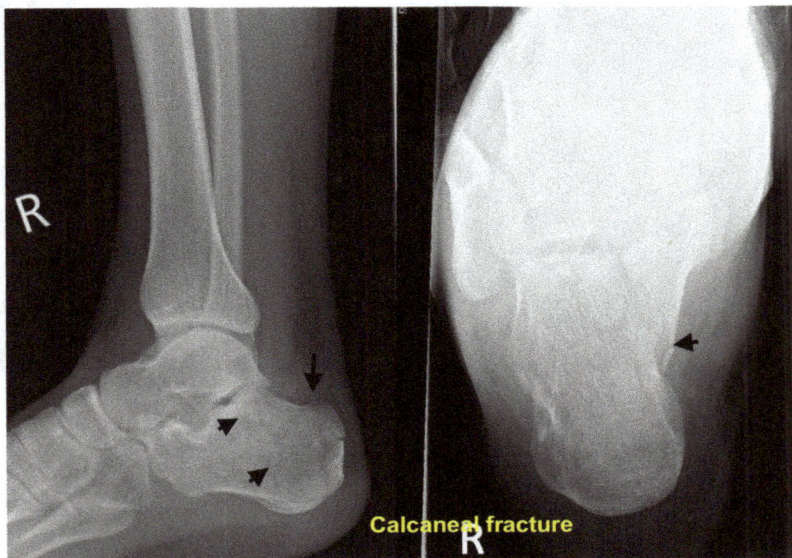

Figure 2.4.21   Acute traumatic calcaneal fractures on X-ray.

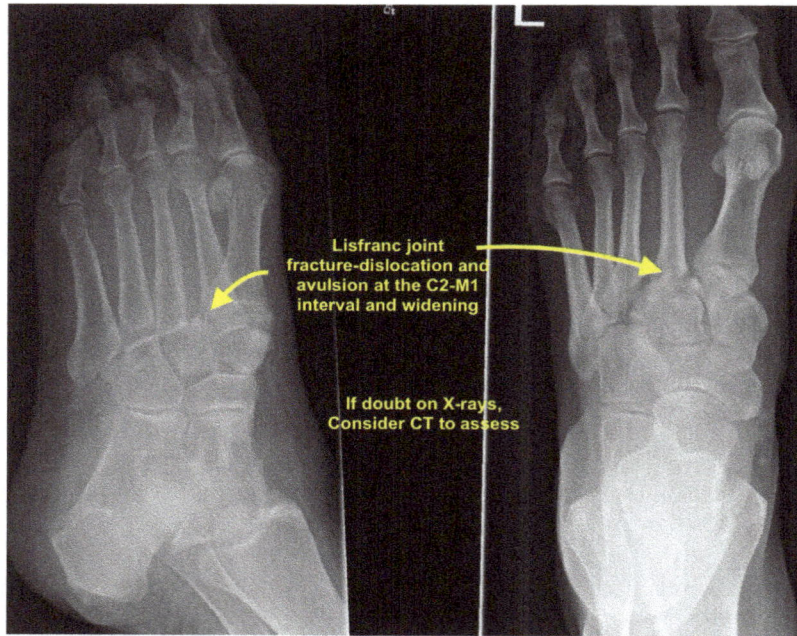

Figure 2.4.22 Lisfranc fracture–dislocation.

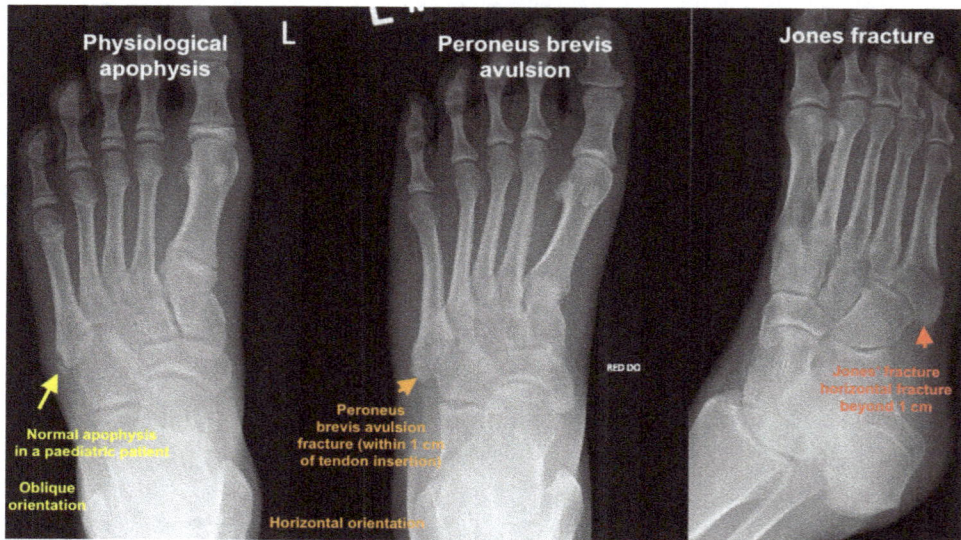

Figure 2.4.23 Fifth metatarsal base appearances (apophysis and fractures).

BONE HEALING IN CHRONIC FRACTURES

Hematoma/Inflammation Phase

- Disruption of the periosteum and separation of bony fragments leads to bleeding.
- The fracture site hematoma acts as a model for callus formation.

- Multiple pro-inflammatory mediators including tumour necrosis factor alpha and interleukins are released at the site, which stimulates blood vessels growth. Within 8 hours, mesenchymal stem cells are recruited that undergo proliferation and differentiation.

Soft Callus Phase

- Fibrin-rich granulation tissue is formed between the fractured ends.
- Progenitor cells differentiate into fibroblasts and chondroblasts, which lay down collagen and cartilage to create a soft tissue callus bridge.
- Revascularisation and neo-angiogenesis help promote bone repair.

Hard Callus Phase

Soft tissue callus undergoes endochondral ossification; fibroblasts differentiated into osteoblasts convert the soft callus into woven bone, which is disorganised immature bone serving as scaffold for immediate support.

Bone Remodeling Phase

Continual breakdown and replacement of bone by osteoclasts and osteoblasts, respectively, promotes woven bone to be replaced by laminar bone, which is a more organised and mature bone. Continual remodeling strengthens bone and reshapes it to the original bone, providing rigidity and stability.

Factors Influencing Bone Healing

• Age	Decreased vascular perfusion of bone
	Reduced pro-inflammatory response, cellular repair and chemosignalling
• Nutrient	Macro- and micro-nutrients are essential for bone healing
• Smoking	Reduces blood flow; delays in fracture union; increased risk of non-union
• Diabetes	Impairs bone formation leading to mal-union and non-union
• Open fractures	Impeding formation of fracture hematoma
• Soft tissue interposition	Prevents callus bridging
• Fracture pattern	Comminuted, butterfly fragment, >3 mm distance between fracture ends
• Medication	Steroids, NSAIDs, and opiates
• Infection	Reduced nutrient and blood flow to the fracture site

Failure of bone healing is described as non-union.

Mal-Union

Fracture healing in a non-anatomical position because of poor alignment due to poor reduction, incomplete immobilisation, and/or absence of reduction. This can impair function and/or cause poor aesthetics. Surgical correction can be performed if the patient is symptomatic.

Table 2.4.2 Atrophic vs Hypertrophic Non-Union

Atrophic non-union	• Radiologically absent callus formation • Influenced by factors as described above • Management involves addressing underlying aetiology • Bone grafts and osteo-inductive agents can be considered to stimulate healing
Hypertrophic non-union (Figure 2.4.24)	• Radiologically excess callus formation • Fracture site instability due to excess movement impairs bone bridging • Management involves internal or external fixation to promote bridging bone

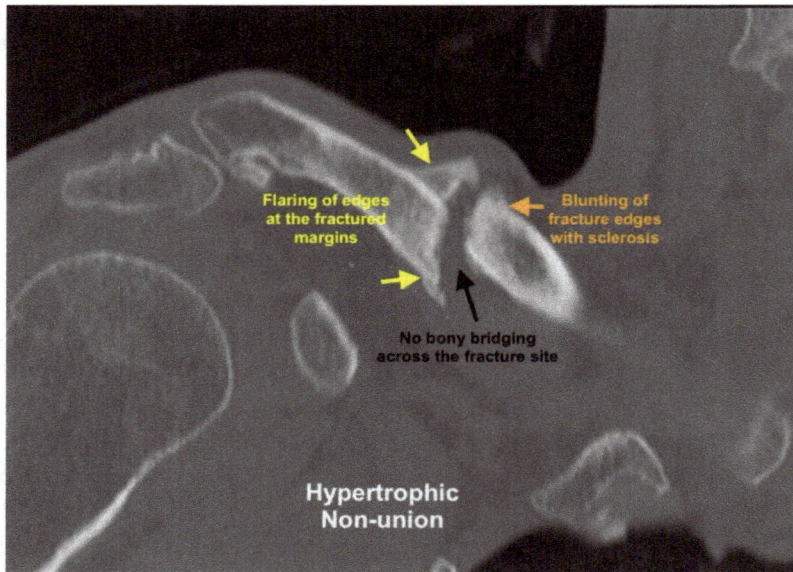

Figure 2.4.24 CT features of hypertrophic non-union.

CONCLUSION

Fractures and dislocations are one of the most common presenting complaints A&E and fracture clinics refer patients for imaging. Relatively simple fractures require at least 2 X-rays in orthogonal planes to make complete diagnosis. Some fractures such as scaphoid fracture require a series of X-ray for complete assessment. Complex fractures or those with potential intra-articular extension requires CT assessment before definitive surgical management.

SUGGESTED READING

- Rogers LF, West OC. *Imaging Skeletal Trauma E-Book*. Elsevier Health Sciences; 2014 Oct 27.

SBA QUESTIONS

1. 40-year-old male presents to ED with swollen knee following a fall in the IRONMAN triathlon race. X-ray of the right knee demonstrates bi-condylar fracture of the tibia. Which classification best describes the fracture?

   A. Neer type I

   B. Neer type II

   C. Schatzker type III

   D. Schatzker type V

   E. Jakob type II

2. 75-year-old male has been referred to the orthopaedic team due to ongoing shoulder pain following a fall 3 years ago. On examination, the shoulder demonstrates limited range of motion in all directions. X-ray indicates mal-union of the head and neck junction with remodelling of the humeral head at the articular surface. Which factor does not influence bone healing?

    A. Nutrition

    B. Smoking

    C. Age

    D. Platelet count

    E. Infection

3. A 25-year-old male was involved in an altercation. The following day, he attends the ED with pain at the base of the thumb. X-ray report reads "intra-articular comminuted fracture at the base of the 1st metatarsal with a Y configuration." Which fracture does this report describe?

    A. Bennett's

    B. Boxer's

    C. Tuft

    D. Mallet finger

    E. Rolando's

Answers: (1) D, (2) D, (3) E

Chapter 2.5
Acute and Chronic Osteomyelitis Including Special Cases

Mark Kong and Raj Chari

LEARNING OBJECTIVES

- To understand the pathophysiology of bone-related infection, including the most common organisms involved

- To know the distribution of osteomyelitis encountered in the paediatric and adult populations

- To understand the appearances of related soft tissue infections and septic arthritis

- To explore typical appearances of both acute and chronic osteomyelitis across various imaging modalities

- To create awareness of atypical infections in the musculoskeletal system

---

INTRODUCTION

- Bone- and joint-related infections can have severe ramifications, sometimes requiring multiple rounds of antibiotic therapy and repeated surgical intervention.

- With the increasing age and morbidity of the general population, it is vital that you have a good understanding of how osteomyelitis is imaged and detected early, as it is a frequent indication for radiological investigation.

The FRCR exam requires an understanding of the mechanisms of infection spread and common organisms of infection alongside the ages and distributions of various acute and chronic presentations of osteomyelitis.

This chapter explores the appearance of acute and chronic osteomyelitis, alongside joint infection (septic arthritis) and involvement of the spine (infectious spondylitis/spondylodiscitis); there is a slight overlap with Chapter 2.2. The chapter also touches on some less common infective agents and their corresponding imaging features.

ROUTES OF INFECTION

- Osteomyelitis is defined as an inflammation of bone and bone marrow caused by an infecting organism.

- Three main routes for bone infections:

  - Haematogenous spread is the most common mechanism for both osteomyelitis and septic arthritis.

  - Direct implantation is also common, particularly after direct trauma and post-surgical intervention.

  - Contiguous spread can be seen from an adjacent focus of infection, such as an infected skin ulcer or soft tissue, with the infection disseminating through tissue to involve nearby bone. This is seen frequently in diabetic foot infection and unhealed pressure sores.

- The anatomical location of infection varies due to their aetiology and should be considered when forming a differential. For example, diabetes-related osteomyelitis and infections of ischaemic ulcers in the setting of peripheral vascular disease, are both conditions most often defined in the lower limb and foot, particularly in the setting of neuropathic arthropathy.

- Intravenous drug abuse is another risk factor, and the resulting sclerosis of veins can lead to subdermal injections that produce severe cellulitis and soft tissue abscesses that involve adjacent bone.

The type of infection is usually defined in the anatomic plane that the infection has predominantly taken hold within. This has implications for whether surgical intervention is required. The terms used to describe the location of infection are listed in Table 2.5.1.

DOI: 10.1201/9781003500247-14

RESPONSIBLE ORGANISMS

- *Staphylococcus aureus* is the most common organism causing skeletal infection and is responsible for between 50% and 70% of cases of osteomyelitis.

  - Haematogenous contamination is the most common route of spread for *S. aureus*.

  - Approximately half of *S. aureus* infections demonstrate methicillin resistance and are particularly challenging to treat due its ability to colonise the osteocyte lacuno-canalicular network of cortical bone, leading to bacterial persistence and sometimes treatment failure in the setting of chronic osteomyelitis.

- Alongside *S. aureus*, other Gram-positive coccal strains such as *Staphylococcus epidermidis* and *Streptococcus pyogenes* can also cause infection.

- Gram-negative rods and anaerobes are less common causative pathogens; however, they can still lead to osteomyelitis. Therefore, fluids collected from a joint (septic arthritis), soft tissue, or osseous lesions are typically sampled through aspiration or biopsy to identify an organism to target anti-microbial therapy.

- Table 2.5.2 highlights the various organisms that can be involved in osteomyelitis across age groups. For the FRCR exams, the most common organisms are the ones to remember.

Table 2.5.1 Infections Based on Anatomic Plane

Anatomic Plane	Infection
Skin	Cellulitis
Fascia	Infective or necrotising fasciitis
Muscle	Pyomyositis
Tendon sheath	Infective tenosynovitis
Bursa	Septic bursitis
Joint	Septic arthritis
Periosteum	Infective periostitis
Bone and marrow	Osteomyelitis
Prosthesis	Prosthetic infection

Table 2.5.2 Organisms Causing Osteomyelitis by Age

Type of Osteomyelitis	Common Causes
Hematogenous	**Usually only one organism**
Infant (<1 year)	• *Staphylococcus aureus* • *Streptococcus agalactiae* (group B *Streptococcus*), *Escherichia coli*
Children (1–16 years)	• *Kingella kingae* (septic arthritis age 1–4 years) • *S. aureus* (age 5 onwards) • *Streptococcus pyogenes* (group A *Streptococcus*) • *Haemophilus influenzae* (now uncommon due to *Haemophilus* vaccine)
Adults (>16 years)	• *S. aureus* • Coagulase-negative staphylococci (e.g. *Staphylococcus epidermidis*) • Gram-negative rod-shaped bacteria (e.g. *E. coli, Pseudomonas, Serratia*)
Direct implantation	**Skin colonisers** • Coagulase-negative staphylococci • Propionibacterium

(Continued)

Table 2.5.2 (Continued) Organisms Causing Osteomyelitis by Age

Type of Osteomyelitis	Common Causes
Contiguous spread	**More likely to be polymicrobial**
Microbiology depends on the primary site of infection	• *S. aureus* (most common) • *Streptococcus pyogenes* (group A *Streptococcus*) *Enterococcus* (i.e. group D *E faecalis* and *E. faecium*) • Coagulase-negative staphylococci (e.g. *S. epidermidis*) • Gram-negative rod-shaped bacteria (e.g. *E. coli, Pseudomonas, Serratia*) • Anaerobes (e.g. *Prevotella, Bacteroides, Fusobacterium, Peptostreptococcus*)
Diabetic foot	• *S. aureus* (most common) • *Streptococcus, Enterococcus*, Gram-negative rod-shaped bacteria (e.g. *Proteus mirabilis, Pseudomonas*) Anaerobes (e.g. *Prevotella, Bacteroides, Fusobacterium, Peptostreptococcus*)

SUPERFICIAL SOFT TISSUE INFECTIONS

- A broad range of soft tissue infections commonly occur alongside osteomyelitis. These are described based on their locations, and they tend to surround the adjacent bone if osteomyelitis is present.

- The epidermal and dermal layers of skin rarely have much relevance in radiological imaging, although they can cause various infectious conditions such as folliculitis, impetigo, furuncles, and carbuncles.

- Erysipelas is a superficial form of cellulitis that is limited to the dermis and is visible on the skin surface. As inflammation extends deeper into the hypodermis and subcutaneous fat, generalised cellulitis becomes the typical descriptor, and imaging starts to demonstrate value in identifying complications such as abscess formation and bony involvement.

- Cellulitis is typically a clinical diagnosis, but imaging features can define its extent.

- On ultrasound, the appearance of cellulitis is characterised by inflamed subcutaneous fat that is of increased echogenicity with indistinct margins, interspersed with generalised hypoechogenic fluid, often called "cobblestone" in appearance, that can confirm a suspicion of cellulitis.

Imaging Appearance

- Ultrasound is useful in assessing the adjacent structures, such as for thrombophlebitis or a foreign body.

- The MRI features of cellulitis include lower normal fat signal on T1W imaging, alongside increased T2 and STIR signal to indicate oedema, as well as diffuse post-contrast enhancement (although contrast is usually not required).

- MRI is then particularly helpful for delineating the deep extension of infection and accurately measure the extent of any underlying abscess, which typically manifests as a focal collection of fluid signal on T2 and STIR, with thick rim enhancement on post-contrast T1W imaging.

- A phlegmon is a conglomerate mass of infection that has not liquefied into an abscess and that replaces the underlying fat or soft tissues.

- Cellulitis is common and can often lead to bone infection through contiguous spread. Frequently seen in the setting of diabetes and diabetic foot infection, the formation of ulceration and sinus tracts can lead to osteomyelitis.

- Sinus tracts are seen on MRI as a thin, discrete line of fluid signal with surrounding high soft tissue signal and enhancement. This often travels from an abscess directly towards the skin surface.

Deep Soft Tissue Infections

- When infection is centred on the underlying muscle, it is described as myositis, or pyomyositis when intramuscular collections of pus form (Figure 2.5.1).

- It can start with non-specific muscle oedema with high T1/STIR signal, and it has a wide differential, although in its suppurative phase, it forms an intramuscular abscess that can lead to sepsis and has a significant risk of mortality.

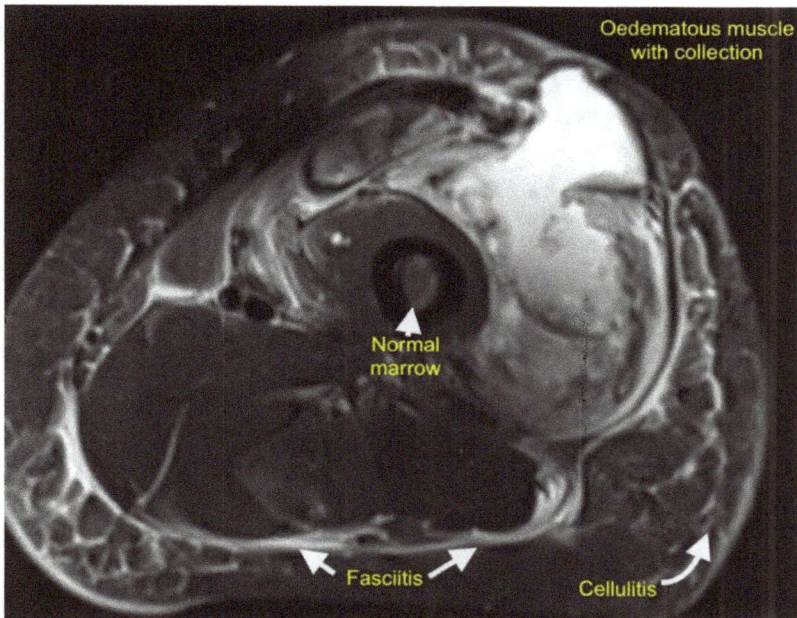

Figure 2.5.1 Intramuscular abscess (pyomyositis) with diffuse cellulitis.

- Other planes of potential infection include the synovial membrane lining the tendon, referred to as infectious tenosynovitis and manifesting as heterogenous, complex fluid signal along the tendon sheath with surrounding soft tissue oedema and enhancement.

- The clinical assessment and history are key to identifying an infectious cause, as the early MRI appearances can be similar to inflammatory tenosynovitis in the absence of surrounding abscess or features of pus or gas.

Septic Arthritis

Early septic arthritis is usually characterised by a joint effusion (Figure 2.5.2).

- It can often be detected on ultrasound, where aspiration of the fluid can prove useful in identifying the infecting organism. The fluid aspirate in an infected joint is often yellow and turbid, although the appearance of the fluid is not typically diagnostic.

- No joint effusion on ultrasound reliably predicts absence of infection.

- As an infection progresses, it causes discrete cortical bone erosion and loss of joint space due to chondrolysis.

- Radiographs only show changes in the late stages of joint infection (bony erosion) and is not usually sensitive in the acute setting. MRI helps with detecting associated complications such as intraosseous abscess and deep soft tissue collections.

- The septic joint requires urgent treatment with initial management involving fluid drainage of the affected joint and initiation of antibiotic therapy. It reduces the risk of irreversible damage to the articular cartilage of the joint, subsequent premature arthropathy, and further risk of potential systemic infection.

Acute Osteomyelitis

Osteomyelitis typically presents across three clinical stages: acute, subacute, and chronic. While there is significant clinical overlap, imaging features can indicate the stage of infection and can help guide management.

- Early osteomyelitis demonstrates subtle bony erosion or periosteal reaction without a discrete intraosseous abscess.

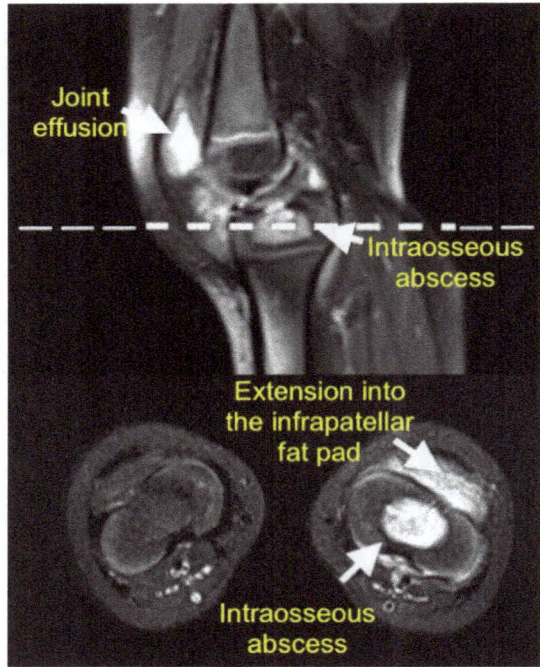

Figure 2.5.2 Septic arthritis and osteomyelitis in the knee of a child.

- It is usually ill defined on radiographs, with MRI signal a more sensitive indicator of early bone marrow replacement.

- On MRI, acute osteomyelitis is characterised by altered bone marrow signal, initially with loss of normal fat signal (reduced T1W) and marrow oedema (increased T2W or STIR signal), with subtle enhancement on post-contrast T1W MRI (Figure 2.5.3).

- Periostitis can be seen as a thin, linear rim of oedema and post-contrast enhancement surrounding the outer bony cortex that then becomes thickened cortical bone in the chronic setting.

- Intra-medullary fat globules are an infrequent presentation but suggest osteomyelitis (Figure 2.5.4).

In adults, bone infection is usually insidious and is often related to adjacent skin ulceration, cellulitis, soft tissue abscess, and sinus tracts, all of which are secondary indicators of potential osteomyelitis and should be identified when assessing any imaging modality. Gas in the soft tissue suggests gas gangrene (clostridial myonecrosis), which can involve the underlying bone; if the gas spreads rapidly along fascial planes, it is more indicative of necrotising fasciitis.

In borderline or surface osteomyelitis, bone marrow oedema on MRI may not have the typical replacement of fat signal on T1-weighted images or cortical erosion (Figure 2.5.5). It has previously been referred to as reactive osteitis, particularly in bone adjacent to a soft tissue defect such as an ulcer. It is now considered as representing a risk of underlying surface osteomyelitis.

Osteomyelitis of the Unfused Skeleton

Age is important in considering the aetiology of a bone infection.

- In the immature skeleton, where the physeal growth plates have not yet fused, infection favours the metaphyseal and epiphyseal regions of the long bones as the open growth plates yield small transphyseal vessels that are a route for haematogenous infection.

- In infants younger than 18 months, these small transphyseal blood vessels make both the metaphysis and epiphysis prone to infection.

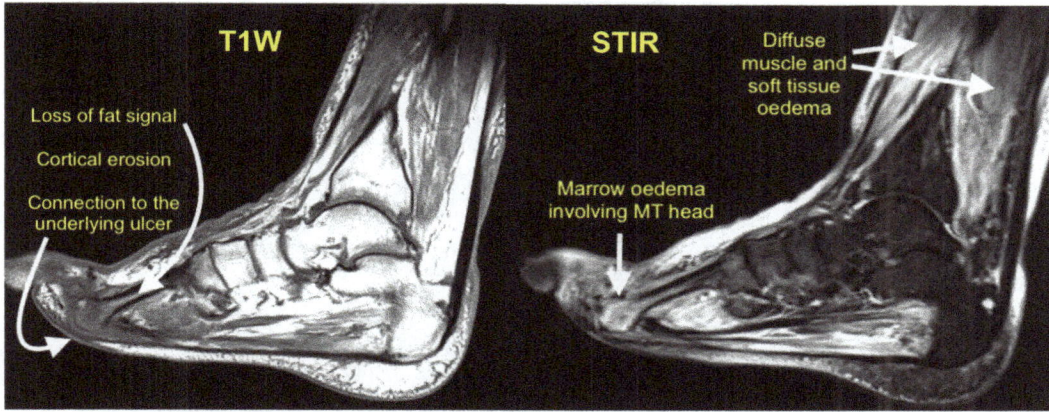

Figure 2.5.3 Acute osteomyelitis of the second metatarsal plantar surface in a patient with diabetic foot. (Image courtesy of Dr Siddharth Thaker, Leicester, UK.)

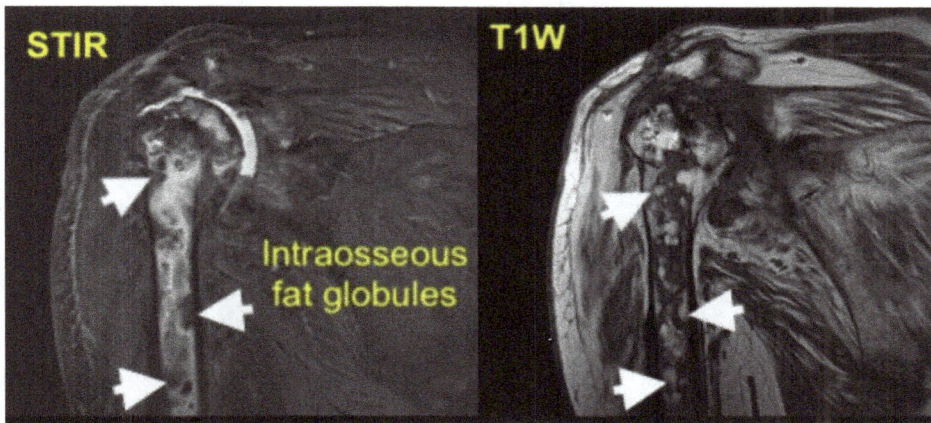

Figure 2.5.4 Osteomyelitis with intraosseous fat globules.

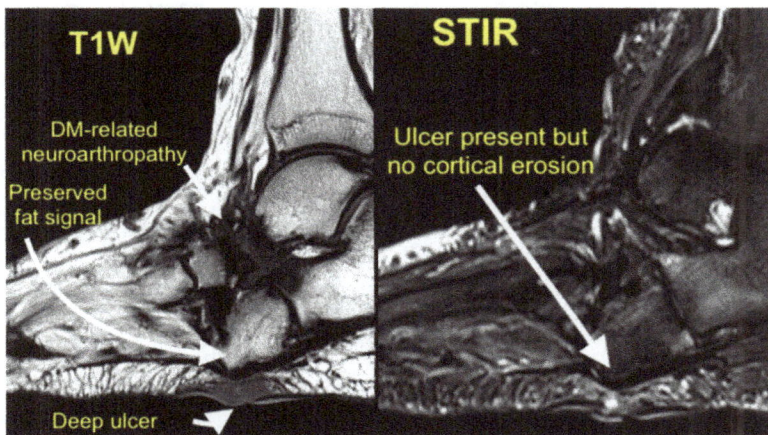

Figure 2.5.5 Deep soft tissue ulceration in diabetic neuroarthropathy and at-risk surface osteomyelitis.

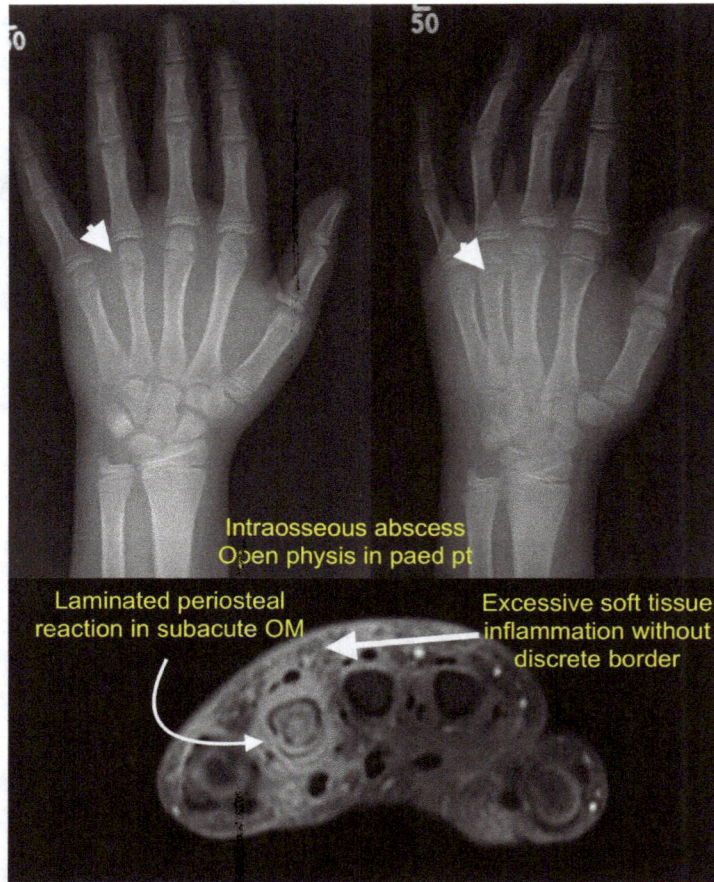

Figure 2.5.6 Subacute osteomyelitis of the 4th metacarpal.

- In those over 18 months, the epiphysis develops its own nutrient vessels and are relatively protected by the developed growth plate, with the metaphysis becoming the predominant focus of infection (Figure 2.5.6).

- The relatively loose attachment of the periosteum can predispose to subperiosteal abscess.

- A subperiosteal abscess is an accumulation of pus beneath an elevated periosteum, which in children is not as firmly adherent to the cortex as it is in adults.

Subacute and Chronic Osteomyelitis

As osteomyelitis develops over days to weeks, signs of chronic disease can emerge. In particular, a lucent intraosseous collection becomes apparent on radiographs.

- The disruption of intraosseous and periosteal blood supply during acute/subacute infection can result in a sequestered fragment of bone within the medullary canal or soft tissues.

- A sequestrum, a devascularised bony fragment, is often a focus of chronic infection and is often resistant to intravenous antibiotics, instead requiring surgical curettage and debridement (Figures 2.5.7 and 2.5.8).

- Diffuse bony sclerosis and cortical remodelling ensue alongside abscess formation in the bone. Thickened periosteal new bone formation around a sequestered fragment is known as an involucrum (Figures 2.5.7 and 2.5.8).

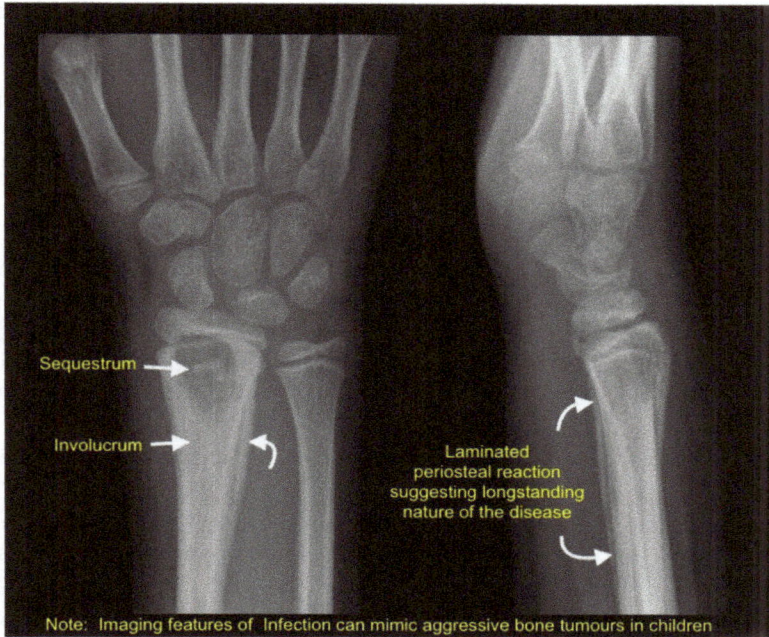

Figure 2.5.7 Chronic osteomyelitis of the distal radius.

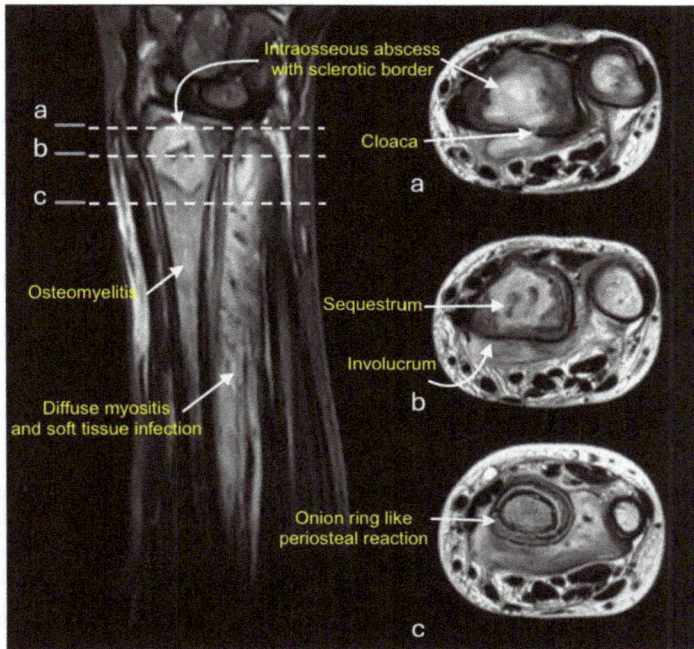

Figure 2.5.8 MRI features of a Brodie's abscess within the distal radius. Coronal STIR (left) and axial T2 images (right) from distal to proximal (top to bottom). Axial image (a) shows the cortical breakthrough (cloaca) and drainage of pus into the surrounding soft tissues, (b) demonstrates sequestrum within the abscess, and (c) highlights the thickened involucrum.

- A cloaca, a tract through the bony cortex for an intra-osseous collection to drain into the soft tissues (Figure 2.5.9), may also be visible. Table 2.5.3 summarises all terms used for subacute and chronic osteomyelitis.

In adults, sinus tracts commonly indicate chronic bone infection, often linked to poorly healing skin defects, especially in cases of venous insufficiency, peripheral arterial disease, or diabetes mellitus. Venous, arterial, and neuropathic ulcers can co-exist and lead to persisting low-grade soft tissue infection and underlying bony involvement.

Brodie's Abscess

An intraosseous cavity of pus walled off by granulation tissue, reactive sclerosis, and inflammation that occurs in children and young adults, with subacute and chronic presentations of osteomyelitis (Figure 2.5.10).

- The most frequent organism associated with Brodie abscesses is *S. aureus*, although cultures are often sterile. Diagnosis can be delayed due to non-specific symptoms, the absence of fever, and normal serum inflammatory markers.

- It usually affects the long bones and occurs twice as often in the metaphysis as in the diaphysis.

- Radiographs usually demonstrate rounded lucency with an ill-defined sclerotic rim that blends into the cancellous bone around it. Sometimes a dense sequestrum can be visualised within the cavity. Differential diagnoses of this appearance include eosinophilic granuloma, Ewing's sarcoma, osteoid osteoma, chondroblastoma (in the epiphysis), and metastasis.

- On T1W MRI, a penumbra—a hyperintense rim of granulation tissue—appears due to the protein-rich contents around the margin of the intraosseous abscess.

- The appearance of the involucrum is sometimes described as a double line effect, where high signal granulation tissue around the cortex is surrounded by a low signal rim due to the marked sclerosis.

Periprosthetic Infection

Due to the metallic artefact associated with prosthetic implants, current cross-sectional imaging techniques make assessing the bone and soft tissue around an implant challenging.

- Plain radiographs remain the first imaging modality in prosthetic imaging, mainly to evaluate for any concomitant issues such as periprosthetic loosening, bone resorption, or fractures.

- MRI can detect infection-related periostitis, abscesses, or surrounding oedema, aided by metal artefact reduction sequences, artefact correction, and lower-ferromagnetic alloys in prostheses (Figure 2.5.11). However, this is still limited in terms of fine detail around any implant.

- With a high clinical suspicion of periprosthetic infection, functional imaging can play a significant role. Techniques such as three-phase bone scintigraphy, FDG-PET, gallium scintigraphy, labelled white cells, and antibodies studies can highlight peri-prosthetic infection. These are highly sensitive studies that if negative can exclude active periprosthetic infection.

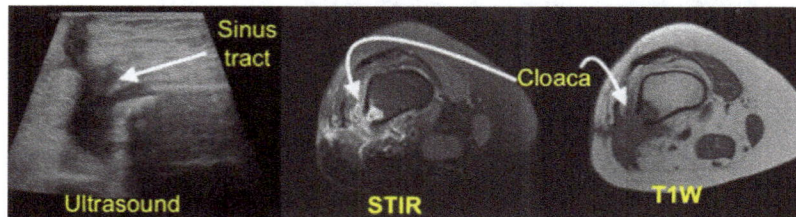

Figure 2.5.9 Intraosseous femoral abscess with a cloaca and soft tissue sinus tract.

Table 2.5.3 Key Terms Used to Describe Osteomyelitis

Key Term	Notes
Bone marrow oedema	Increased signal on fluid-sensitive sequences within the medullary canal. This is usually prior to abscess formation, and the replacement of T1 fat signal increases the risk of underlying osteomyelitis.
Intraosseous abscess	Intramedullary collection of pus, with surrounding cortical bone reaction.
Brodie's abscess	Intramedullary pus collection, typically within the metaphyseal region in the unfused skeleton of a child.
Subperiosteal abscess	Lifting of the periosteum in a child, with pus tracking beneath it.
Cloaca	Cortical defect of bone, allowing pus to drain from the medullary canal into the surrounding soft tissue.
Sequestrum	Fragment of necrotic bone within an intramedullary collection of pus, that has separated from the underlying bone.
Involucrum	Reactive periosteal new bone formation with expansion and sclerosis of the bony cortex in response to infection.
Sinus tract	A soft tissue channel allowing pus to drain that can extend from the bone to the skin surface.

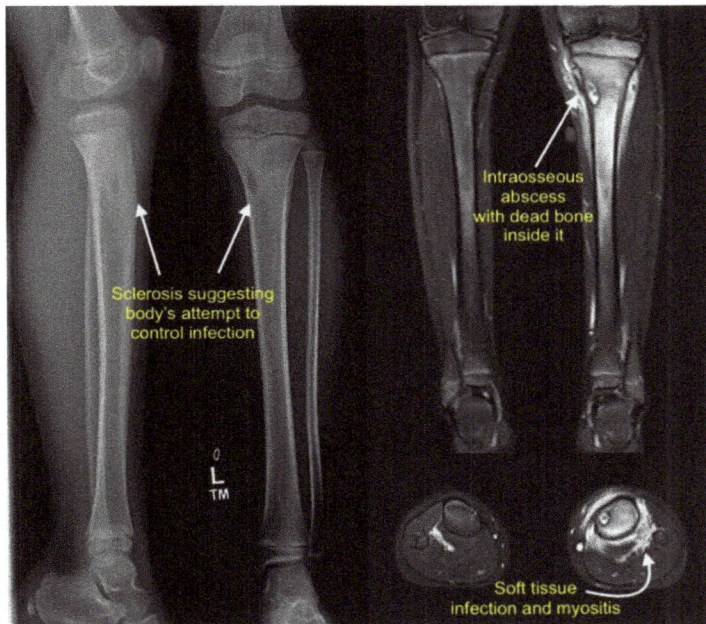

Figure 2.5.10 Brodie's abscess on X-ray and MRI.

Differential Diagnoses to Osteomyelitis

- Inflammatory arthritis, e.g. rheumatoid
- Langerhans cell histiocytosis
- Osteoid osteoma
- Neuropathic arthropathy
- Crystalline disease, e.g. gout
- Malignancy, e.g. lymphoma, leukaemia, or Ewing's sarcoma

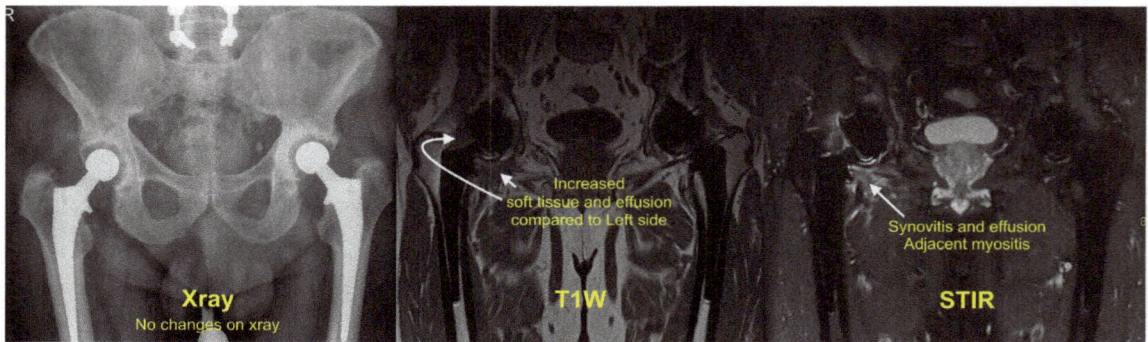

Figure 2.5.11 Periprosthetic infection.

SPECIAL CASES

Infected Osteonecrosis

Osteonecrosis refers to an avascular bone infarct, typically within an epiphysis or metaphysis of a long bone, most commonly the femur or tibia.

■ Aetiologies of osteonecrosis include sickle cell disease, septic emboli, steroid use, excess alcohol intake, systemic lupus erythematous, chemotherapy, radiotherapy, and trauma.

■ Osteomyelitis related to such bone infarcts is sometimes known as a giant sequestrum because the infarct acts as a large necrotic bone fragment—a nidus prone to colonisation and subsequent osteomyelitis (Figure 2.5.12).

■ In the setting of bone infarction due to sickle cell disease, there is an increased tendency for *Salmonella* to be the infecting agent. Otherwise, *S. aureus* is the most likely organism, much as in typical osteomyelitis.

Sclerosing Osteomyelitis of Garré

This is a rare type of chronic osteomyelitis that has been frequently described in dental radiology, mostly in respect to chronic jaw infection. It tends to affect children and young adults and is seen as asymmetric cortical thickening of the mandible.

■ It can occasionally occur in the appendicular skeleton, manifesting as a reactive, non-suppurative, proliferative periostitis that appears as a diffusely irregular thickened bony cortex on plain film (Figure 2.5.13).

■ Sometimes mistaken for a malignancy, the history is key, as this usually results from an insidious, chronic reaction to bony infection over a period of months to years.

Infective Spondylodiscitis

Spondylodiscitis is an infection of the vertebral body, intervertebral disc, paraspinal soft tissue, or epidural space. While discitis is commonly considered to be limited to the intervertebral disc itself, it often involves the bony endplate of the adjacent vertebra and has the same spectrum of severity as osteomyelitis elsewhere in the body.

■ Much like any other bone, spinal infections can arise from haematogenous seeding, contiguous spread of infection from adjacent soft tissues (e.g. infected facet joint or psoas major collection), or direct inoculation during spinal procedures such as surgery or an epidural.

■ MRI is the primary modality for the diagnosis of infectious spondylitis, where low T1 signal and high T2 signal of the intervertebral disc and endplates highlight the increase in internal water content corresponding to endplate oedema (Figure 2.5.14). See Chapter 2.2 for a detailed assessment of infective spondylodiscitis.

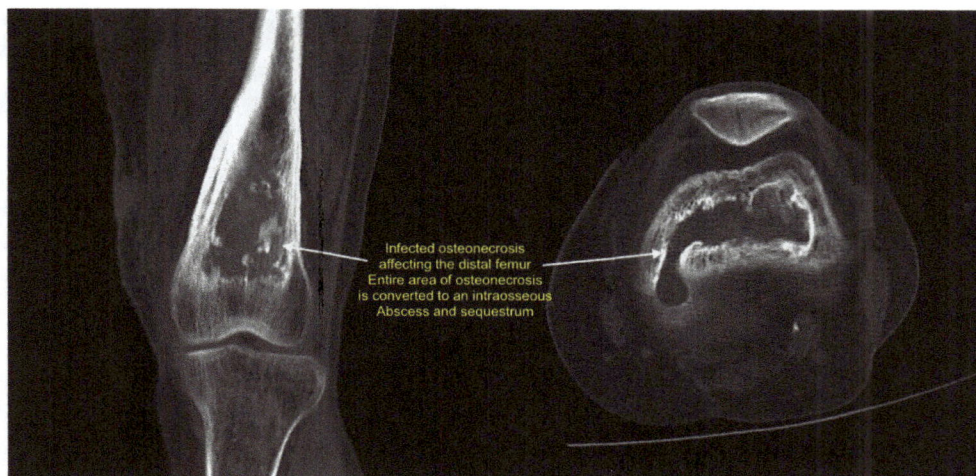

Infected osteonecrosis affecting the distal femur Entire area of osteonecrosis is converted to an intraosseous Abscess and sequestrum

Figure 2.5.12 Infected bone infarction.

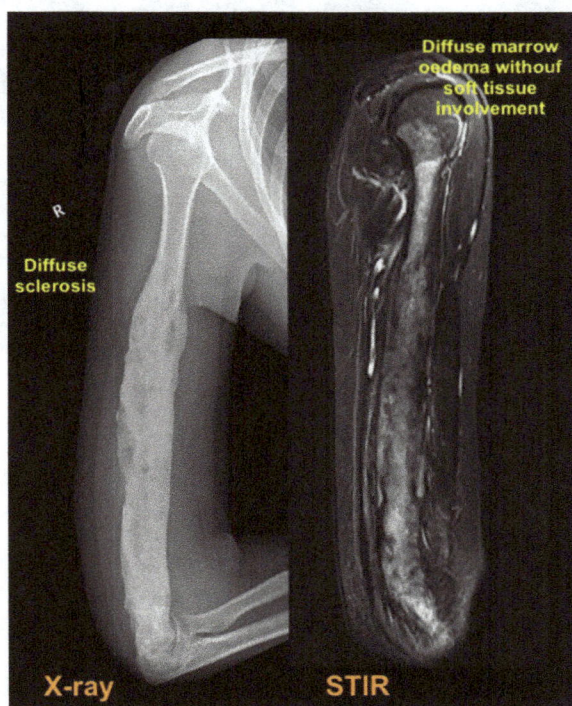

Diffuse marrow oedema withouf soft tissue involvement

Diffuse sclerosis

X-ray   STIR

Figure 2.5.13 Sclerosing chronic osteomyelitis of Garré.

Atypical Organisms

Numerous atypical organisms can also affect the bone and soft tissues. Most cases of osteomyelitis are bacterial and due to *Staphylococcus* or *Streptococcus*. Osteomyelitis can also arise from atypical bacterial, fungal, viral, and parasitic infections including:

■ Brucellosis

■ Mycobacterial tuberculosis (extrapulmonary)

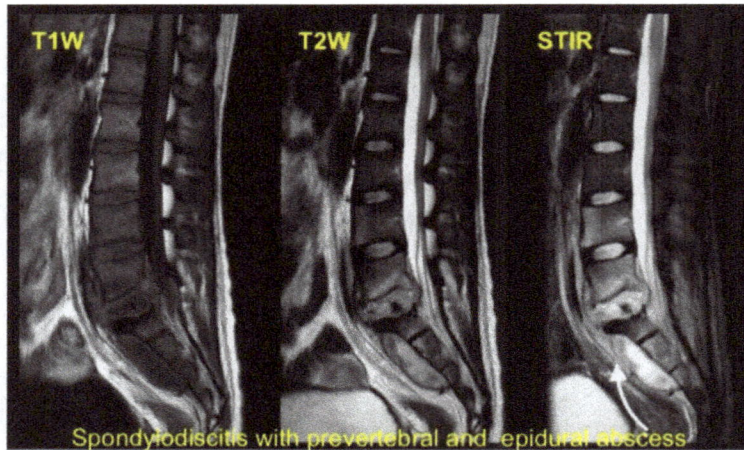

Figure 2.5.14   Infective spondylodiscitis.

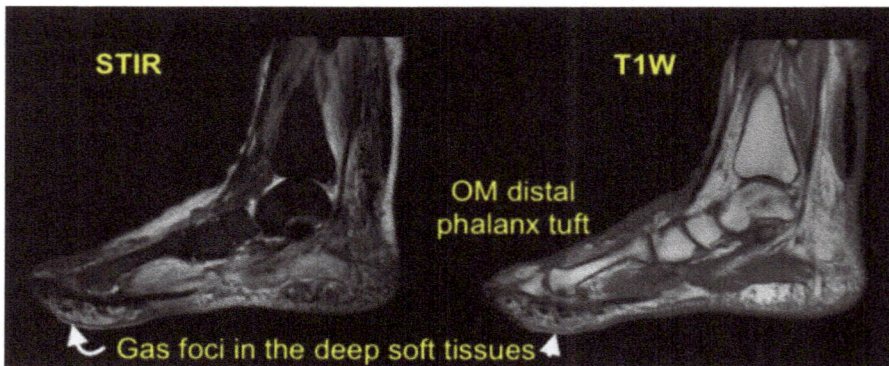

Figure 2.5.15   Gangrenous infection of diabetic foot.

- Gas-forming organisms including Gram-negative pathogens (Figure 2.5.15)
- Hydatid disease (Figure 2.5.16)
- Cysticercosis

Chronic Non-Bacterial Osteomyelitis

A rare auto-inflammatory disease that usually occurs in children and young adolescents and causes intermittent pain.

- It can mimic osteomyelitis and demonstrate increased bone marrow signal within the metaphyses of the femur and tibia, medial clavicles, and sternoclavicular joints.
- MRI features are those of subacute to chronic osteomyelitis. CNO involves multiple sites with predominant affinity to metaphyses (Figure 2.5.17). Long-standing cases produce marked sclerosis.
- CNO is a diagnosis of exclusion when no consistent pathogen or biopsy cultures have identified a causative organism.

CONCLUSION

For the FRCR exam, the topic of acute and chronic osteomyelitis requires awareness of the underlying structure of bone and soft tissue, the propensity for metaphyseal involvement in children, and the behaviour of

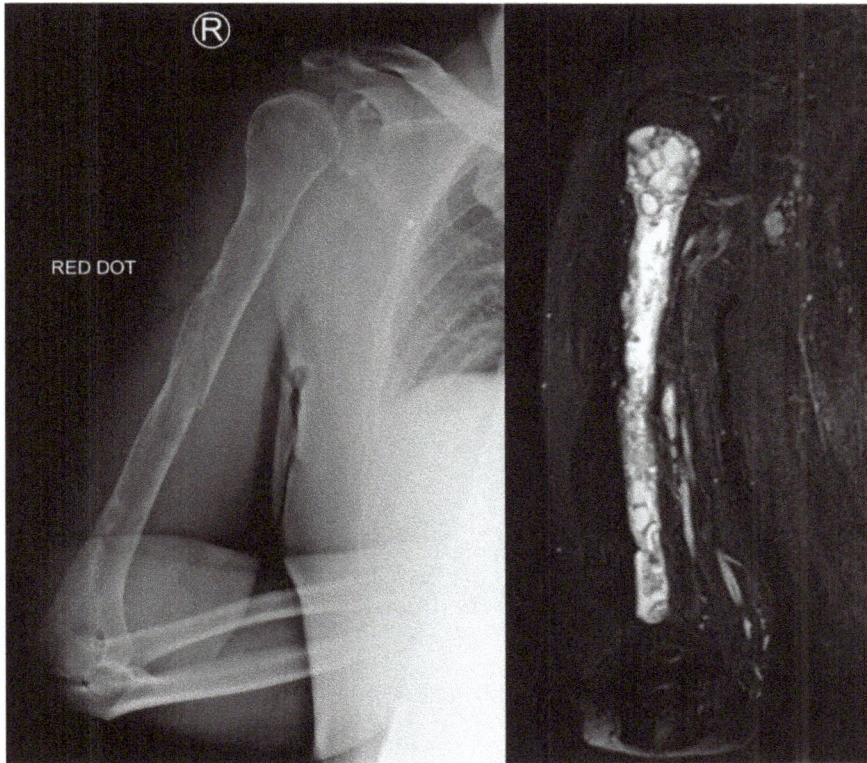

Figure 2.5.16 Diffuse hydatid infection of the right humerus.

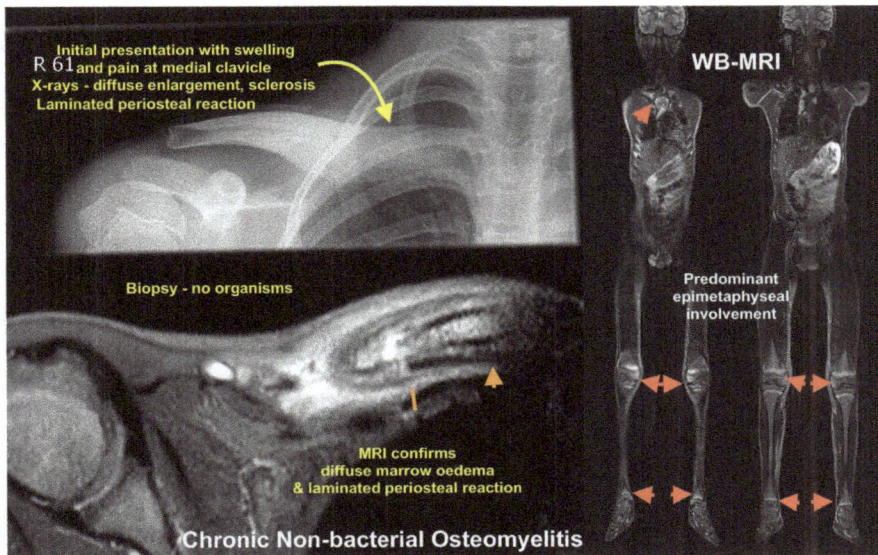

Figure 2.5.17 Classic X-ray and MRI features of chronic recurrent non-bacterial osteomyelitis. (Image courtesy of Dr Siddharth Thaker, Leicester, UK.)

bone in response to chronic inflammation. The soft tissue features are key, particularly if underlying diabetic neuropathy or peripheral arterial disease is suspected.

SUGGESTED READING

- Chin TY, Peh WC. Imaging update on musculoskeletal infections. *Journal of Clinical Orthopaedics and Trauma*. 2021 Nov 1;22:101600.

SBA QUESTIONS

1) A 33-year-old man with history of previous motorbike accident and metalwork fixation presented with a chronically discharging wound along the shin. X-ray and MRI showed thickened periosteal new bone formation with a central track of dead bone. Histopathology confirmed osteomyelitis. What is the thickened new bone formation called?

   A. Involucrum

   B. Cloaca

   C. Sequestrum

   D. Periosteoma

   E. None of the above

2) A 25-year-old immunocompromised woman presented with pain of the upper arm. The X-ray showed ill-defined lucency with no geographical border, and the reporting radiologist reported it as permeative lesion. Which of the following is not in the differential diagnosis for the permeative appearance on an X-ray?

   A. Lymphoma

   B. Osteomyelitis

   C. Fibrous dysplasia

   D. Ewing's sarcoma

   E. Leukaemia

3) Erysipelas refers to which type of soft tissue infection?

   A. Infection limited to hypodermis

   B. Infection limited to subcutaneous fat

   C. Infection related to dermis

   D. Infection related to maxillofacial soft tissue

   E. Infection spreading along the deep fascia

Answers: (1) A, (2) C, (3) C

Chapter 2.6
Soft Tissue Tumours—Approach and Role of Radiology in the Management

Moomal Rose Harris and Harun Gupta

LEARNING OBJECTIVES

- To understand various imaging appearances of soft tissue tumours on multimodality imaging

- To appreciate differences of benign and indeterminate/aggressive soft tissue neoplasms on imaging and advise on appropriate onwards referral

- To know national guidelines underpinning the imaging referrals from primary or secondary care for soft tissue lumps and bumps

---

INTRODUCTION

Soft tissue lesions arise from mesenchymal tissues such as fat, cartilage, muscles, nerves, blood vessels, and fibrous tissues; they are very common in clinical practice, and the vast majority reflect benign aetiology. Soft tissue sarcomas, in contrast, are rare, accounting for less than 1% of all malignancies in adults. Due to their rarity, they can be associated with delayed diagnosis and initiation of treatment. These lesions manifest with poor clinical outcomes including low 5-year survival rates (estimated around 50%), so it is important that such lesions are identified and treated early.

Radiology plays an important role in the diagnosis and biopsy of soft tissue lesions as well as in follow-up staging and post-treatment assessment of soft tissue sarcomas.

- Different imaging modalities including radiographs, ultrasound, CT, and MRI are used to variable degrees dependent on what type of soft tissue lesion is suspected.

- Despite significant advancements in imaging and modifications in imaging techniques and sequences, it is often only possible to make a definite imaging diagnosis in up to one-third of cases. It leaves many indeterminate lesions, which will often need either biopsy for histological diagnosis or close clinical and imaging follow-up if biopsy is not possible.

NICE GUIDANCE

Please see Chapter 1.4 for the British Sarcoma Group, NICE, and RCR guidelines that underpin the imaging and referral standards for soft tissue lumps and bumps that present to primary and secondary care in the UK NHS. Here, the most up-to-date NICE guideline with regards to soft tissue lumps is that if the GP is concerned regarding the possibility of soft tissue sarcoma, then they may request a fast-track ultrasound (within 2 weeks) to assess for this. Clinical features that warrant fast-track scans include lumps >5 cm, lesions seated below deep fascia, and rapidly growing lumps.

NICE recommends all patients with bone or soft tissue sarcoma have their management plan determined by agreement of a tertiary centre sarcoma MDT. Radiologists in a non-tertiary centre should be familiar with local and regional guidelines for sarcoma MDT referral for indeterminate and malignant lesions. Unsurprisingly, there is often significant variation in referral guidelines throughout the UK; see Chart 2.6.1.

IMAGING OF SOFT TISSUE TUMOURS

When a benign clinical diagnosis cannot be confidently provided, further evaluation of a soft tissue lump with imaging is required. Imaging modalities are often combined to determine staging and obtain a diagnosis.

Radiographs

- Initial assessment of a soft tissue mass often begins with radiographs, and this is supported by the European Society for Medical Oncology.

DOI: 10.1201/9781003500247-15

CHART 1

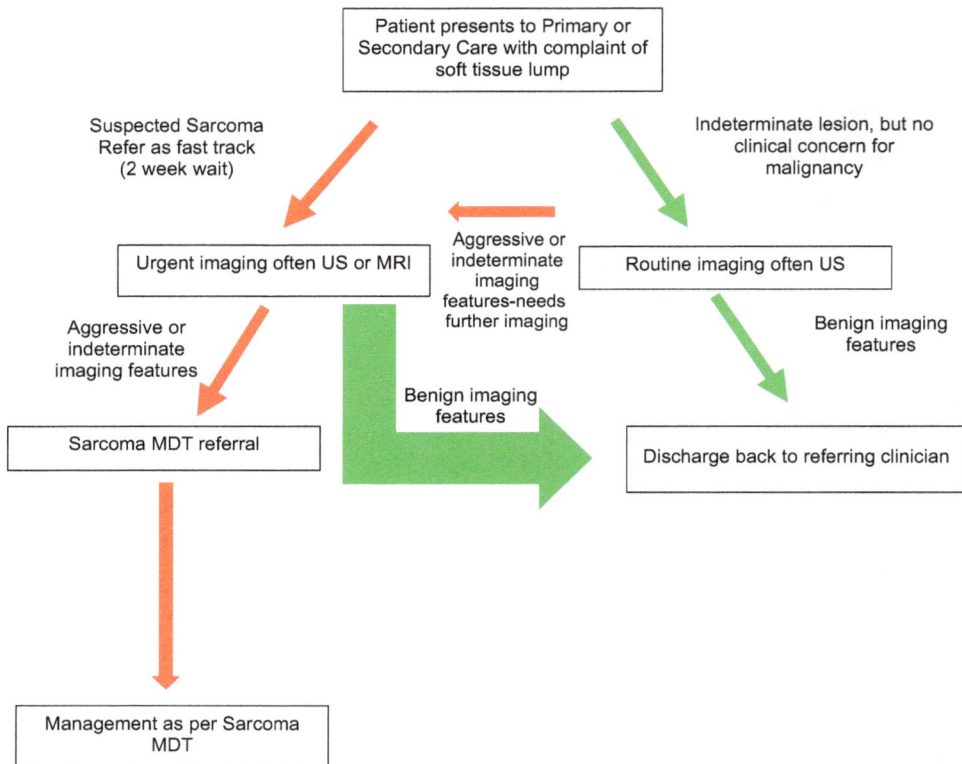

Chart 2.6.1   A potential referral pathway for presentation of soft tissue lumps.

■ Radiographs can demonstrate soft tissue mineralisation based on specific patterns. For instance, phlebo-liths are often seen within haemangiomas (Figure 2.6.1), peripheral mature ossification often occurs in myositis ossificans (Figure 2.6.2), and osseocartilaginous masses are often seen with synovial osteochon-dromatosis (Figure 2.6.3).

■ Radiographs can also show if there is any secondary involvement of bone by a soft tissue mass lesion or primary bone lesions which can mimic soft tissue lesions such as osteochondromas (Figure 2.6.4). Note that MRI is the best technique for assessing the cartilage cap of the lesion.

■ It is important to note that radiographs may not demonstrate any abnormality; this should not provide false reassurance that a soft tissue mass lesion is not present.

Ultrasound

■ The most commonly used imaging technique for fast-tracked (2-week wait) patients referred from primary or secondary care.

■ Inexpensive, non-invasive imaging modality with additional benefit of no radiation, which makes it especially appealing in the paediatric masses.

■ US can evaluate depth of a lesion, differentiate solid and cystic masses, and assess vascularity and pattern of vascularity through Doppler.

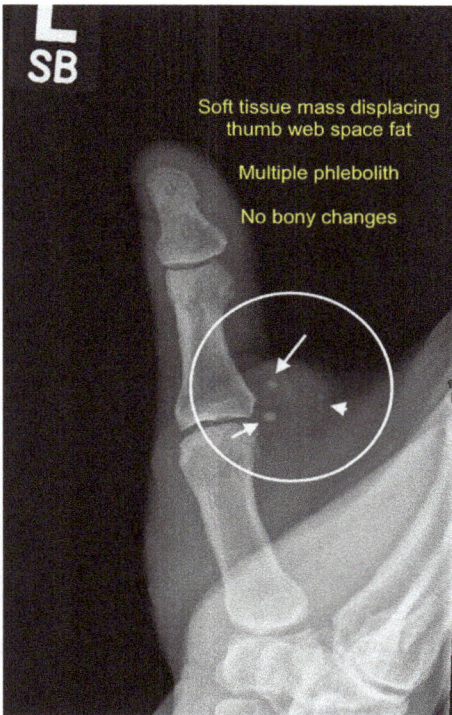

Figure 2.6.1 Soft tissue haemangioma with phlebolith on X-ray.

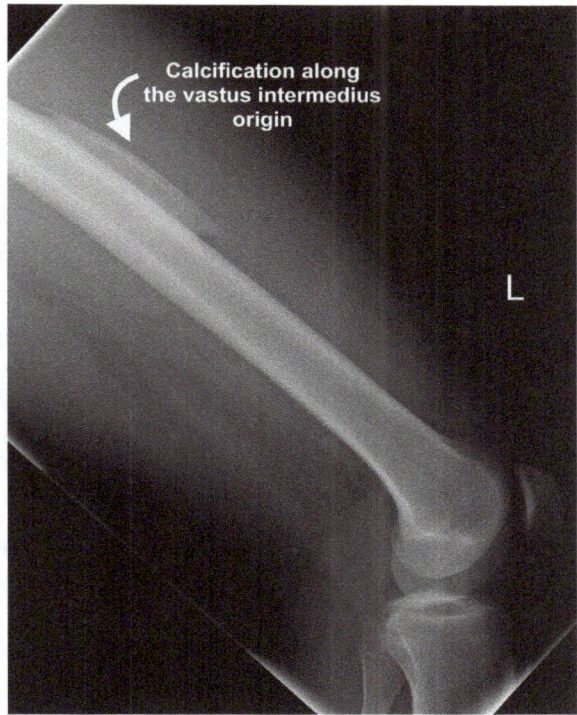

Figure 2.6.2 Myositis ossificans along the vastus intermedius origin on X-ray.

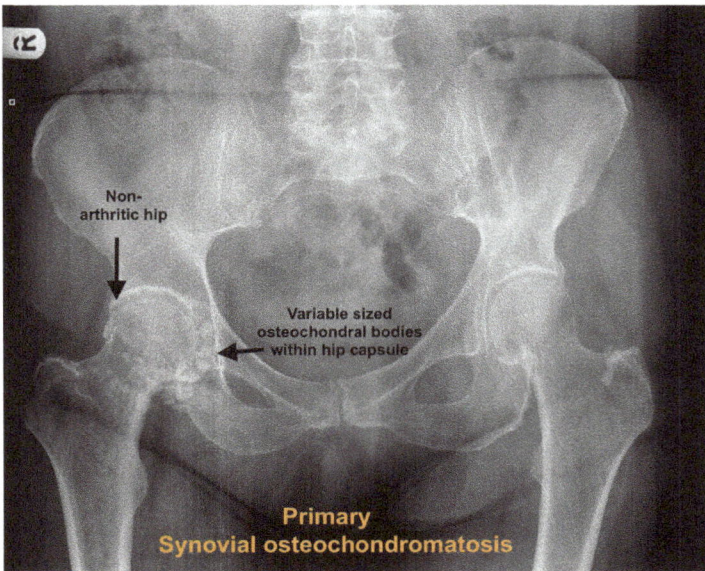

Figure 2.6.3 Primary osteochondromatosis of the right hip.

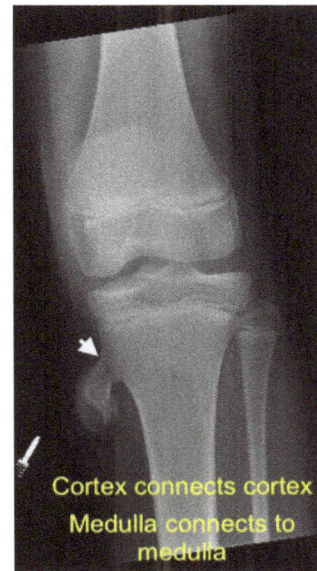

Figure 2.6.4 Sessile osteochondroma.

107

- US is excellent for discriminating benign from malignant lesions. Lesions with indeterminate features need biopsy or additional imaging), whilst benign lesions can be confidently identified with no further imaging confirmation needed.

- US is the tool of choice for image-guided biopsies for indeterminate soft tissue lesions (see Figure 2.6.1).

Computed Tomography

- CT does not typically play a role in the initial evaluation of a soft tissue mass. It can be useful when further information is needed; for instance, with mineralisation, CT is superior to radiographs in detecting zonal patterns.

- CT can also differentiate soft tissue masses based upon intrinsic density such as fat.

- CT can be used when radiographs are limited due to complex osseous anatomy.

- Modern dual-source CT scanners enable the acquisition of single post-contrast scans with the ability to reconstruct virtual non-contrast images; this reduces the need for a separate pre-contrast scan, which reduces radiation exposure.

- CT is considered more accessible than MRI and is often preferred in patients in whom MRI is contra-indicated or those who are claustrophobic.

- CT is also helpful in guiding biopsies in deep lesions inaccessible to ultrasound, e.g. beneath the scapula.

Magnetic Resonance Imaging

- MRI is the gold standard imaging modality for evaluation of soft tissue lesions given its superior soft tissue contrast resolution capability relative to other imaging modalities.

- The multiplanar capability of MRI also improves lesion detection, intrinsic tumour characterisation, and local staging.

- Vascular and neurovascular involvement are better demonstrated on MRI than with CT. Contrast-enhanced MRI is controversial but allows better delineation between viable tumour and muscle, oedema, haemorrhage, and tumour necrosis.

- Post-contrast imaging can also help characterise certain soft tissue lesions such as nerve sheath tumours as well as differentiating cystic from solid areas. It is especially helpful in the assessment of post chemo- or radiotherapy changes and in the differentiation of scar tissue and recurrence during post-surgical follow-up.

- Diffusion-weighted imaging and Dixon sequences are increasing used in clinical practice due to their potential to detect intracellular fat concurrent with benignity of the lesion. It can provide more homogenous fat suppression than T2W fat saturation sequences and better resolution than inversion recovery sequences. Dixon also helps to reduce imaging time as the water-only and fat-only images are acquired simultaneously.

- MRI can provide diagnostic certainty in conditions such as lipomatous lesions and diffuse tenosynovial giant cell tumours with GRE sequences.

PET-CT

- The most common radioisotope currently used for PET is fluoro-2-dexoy-glucose (FDG). FDG behaves like glucose within the body and is a mean of quantifying glucose metabolism.

- PET-CT imaging is already established for use in staging of various malignancies such as lymphomas and non-small cell lung cancers.

- The maximum standard uptake value on PET can be useful for differentiating between benign and malignant soft tissue masses and when combined with the CT component can distinguish aggressive soft tissue from benign lesions.

- PET-CT is an excellent modality for detecting metastatic disease and assessing treatment response especially myxoid liposarcoma and malignant peripheral nerve sheath tumour (MPNST).

- However, the low-dose CT component of PET-CT is of lower resolution than conventional CT and is not optimal for characterising soft tissue mineralisation.

- PET-CT cannot differentiate inflammatory and infectious lesions from malignant lesions in all cases as they can demonstrate increased standard uptake values.

SELECTED SOFT TISSUE TUMOURS

The WHO classification of soft tissue tumours is the most widely and commonly accepted pathology-based classification system for such disorders; see Box 2.6.1 for some abridged content from the most up-to-date version (5th Edition, Volume 3, 2020).

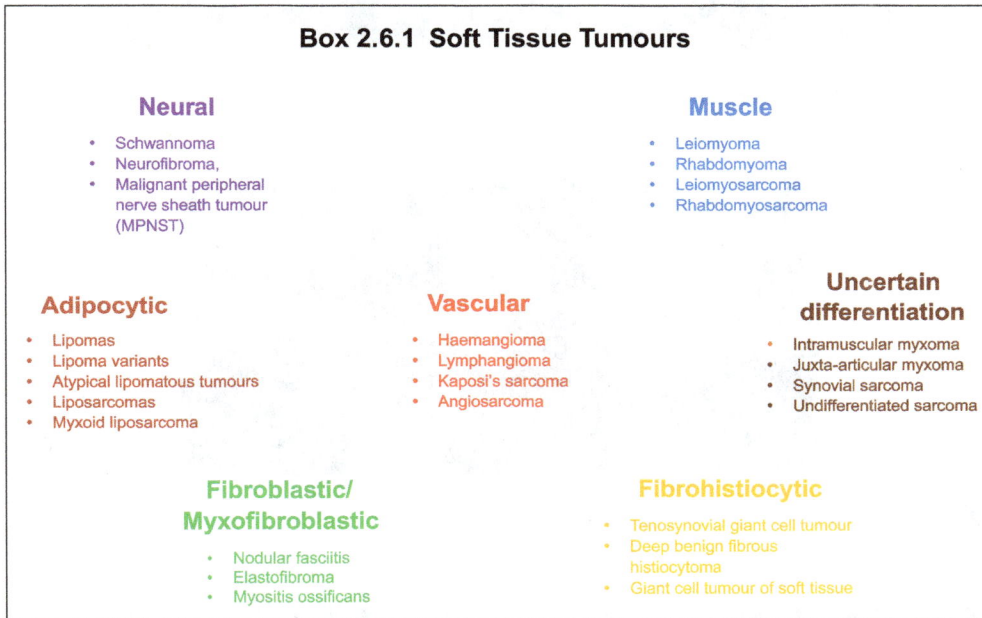

Box 2.6.1 Soft Tissue Tumours

Neural
- Schwannoma
- Neurofibroma,
- Malignant peripheral nerve sheath tumour (MPNST)

Muscle
- Leiomyoma
- Rhabdomyoma
- Leiomyosarcoma
- Rhabdomyosarcoma

Adipocytic
- Lipomas
- Lipoma variants
- Atypical lipomatous tumours
- Liposarcomas
- Myxoid liposarcoma

Vascular
- Haemangioma
- Lymphangioma
- Kaposi's sarcoma
- Angiosarcoma

Uncertain differentiation
- Intramuscular myxoma
- Juxta-articular myxoma
- Synovial sarcoma
- Undifferentiated sarcoma

Fibroblastic/Myxofibroblastic
- Nodular fasciitis
- Elastofibroma
- Myositis ossificans

Fibrohistiocytic
- Tenosynovial giant cell tumour
- Deep benign fibrous histiocytoma
- Giant cell tumour of soft tissue

ADIPOCYTIC TUMOURS

- Also called lipomatous or fatty tumours

- Very common (1 in 1000 people)

- The majority of such lesions are benign (lipomas) and can be confidently diagnosed by radiological evaluation.

- Seen in adults aged 40–60 but can develop at any age.

Benign Lipomas

- Variably homogenous echogenic masses on ultrasound with no or minimal vascularity.

- They can be encapsulated or unencapsulated where measurements can be difficult to obtain (Figure 2.6.5).

- On CT, lipomas appear as homogenously low-density lesions, as fat is less dense than water. Typically, internal density of lipomas ranges from −60 to −120 Hounsfield units (Figure 2.6.6).

- On MRI, lipomas are homogenously hyperintense (bright) on T1W imaging and demonstrate homogenous loss of signal on fat saturated or supressed (STIR or Dixon) imaging sequences (Figure 2.6.7).

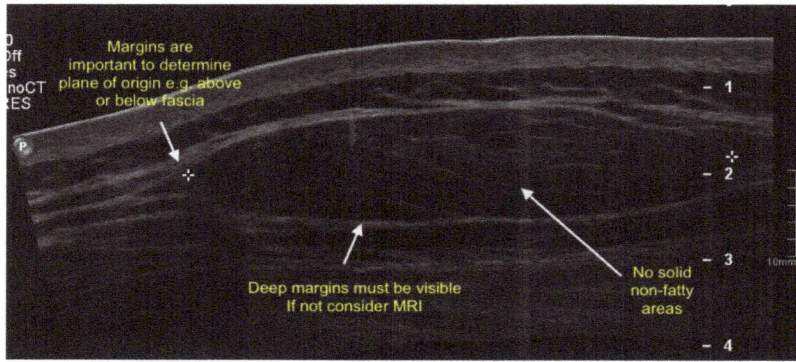

Figure 2.6.5 Encapsulated lipoma on ultrasound.

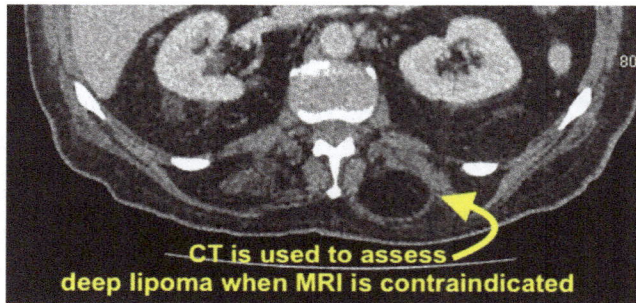

Figure 2.6.6 CT features of benign lipoma.

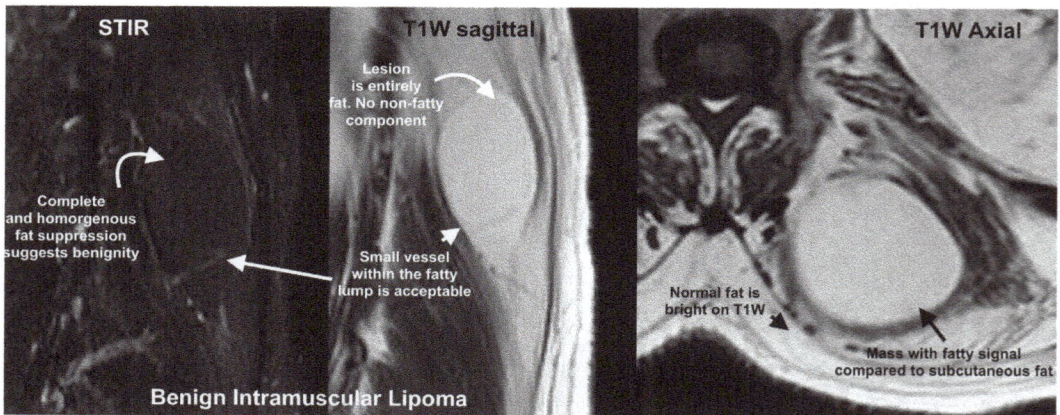

Figure 2.6.7 MRI features of benign lipoma.

Key Points to Remember

- Benign lipomas do not have solid non-fatty soft tissue component on US or MRI or disorganised vascularity on US.

- The fatty component is directly proportional to the benignity of the lesion: Fatty component decrease and non-fatty components increase as lipomatous lesions become indeterminate or more aggressive.

- Dedifferentiated liposarcoma or myxoid liposarcoma can virtually be devoid of fatty components (Figure 2.6.8).

- Imaging cannot differentiate between lipoma variant, mechanical changes including fat necrosis in lipomatous lesion, or atypical lipomatous tumour. When in doubt, discuss in the locoregional sarcoma triage MDT and biopsy if needed (Figure 2.6.9).

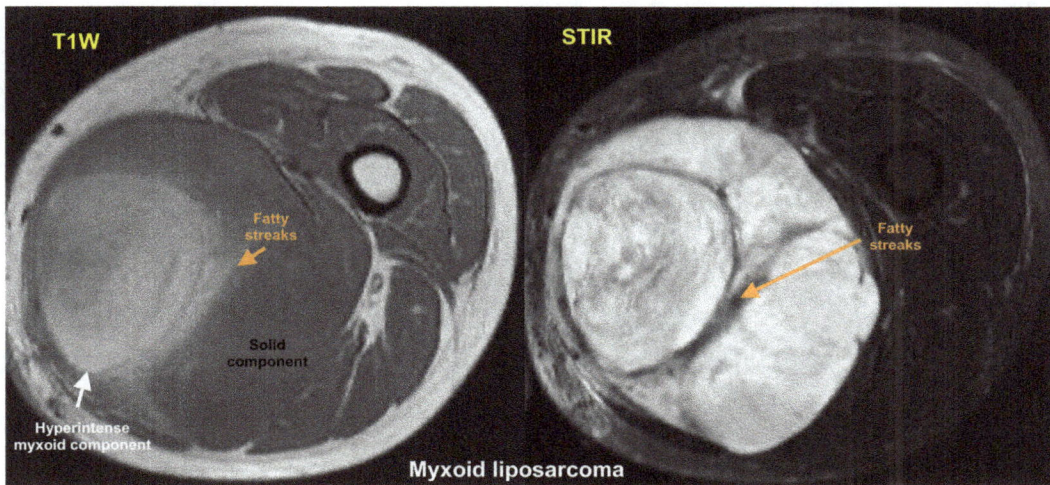

Figure 2.6.8 Myxoid liposarcoma on MRI.

For the tumours shown in Figure 2.6.9, biopsy is beneficial for confirming diagnosis. The following US or MRI appearances require discussion in the locoregional sarcoma triage MDT:

- Heterogenous internal appearances

- Increased and/or disorganised internal vascularity (septal vascular flow is okay)

- Deep-seated, large (>5 cm) subfascial, inter- or intramuscular lesions, especially in male patients over age 60

MYXOID TUMOURS

- These mesenchymal tumours are characterised by their abundant extracellular myxoid matrix.

- They reflect a wide group of benign and malignant lesions.

- Some myxoid lesions are harmless, others can be locally aggressive, and a further subset can act as aggressive malignant tumours that metastasise.

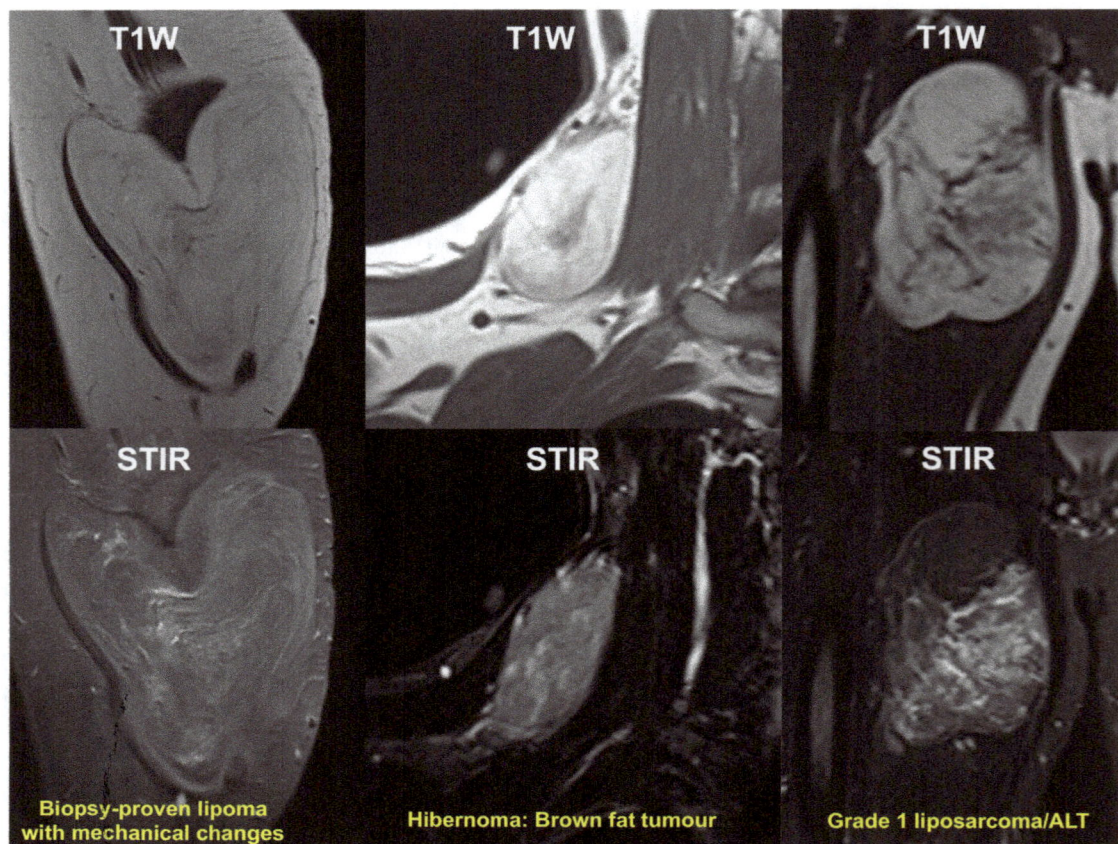

Figure 2.6.9 Diagnostic conundrum: Lipoma with mechanical changes, hibernoma (brown fat tumour), and grade 1 liposarcoma showing lesions with both fatty and non-fatty areas.

Intramuscular Myxomas

- These are the most common benign myxoid soft tissue tumours.

- They are often seen in adults aged 40–70 with a slight female predominance.

- The thigh, shoulder girdle, and buttock in descending order are the most common sites of occurrence. They typically present as slow-growing masses.

- Intramuscular myxomas can also occur in association with polyostotic fibrous dysplasia in a condition known as Mazabraud syndrome.

- Ultrasound demonstrates a well-defined hypo or an echoic lesion with intrinsic "whorled" appearance and minimal to no internal vascularity. Posterior acoustic enhancement is often evident.

- On MRI, intramuscular myxomas demonstrate homogenous low to intermediate signal on T1W sequences, hyperintense signal on T2W, and fluid-sensitive sequences secondary to their high myxoid content. They can also show local leakage of myxomatous material at their margins along the muscle axis (Figure 2.6.10).

- A thin rim of fat can be seen in up to 89% of intramuscular myxomas, and this finding is often referred to as a "fat cap" sign.

- Contrast is not considered necessary for diagnosis of an intramuscular myxoma.

- Contrast enhancement pattern is non-specific and shows mild to moderate, diffuse, peripheral, and septal patterns of enhancement.

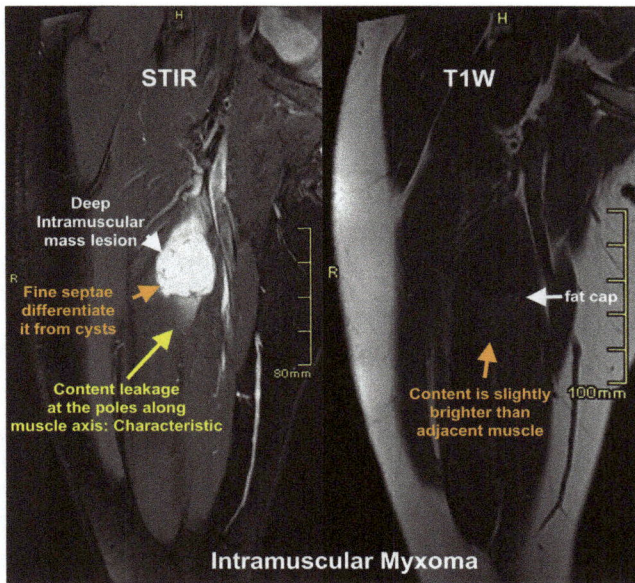

STIR

T1W

Deep
Intramuscular
mass lesion

Fine septae
differentiate
it from cysts

Content leakage
at the poles along
muscle axis: Characteristic

fat cap

Content is slightly
brighter than
adjacent muscle

80mm

100mm

Intramuscular Myxoma

Figure 2.6.10 Classic MRI features of intramuscular myxoma.

FIBROHISTIOCYTIC TUMOURS

Tenosynovial giant cell tumours (tGCTs) are benign fibrohistiocystic tumours which most often arise from the synovium of joints, bursa, or tendon sheaths and show synovial differentiation.

- Can be localised or diffuse.

- In diffuse form, previously known as pigmented villonodular synovitis.

- Localised tGCTs characteristically present as slow-growing, painless masses and are the second most common tumour of the hands and fingers (after ganglions) in patients in their 30s to 50s.

- There is a slight predominance in females.

- The knee is, the most commonly affected large joint.

On radiographs, localised tGCTs can appear as a localised periarticular soft tissue density with associated pressure erosions relating to the adjacent bone. Rarely they can invade the bone mimicking an intraosseous lesion. Periosteal reaction and calcification are uncommon, but their presence does not exclude the diagnosis.

Ultrasound typically demonstrates solitary, homogenously, hypoechoic subcutaneous soft tissue nodules associated with the volar surface of the digits. Most nodules show some internal vascularity on Doppler imaging (Figure 2.6.11). The nodule does not move with the underlying flexor tendon.

On MRI, these lesions are typically low signal intensity on both T1W and T2W sequences. Gradient echo sequences can demonstrate blooming artefact due to intrinsic haemosiderin deposition (Figure 2.6.12). Contrast is not considered necessary for diagnosis, but if given, it generally shows moderate enhancement.

NEURAL TUMOURS

Tumours of neurogenic origin are estimated to reflect approximately 12% of all benign soft tissue tumours; they include schwannomas, neurofibromas, and neuromas.

- Schwannomas and neurofibromas are benign peripheral nerve sheath tumours (PNSTs).

- Schwannomas are slightly less common, and the vast majority are solitary lesions, which typically are eccentric and displace the nerve.

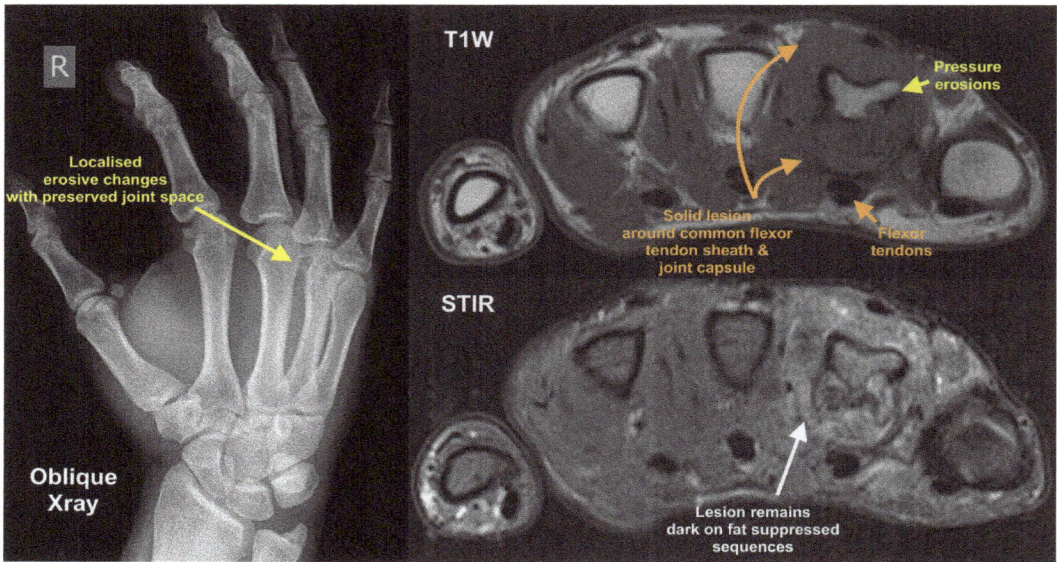

Figure 2.6.11 tGCT arising from the common flexor tendon sheath with pressure erosions in adjacent bones.

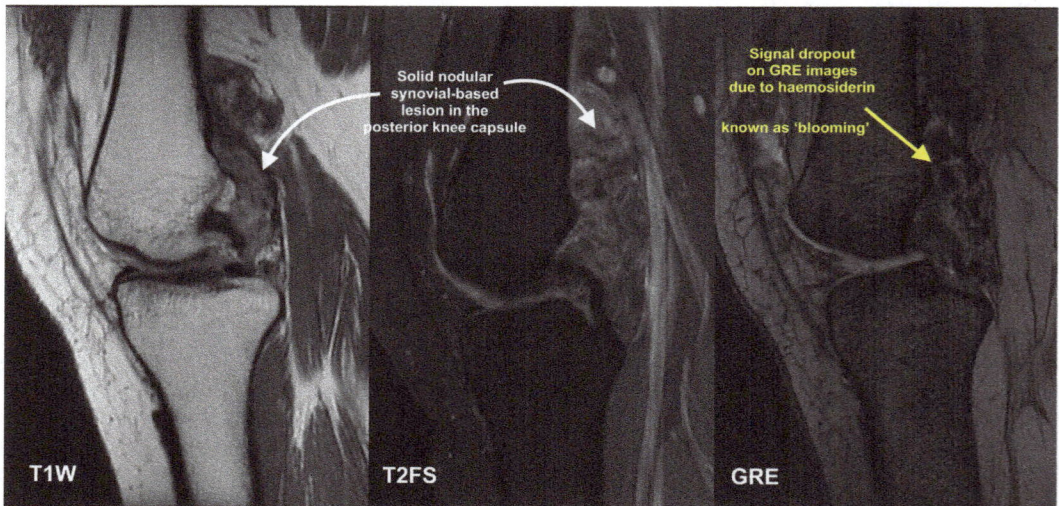

Figure 2.6.12 Diffuse tGCT of the knee with blooming artefact on GRE-MRI.

- Cystic change, haemorrhage, and/or calcification can occur in "ancient" schwannomas.

- Neurofibromas are more common; 90% are solitary and occur in young adults with no association with neurofibromatosis 1 (NF1).

- Neurofibromas are often located in the superficial tissue, and unlike schwannomas, they are often unencapsulated with the nerve entering and exiting a fusiform mass.

- Plexiform neurofibromas are pathognomonic of NF1.

114

- They involve a long segment of the nerve in a diffuse manner and can also extend into its branches and the surrounding fat, muscle, and subcutaneous tissues.

- MRI in PNSTs is often diagnostic, with the tumour seen in close relation to the neurovascular bundle. A nerve detected entering and exiting a fusiform mass oriented along the axis of the nerve is considered pathognomonic, though this may be difficult to appreciate in smaller nerves.

- It is possible to differentiate schwannomas and neurofibromas on MRI based upon aforementioned information regarding displacement of the nerve with eccentrically positioned schwannomas and fusiform central mass related to the nerve with neurofibromas.

- Additional imaging features of PNST include the "split-fat" sign, which indicates origin in the intermuscular plane and the "fascicular" sign relating to hypointense (dark) ringlike structures on T2W imaging corresponding to nerve fascicles.

- Distal muscle denervation is sometimes a secondary sign.

- Contrast enhancement is often intense, homogenous, or targetoid in smaller lesions and predominantly peripheral, central, or heterogeneously nodular in larger lesions (Figure 2.6.13).

ELASTOFIBROMAS

- Uncommon

- Almost exclusively occur in the infra- or sub-scapular region

- Presents in elderly, predominantly female, patients

- Typically appear on MRI as ill-defined masses adjacent to the rib cage with displacement of adjacent muscles

- Typically isointense to skeletal muscle on both T1W and T2W images with some interspersed streaks of fatty signal (Figure 2.6.14)

- Bilateral in up to two-thirds of cases

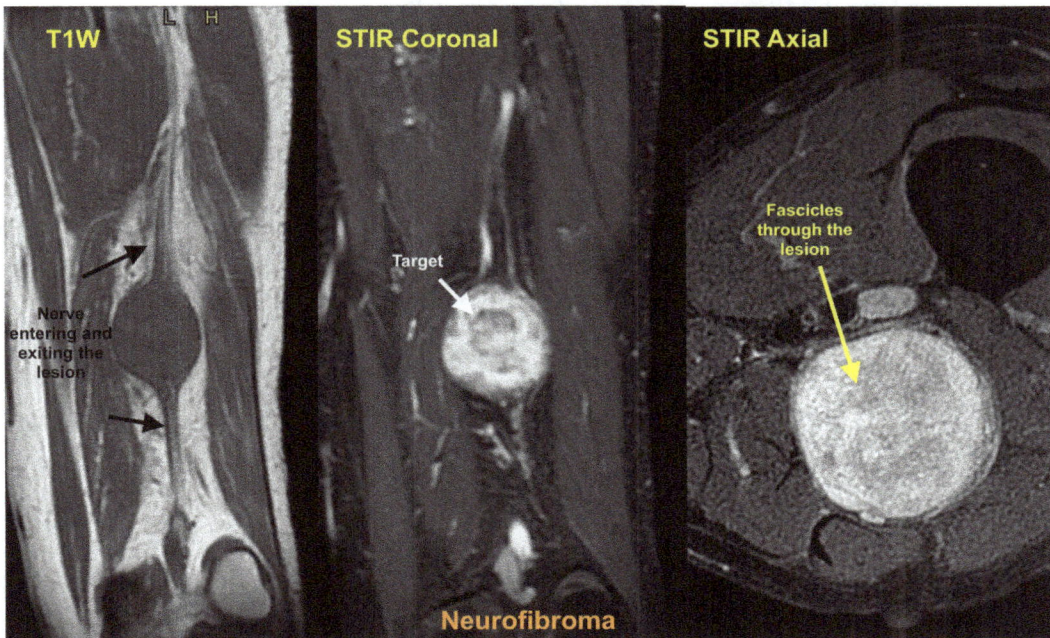

Figure 2.6.13   MRI characteristics of a peripheral nerve sheath tumour.

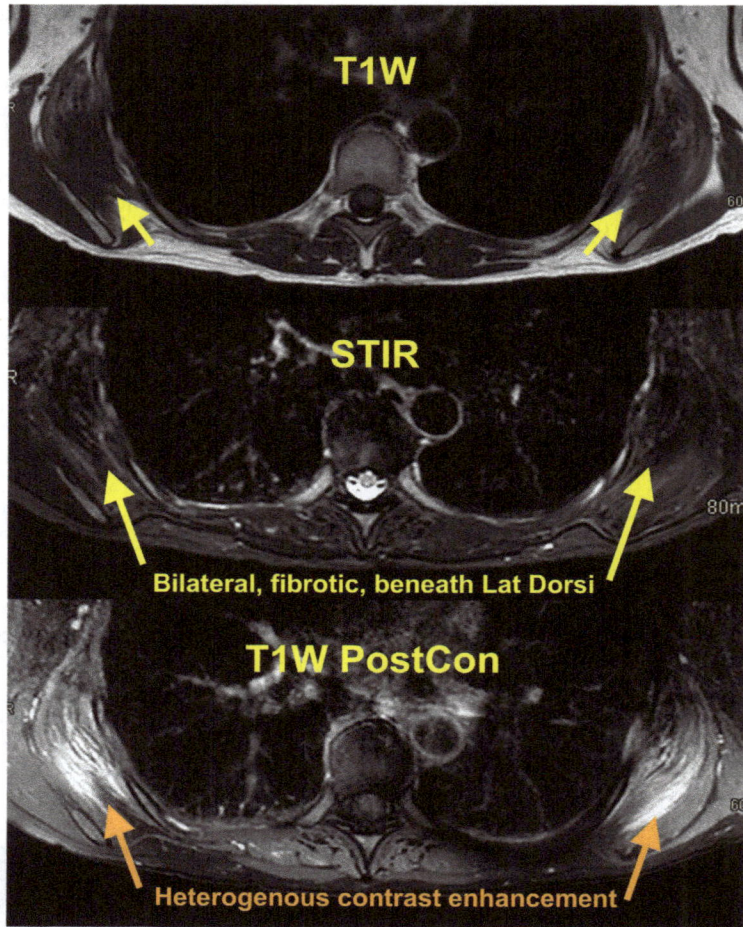

Figure 2.6.14 MRI characteristics of bilateral elastofibroma dorsi.

EPIDERMAL INCLUSION CYSTS

- Also known as sebaceous cysts.

- Formed by the implantation of various epidermal components in the dermal and subcutaneous tissues.

- The most common cutaneous/subcutaneous cysts and can occur anywhere on the body.

- Typically clinically diagnosed and appears as fluctuant nodules of variable size with a visible central punctum.

- Can become inflamed and cause localised erythema and pain.

- Rarely can develop into squamous cell carcinoma, with neoplastic changes associated with pain, rapid growth, or ulceration.

- On ultrasound, typically shows as encapsulated and ovoid with pseudotestis appearance and posterior acoustic enhancement secondary to cystic content with an anechoic tract visible at the superficial aspect extending towards the skin surface (Figure 2.6.15).

- Variable vascularity possible when the lesion is inflamed, infected, or ruptured.

- Ruptured cysts can have adjacent hypoechoic fluid accumulation.

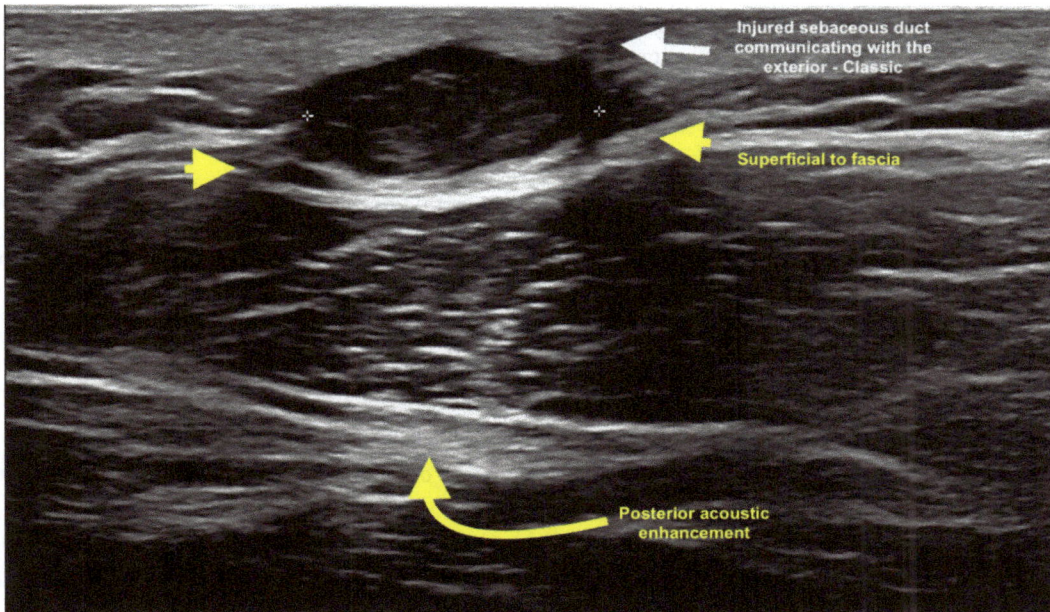

Figure 2.6.15   Ultrasound features of an epidermoid inclusion cyst.

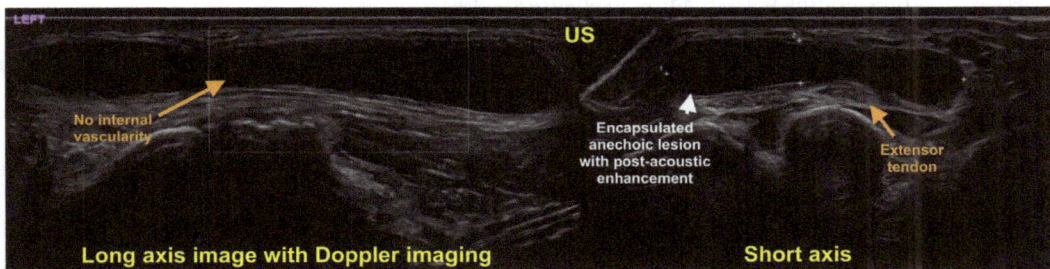

Figure 2.6.16   Imaging appearances of a ganglion.

Ganglions

- One of the most common soft tissue lumps encountered in practice

- Associated with underlying joint degeneration, most commonly around wrists and feet

- Can be related to the finger pulleys; flexor tendons; menisci; glenoid and hip labrum; cruciate ligaments; and sometimes bone, muscles, and nerves

- Unilocular or multiloculated

- Can traverse or insinuate many compartments and produce mass effect

- Can affect any age

- Appear on US as hypoechoic structures with posterior acoustic enhancement without any internal vascularity; sometimes can be septated and show internal debris and septal vascular flow (Figure 2.6.16)

- Appear bright on STIR or fat-suppressed images and dark (hypointense) on T1W on MRI and show no or septal enhancement on post-gadolinium images

- Usually managed conservatively with observation

- With symptoms present, can require image-guided aspiration and/or fenestration or injection with steroid and local anaesthetic

- Require excision if refractory

CONCLUSION

This chapter has provided the reader with a good understanding of the most common soft tissue tumours based on the WHO classification. US and MRI appearances of benign tumours such as lipomas, epidermal inclusion cysts, ganglia, and bursae require no additional imaging. Any indeterminate or malignant appearing pathologies require further discussion in the locoregional sarcoma triage MDT, potentially a biopsy, and further management planning. When in doubt, always seek help of a colleague to make sure no potentially sinister lesion is missed.

SUGGESTED READING

- Gupta H, Thaker S, eds. *Practical Guide for Imaging of Soft Tissue Tumours*, 1st edition. CRC Press; 2023.

- Goodwin RW, O'Donnell P, Saifuddin A. MRI appearances of common benign soft-tissue tumours. *Clin Radiol.* 2007;62(9):843–853.

- Soft Tissue Tumors. *A Practical and Comprehensive Guide to Sarcomas and Benign Neoplasms.* Simone Mocellin. Springer; 2021.

SBA QUESTIONS

1) Ultrasound and MRI were performed on a 5 cm soft tissue lesion within the left upper thigh. The lesion was labelled indeterminate on imaging. What is the most appropriate next step?

   A. Follow-up in 3 months with imaging to ensure stability

   B. Refer the patient with imaging to the soft tissue sarcoma MDT

   C. Perform a biopsy of the lesion

   D. Discharge the patient back to the referring clinician for them to decide onward management

2) Ultrasound and MRI have been performed for an intramuscular lipoma. The lipoma shows no concerning imaging features. What is the most appropriate next step?

   A. Fast-track referral to the soft tissue sarcoma MDT

   B. Discharge patient back to the referring clinician

   C. Non-urgent referral to the soft tissue sarcoma MDT

   D. Refer to general surgeon for removal

3) Ultrasound demonstrates a 5 cm well-encapsulated subcutaneous lipoma with no concerning imaging features. The patient states the lesion has been gradually increasing over time. What is the most appropriate next step?

   A. Recommend MRI for further evaluation

   B. Fast-track referral to the soft tissue sarcoma MDT

   C. Non-urgent referral to the soft tissue sarcoma MDT

   D. Discharge patient back to the referring clinician

Answers

(1) B. Any lesion which cannot be characterised as a benign entity should be referred to the sarcoma MDT. In many cases, indeterminate lesions will need biopsy to exclude malignancy, but this

is preferably done in a centre with soft tissue sarcoma biopsy experience to minimise risk of seeding.

(2) C. The British Sarcoma Group recommends non-urgent referral to a soft tissue sarcoma MDT for any lipoma which is deep to the fascia.

(3) D. Benign, superficial lipomas measuring less than 7 cm (some centres cut off at 10 cm) do not need additional imaging and can be discharged back to the referring clinician. If the referring clinician or patient remains concerned, surgical excision can be discussed.

Chapter 2.7
Bone Tumours—Approach and Role of Radiology in the Management

Kirran Khalid and Ganesh Hegde

LEARNING OBJECTIVES

- Learn the imaging approach and parameters used to assess bone lesions
- Learn to differentiate aggressive versus non-aggressive bone lesions based on imaging features
- Learn the imaging features of common bone tumours and pathologies
- Understand the need for prompt referral to a bone tumour unit for further investigation

---

INTRODUCTION

Bone tumour is an umbrella term that encompasses both benign and malignant pathologies as well as reactive focal abnormalities, metabolic abnormalities, and "tumorlike" conditions. Imaging plays a vital role in identification, characterisation, local and distant staging, and image guidance for biopsies when necessary. The role of imaging does not stop at diagnosis and is paramount in post-treatment follow-up to assess the effectiveness of treatment such as chemotherapy, complications related to surgery, and local recurrence.

IMAGING MODALITIES

Radiographs

Despite significant advances in imaging techniques, radiographs still play the central role in the evaluation of bone lesions. They are the primary imaging modality used to assess location, tumour matrix, zone of transition, and periosteal reaction. Many lesions have characteristic appearances on radiographs, and hence it should always be obtained even when a lesion is identified on other modalities such as MRI.

CT Scan

CT is useful for evaluating subtle mineralisation in a lytic lesion, for demonstrating radiographically occult bone destruction, or for demonstrating the lucent nidus of an osteoid osteoma amid a large area of reactive sclerosis.

MRI

Primarily used to further characterise lesions seen on other modalities; excellent for evaluating the extent of the lesion, characterising the matrix by evaluating the internal components of the lesion such as cartilage, vessels, fat, liquid, and hemosiderin. MRI is particularly useful in evaluating the local extent of a malignant process for the purposes of staging, surgical planning, and assessing tumour response to radio and chemotherapy. However, some lesions have a non-specific appearance on MRI, and sometimes the aggressiveness of some benign tumours can be overestimated secondary to the extensive bone marrow and soft tissue oedema, making them appear more aggressive than they are, resulting in unnecessary increased suspicion and potentially subjecting the patient to invasive investigations such as a biopsy. Thus, a multimodality approach is necessary.

A typical bone tumour protocol involves T1, T2, and fluid-sensitive sequences. Diffusion images and chemical shift imaging are used as problem-solving tools where necessary. Routine MSK tumour protocols do not involve the use of gadolinium-based contrast medium; rather, it is used judiciously to differentiate a cystic lesion from a solid one or to demonstrate viable tumour tissue in a large heterogenous lesion for tissue sampling.

Nuclear Imaging

This is not required in all cases; however, nuclear imaging studies such as bone scans are useful for identifying a multiplicity of bone lesions. Aggressive processes are metabolically active, and nuclear imaging helps

DOI: 10.1201/9781003500247-16

in differentiating non-aggressive from aggressive lesions. PET-CT is used for staging and also to identify metabolically active areas in a lesion for biopsy planning.

Assessment of Bone Lesions

To reach a confident diagnosis of a bone tumour, one must employ an organised and systematic approach, paying attention to certain imaging features:

■ Tumour location

■ Tumour margins

■ Zone of transition

■ Periosteal reaction

■ Matrix mineralisation

■ Size of lesion

■ Number of lesions

■ Presence of a soft tissue component

Various bone tumours have a predilection for certain age groups, making age important in diagnosis, as well as the location: Both are indispensable.

Age

Most bone tumours have a predilection for a specific age group, and it is a vital piece of clinical information to narrow down the differential diagnosis while assessing a bone tumour. Although exceptions exist, typical age groups pertaining to various bone tumours are listed in Table 2.7.1.

Common bone lesions such as simple cysts and chondroblastoma occur in skeletally immature patients, whereas giant cell tumours occur in skeletally mature patients. Ewing sarcoma typically occurs in patients between 10 and 20, and a malignant bone tumour in an adult patient over 40 is likely to be a metastatic carcinoma, myeloma, or lymphoma rather than a primary bone sarcoma.

Table 2.7.1 Bone Tumours by Age

Age (in years)	Benign	Malignant
0–10	• Simple bone cyst • Eosinophilic granuloma • Infection	• Ewing sarcoma • Leukaemia • Metastasis (neuroblastoma)
0–20	• Non-ossifying fibroma/fibroxanthoma • Fibroid dysplasia • Simple bone cyst • Aneurysmal bone cyst • Osteochondroma • Osteoid osteoma • Osteoblastoma • Chondroblastoma • Chondromyxoid fibroma • Infection	• Osteosarcoma • Ewing sarcoma
20–40	• Enchondroma • Giant cell tumour • Osteoid osteoma • Osteoblastoma • Fibrous dysplasia • Brown tumour (hyper-parathyroidism)	• Parosteal osteosarcoma • Adamantinoma
≥40	• Fibrous dysplasia • Paget disease • Osteoma • Geode	• Metastasis (most common) • Multiple myeloma • Chondrosarcoma • Osteosarcoma (secondary to Paget disease)

Location

Most bone tumours occur in a typical location in the skeleton (for example, the axial versus appendicular skeleton or long versus flat bone). See Table 2.7.2 for a comprehensive list of tumours and their typical locations. While assessing the lesion, it's important to note both the longitudinal and transverse location of the lesion in the bone. In the longitudinal direction, lesions can be epiphyseal, metaphyseal, or diaphyseal. In the transverse location, they can be medullary, cortical, or juxtacortical.

Tumours like osteosarcoma have a propensity for sites of rapid bone growth, usually the metaphyseal region, while Ewing sarcoma usually follows red marrow distribution. Simple bone cysts and non-ossifying fibromas, although seen in the same longitudinal location (metaphysis), do not share the same transverse location. A simple bone cyst is an intramedullary process, whereas the latter is cortical. The simple cysts are usually central, whereas aneurysmal cysts have eccentric locations.

An apophysis, a growth centre that does not contribute to bone length, is the equivalent of an epiphysis, a growth centre at the end of a bone that also does not contribute to length. Therefore, lesions that have a predilection for epiphysis can be seen in an apophysis as well. Common sites of apophyse include the

Table 2.7.2 Locations of Bone Tumours

Location	Benign	Malignant
Epiphyseal (end of bone)	• Chondroblastoma (skeletally immature patient) • Giant cell tumour (skeletally mature patient) • Osteomyelitis (pyogenic: starts in metaphysis and may spread to epiphysis if the patient is less than 18 months old; tuberculosis or fungus at end of bone in skeletally mature patients) • Paget's disease • Intraosseous ganglion/geode (should have associated arthritis) • Osteochondral injury	• Clear cell chondrosarcoma (exceedingly rare)
• Metaphyseal • Medullary • Cortical • Juxtacortical	• Simple (unicameral) bone cyst (central location) • Aneurysmal (multicameral) bone cyst (eccentric location) • Secondary formation maybe seen giant cell tumour and chondroblastoma) • Enchondroma (central location) • Fibrous dysplasia • Osteomyelitis (typical location for pyogenic infection in children less than 18 months of age and adults) • Localised Langerhans cell histiocytosis • Chondromyxoid fibroma (eccentric location) • Fibrous cortical defect and non-ossifying fibroma (lytic in children, fills in and involutes in adults) • Osteoid osteoma (small lucent nidus with surrounding reactive sclerosis) • Juxtacortical chondroma (arises from periosteum)	• Conventional osteosarcoma • Chondrosarcoma • Metastatic disease • Myeloma (over age 40) • Lymphoma • Malignant vascular tumours (exceptionally rare; angiosarcoma, hemangiopericytoma) • Metastatic disease (especially lung) • Periosteal osteosarcoma (arises from the deep layer of the periosteum) • Parosteal osteosarcoma (arises from the superficial layer of the periosteum) • Juxtacortical chondrosarcoma (arises from the periosteum)
• Diaphyseal (shaft) • Medullary • Cortical	• Fibrous dysplasia • Localised Langerhans cell histiocytosis (also occurs in metaphysis and flat bones: calvarium, pelvis, mandible, ribs) • Ossifying fibroma (osteofibrous dysplasia or Campanacci lesion, which is part of the Jaffe–Campanacci syndrome)	• Ewing sarcoma (occurs in the metaphysis and in the flat bones following red marrow distribution) • Lymphoma • Myeloma (at sites of red marrow, e.g. axial skeleton and proximal aspects of humerus and femur) • Metastatic disease (medullary or cortical) • Malignant vascular tumours (exceedingly rare; angiosarcoma, haemangiopericytoma) • Adamantinoma (mixed lytic and sclerotic lesion occurring almost exclusively in anterior cortex of tibia; tibia may be bowed; look for satellite lesion in tibia or adjacent fibular involvement) • Metastatic disease (especially lung)

greater trochanter of the femur; the tibial tubercle; the patella, carpal bones, hindfoot, and midfoot; and the subarticular portion of the flat bones, such as around the sacroiliac joints, acetabulum, glenoid, and scapula.

ZONE OF TRANSITION/MARGIN

The type of margin/transition zone between the tumour and adjacent normal bone helps in determining the aggressiveness of the lesion.

Radiographically sharp margins/narrow transition or geographic lesion (Type 1) is considered a non-aggressive lesion (see Figure 2.7.1). These margins can be well defined and sclerotic (Type 1a), well defined and non-sclerotic (Type 1b), or they could be a lytic lesion with ill-defined borders (Type 1c). Aggressive lesions (see Figure 2.7.2) have a broad zone of transition that can be ill-defined (Type 2, moth-eaten) or permeative (Type 3), where a lesion is so ill-defined that it appears as multiple small lucencies.

Non-aggressive imaging features suggest a benign process, and an aggressive imaging feature usually suggests a malignant process; however, this does not always hold true:

- Osteomyelitis and localised Langerhans cell histiocytosis are benign processes but can demonstrate permeative aggression on imaging.

- Giant cell tumours may appear well defined on imaging but be locally aggressive and on rare occasions even metastasise.

- Permeative appearance is typical of a class of malignant lesions called the "small round blue cell group" owing to their histologic appearance on haematoxylin and eosin-stained specimens.

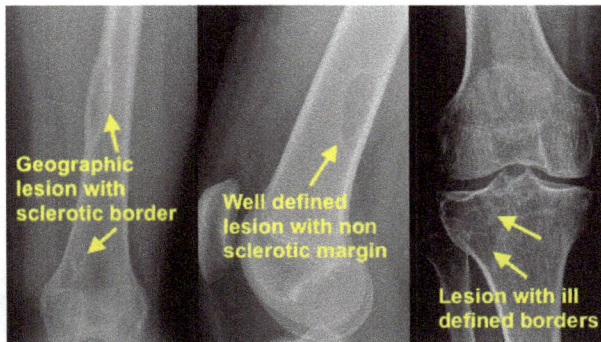

Figure 2.7.1   Margin of bone nonaggressive lesions.

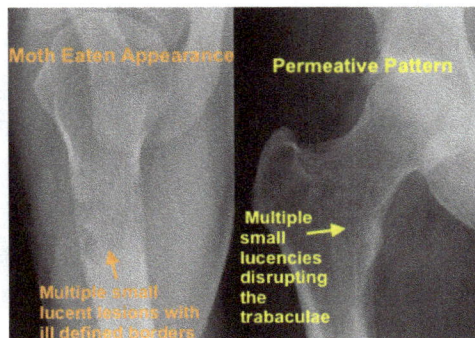

Figure 2.7.2   Margin of bone aggressive lesions.

123

PERIOSTEAL REACTION

This is host bone's response to tumour tissue, and the type of periosteal reaction is a marker of the aggressiveness of the lesion (Figure 2.7.3):

- Solid or unilamellated periosteal reaction: Non-aggressive appearance indicating that the underlying lesion is slow-growing and is giving the bone the opportunity to wall the lesion off.

- A multilamellated or onion-skin appearance: An intermediate aggressive process that waxes and wanes or one where the bone is continually trying to wall off but fully unable to, leading to regional disruption

- A spiculated, or "hair-on-end" (perpendicular to the cortex) or sunburst pattern is the most aggressive imaging appearance and is highly suggestive of malignancy.

A Codman triangle is the elevation of the periosteum away from the cortex with an angle formed where the elevated periosteum and bone come together. Codman triangle, although often associated with conventional osteosarcoma, can also be seen with other aggressive processes that elevate the periosteum. Benign entities such as infection and subperiosteal haematoma can produce a Codman triangle.

MATRIX MINERALISATION

Matrix refers to internal tumour tissue. It can be osteoid, chondral, fibrous, or adipose. The matrix defines the histological lesion type and aids in tumour diagnosis as osteoid or chondroid, mainly based on mineralisation within the lesion:

- Chondral: Punctate, comma-shaped, arc, or ring-like mineralisation (enchondroma, chondrosarcoma, or chondroblastoma)

- Osteoid: Fluffy, amorphous, cloud-like mineralisation pattern; opaque on radiograph

- Fibrous: Intermediate or ground-glass appearance

Matrices are primarily assessed on radiographs; however, faint mineralisation is best investigated using CT, which is more sensitive.

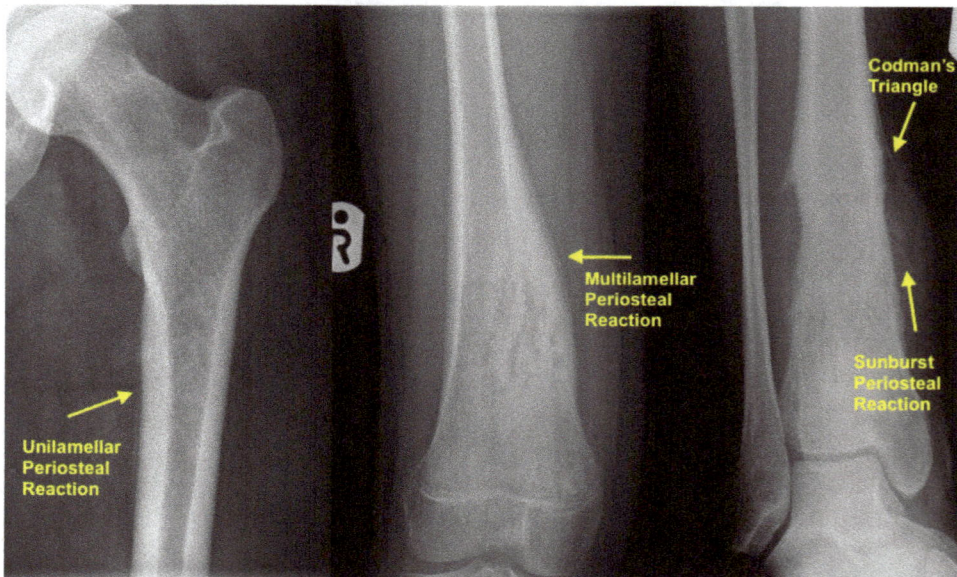

Figure 2.7.3 Types of periosteal reactions.

Size and Number

Some entities have size criteria, and thus size can help in differentiating them. For example, osteoid osteoma and osteoblastoma are similar histological entities but the nidus of an osteoid osteoma is less than 1.5 cm in diameter, while the osteoblastoma nidus is larger than 2 cm. Similarly, fibrous cortical defect and non-ossifying fibroma appear similar on imaging, but "fibrous cortical defect" is used when the lesion is less than 3 cm in craniocaudal length, and a lesion is called a non-ossifying fibroma if it is longer than 3 cm in the maximum craniocaudal dimensions.

Note that lesion size does not necessarily indicate aggressiveness; however, it always needs to be noted, as it can be used to assess the interval changes in follow-up imaging. Primary bone tumours are usually solitary, while multiplicity indicates processes such as metastatic carcinoma, multiple myeloma, and metastatic non-Hodgkin lymphoma; please note, benign entities such as multiple brown tumours and fibrous dysplasia demonstrate multiplicity on imaging.

Cortical Involvement

The cortex is affected by internal pathologies but also by processes originating from the medullary canal, the periosteum, and even the surrounding soft tissue. Cortical involvement is another marker of the aggressiveness of the lesion and takes the following forms:

- Endosteal scalloping: Erosion of the inner surface of the cortex by a slow-growing intramedullary process.

- Cortical destruction: Aggressive intramedullary or cortical lesion destroying the cortex.

- Soap bubble appearance: New bone formation along the periosteum as the inner surface is being eroded by an intermediate aggressive lesion that results in expanded bone with outward ballooning of the cortex, giving rise to lytic, expansile, and "soap bubble" lesions.

- Saucerisation: Secondary to a process that starts on the outer surface of the cortex, either in the periosteum or adjacent soft tissue, eroding the outer surface of the cortex, resulting in an indentation.

Occasionally, the periosteum reacts at the site adjacent to the saucerisation, resulting in a buttressed appearance that is not specific for a benign versus malignant lesion. Buttressing is also seen with slow-growing intramedullary processes that become aggressive and break through or interrupt a solid area of periosteal reaction.

Soft Tissue

A soft tissue component associated with a bone tumour invariably indicates malignancy.

APPROACHES TO BONE TUMOURS

A list of tumours and tumour-like conditions of bone is exhausting, and a systematic approach is needed to arrive at a diagnosis. While some lesions can be "Aunt Minnie's" with classical appearances and straightforward to diagnose, others can be complex and require multiple imaging modalities, correlation with metabolic parameters, pre-existing clinical conditions, and clinical findings. This section discusses paths to approaching a bone tumour.

Narrow Down the Differentials

The first step in the characterisation of a bone lesion is to narrow down the differentials. Many parameters described here can be used for this purpose, with age and lesion location being the most helpful. As has been discussed, many bone lesions are seen in defined age groups and tend to affect specific locations in the bony skeleton.

Aggressive vs Non-Aggressive

Often this is the most important step in bone lesion characterisation. Sometimes it's difficult to definitively diagnose a lesion based on imaging. However, characterising them as aggressive or non-aggressive is often enough to guide further referral, definitive treatment, or follow-up imaging. Parameters such as type of margin, zone of transition, presence or absence of periosteal response and its type, and integrity of cortex and surrounding soft tissues are helpful in differentiating a non-aggressive process from an aggressive one.

Definitive Diagnosis

Wherever possible, an attempt should be made to definitively diagnose a bone lesion. However, it should be noted that this often requires the help of histopathology rather than imaging alone.

While multiple parameters are required for a definitive diagnosis, characterisation of the matrix often helps. For example, a lesion with osteoid matrix with aggressive features in the metaphysis of long bone in a child is likely to be osteosarcoma. Similarly, a lesion with a ground glass matrix with no aggressive features in the bone is likely to be a fibrous dysplasia.

Multiplicity also helps; multiple aggressive-appearing bone lesions can be metastatic, whereas multiple non-aggressive bone lesions are seen in fibrous dysplasia. Please note here that lesion aggressiveness does not always indicate malignancy. Infections and benign lesions such as osteoid osteoma, Langerhans cell histiocytosis, and chondroblastomas can appear aggressive on imaging.

REFERRAL PATHWAY

NICE guidelines call for an X-ray within 48 hours if there is clinical suspicion of a bone tumour in children and young adults with unexplained bone swelling and pain, and if the X-ray suggests a bone sarcoma, an urgent specialist appointment. In adults, the cancer pathway referral should take place within 2 weeks.

However, bone lesions present a variety of clinical features that are identified on other imaging modalities. As a result, radiologists in non-tertiary centres should be aware of Trust guidelines and work closely with regional sarcoma centres for appropriate evaluation and management of bone lesions. Although variations exist, the next section describes a usual pathway for referral and evaluation of bone tumours.

COMMON BONE LESIONS

Osteoid Osteoma (Figure 2.7.4)

- Benign lytic osteoblastic tumour
- Long bones are usually involved:
  - 2/3 are extra-articular, involving femur and tibia diaphysis
  - 10% are intra-articular
- Can be seen in the vertebrae, typically lumbar
- Seen in all age groups, typically in the first 3 decades of life

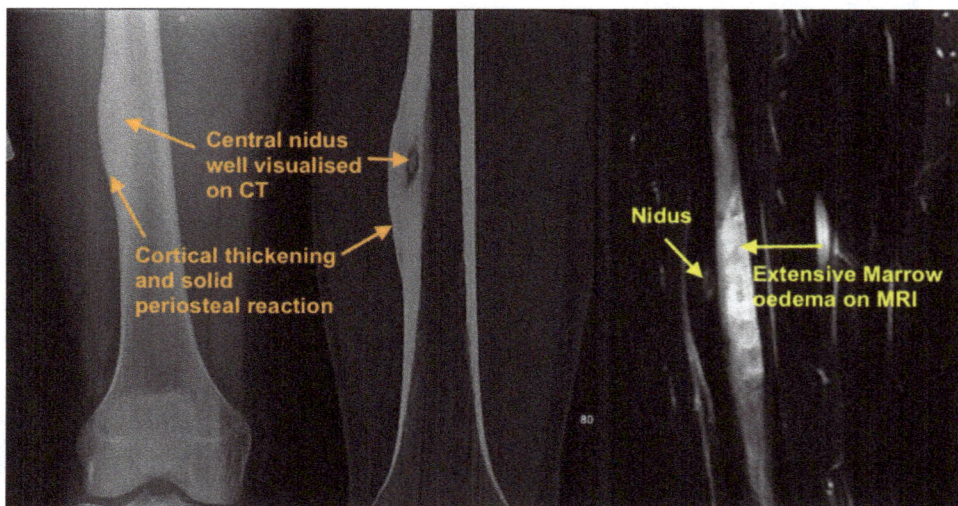

Figure 2.7.4 Imaging features of osteoid osteoma.

- Presents with a dull ache that is worse at night and relieved by non-steroidal anti-inflammatory drugs (e.g. aspirin)
- Monoarthropathy, joint effusion, and synovitis can be seen with an intra-articular tumour
- Radiograph
- Cortical thickening, sclerosis, and solid periosteal reaction. Lucent nidus may or may not be visible

CT

- Best for visualising a central ovoid lucent nidus (less than 1.5 cm)
- Reactive sclerosis with cortical thickening and expansion

MRI

- T1W intermediate signal nidus
- T2W/STIR variable signal nidus (depends on degree of mineralisation/fibrosis)
- Intense enhancement of the nidus following contrast

Three-quarters of cases exhibit reactive changes that are more pronounced in younger patients. Medullary sclerotic lesions give a low signal on T1W and T2W. Extensive oedema gives a low signal on T1W and high T2W/STIR, and periosteal reaction is also possible.

Osteoblastoma (Figure 2.7.5)

- Benign, locally aggressive lytic osteoblastic tumour
- Histologically the same as osteoid osteoma, but the nidus is >2 cm
- Seen in young adults, male > female
- Any bone can be affected, typically seen in femoral diaphysis
- Local extension through the cortex may be seen with surrounding reactive oedema and sclerosis
- Secondary aneurysmal bone cyst can form
- Aggressive lesions seen in older patients with larger tumours
- <1% undergo malignant transformation

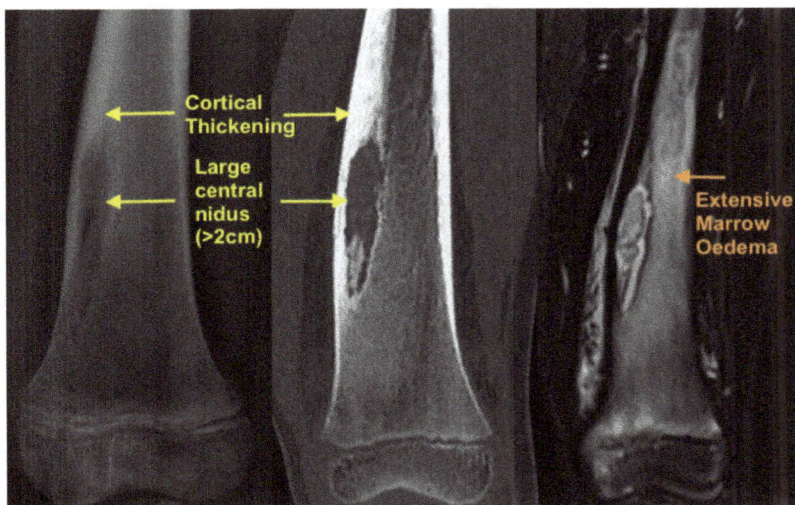

Figure 2.7.5 Imaging features of osteoblastoma.

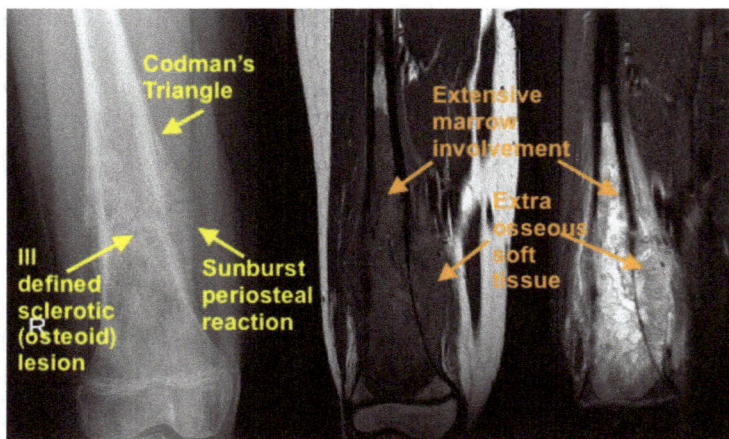

Figure 2.7.6 Imaging features of osteosarcoma.

Osteosarcoma (Figure 2.7.6)

- Malignant osteoblastic tumour
- Most common primary bone malignant tumour
  - Primary: Typically <age 30 (2nd decade of life common)
  - Secondary: Elderly (e.g. malignant degeneration of Paget's disease)
- Presents with pain
- Metaphysis of long bones typically affected:

  - Distal femur > proximal tibia > proximal humerus > proximal femur
  - Diaphyseal and epiphyseal extension not uncommon

Radiograph/CT

- Aggressive tumour with a wide zone of transition
- Sclerosis appears due to osteoblastic tumour or is reactive
- Cortical destruction is typical
- "Sunburst" type of periosteal reaction and Codman triangle

MRI

- Tumour is mixed intermediate T1W signal and intermediate/increased T2W/STIR signal
- Foci of low T1W signal within the tumour can indicate osteoblastic activity or fibrosis, and foci of high signal can indicate blood
- Tumour extension across the growth plate is common
- Skip metastases occur in 10% of cases and have a similar SI to the original tumour but are separated by normal marrow
- Extraosseous tumour can be seen

CARTILAGINOUS LESIONS

Osteochondroma (Figure 2.7.7)

- Most common benign bone tumour
- Can be pedunculated with a stalk connecting the native bone or sessile

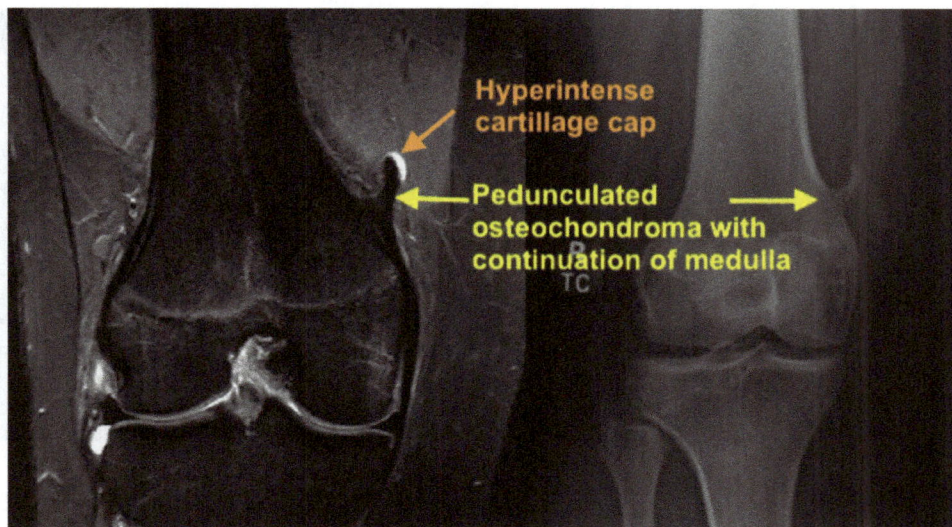

Figure 2.7.7 Imaging features of osteochondroma.

- Typically extends away from the joint
- Medulla of the host bone continues with the osteochondroma
- Lesion contains a cartilage cap that is generally thin and less than 2 cm in thickness
- Most commonly seen around the knee joint
- Most are asymptomatic, but they can produce symptoms due to pressure on adjacent structures, impingement of neurovascular structures, bursa formation or fracture, and malignant degeneration to chondrosarcoma
- Multiple osteochondromas are seen in diaphyseal aclasis.

Radiographs/CT

- A pedunculated or sessile growth from the bone projecting away from the metaphysis
- Continuation of medullary cavity, better appreciated on CT or MRI
- Metaphyseal widening at the site of osteochondroma

MRI

- Best for assessing medullary continuity and cartilage cap
- Modality of choice for evaluating complications

Enchondroma (Figure 2.7.8)

- Benign lytic intramedullary lesion
- Second most common benign bone tumour after osteochondroma
- Typically seen in the phalanges (tubular bones) as well as in the humerus, femur, and tibia
- Usually asymptomatic and discovered incidentally
- Symptomatic cases are usually secondary to a pathological fracture

CT/Radiographs

- Well-defined with a narrow zone of transition
- Slightly expansile and lobulated

129

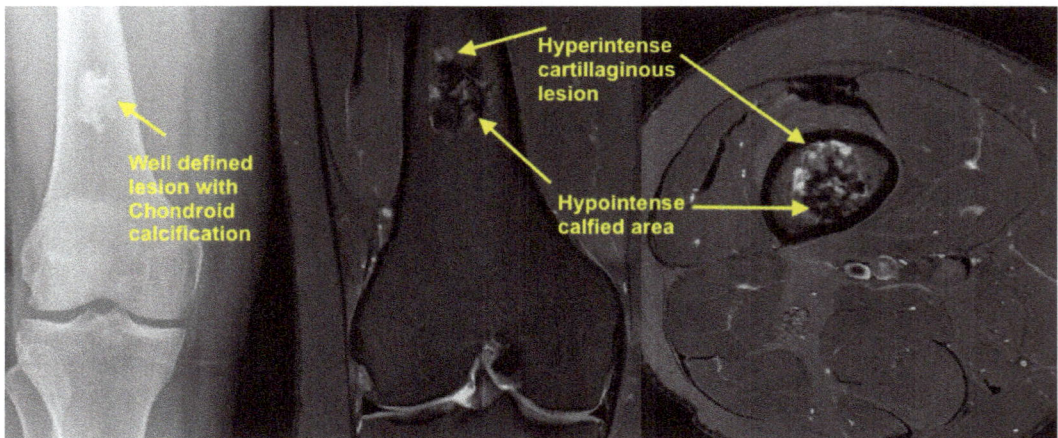

Figure 2.7.8 Imaging features of enchondroma.

- Endosteal scalloping and cortical thinning
- Contain calcified chondroid matrix (irregular, speckled) when located away from phalanges

MRI

- Well-defined lobular lesion
- Intermediate T1W signal and variable increased PDW/T2W signal
- Low signal foci on all pulse sequences represent calcification
- Foci of T1W high signal is normal intervening yellow marrow
- Ollier's disease = multiple enchondromas
- Maffucci's syndrome = multiple enchondromas with soft tissue haemangiomas

Chondroblastoma (Figure 2.7.9)

- Benign chondral tumour
- Male > female (2.7:1)
- Most cases occur between ages 5 and 25, with a mean age of 18
- Tumours are rare over the age of 30; if present, they are usually seen in flat bones
- Presents with joint pain, stiffness, swelling, and effusion
- Typically seen in the epiphysis of a long bone (eccentrically located), mainly the proximal femur and the knee
- With partial closure of the growth plate, a tumour can extend from the epiphysis to the metaphysis in around half of cases
- Epiphyseal equivalents include apophysis and sesamoid bones, e.g. the greater trochanter, greater tuberosity, acromion and patella, calcaneum, and talus

MRI

- Well-defined tumour with lobular margins
- Intermediate T1W signal and high signal on FS PDW/T2W/STIR
- Low T2 signal may be seen due to immature chondroid matrix
- Fluids can accumulate secondary to ABC change

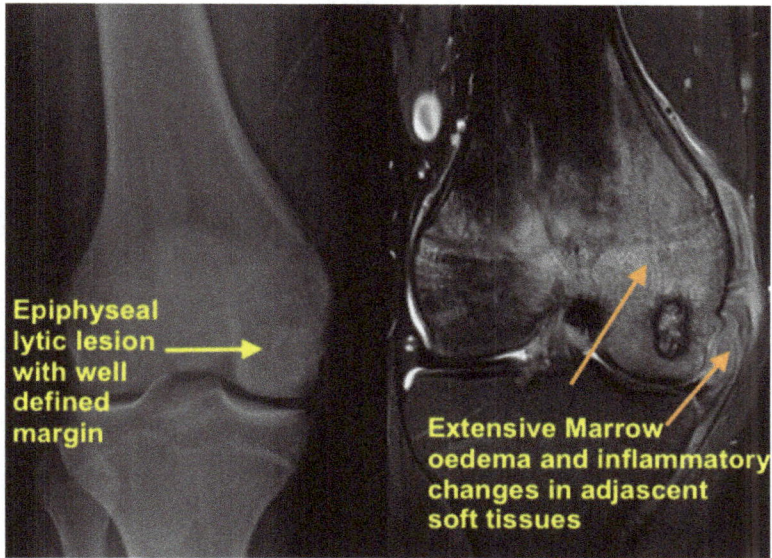

Figure 2.7.9 Imaging features of chondroblastoma.

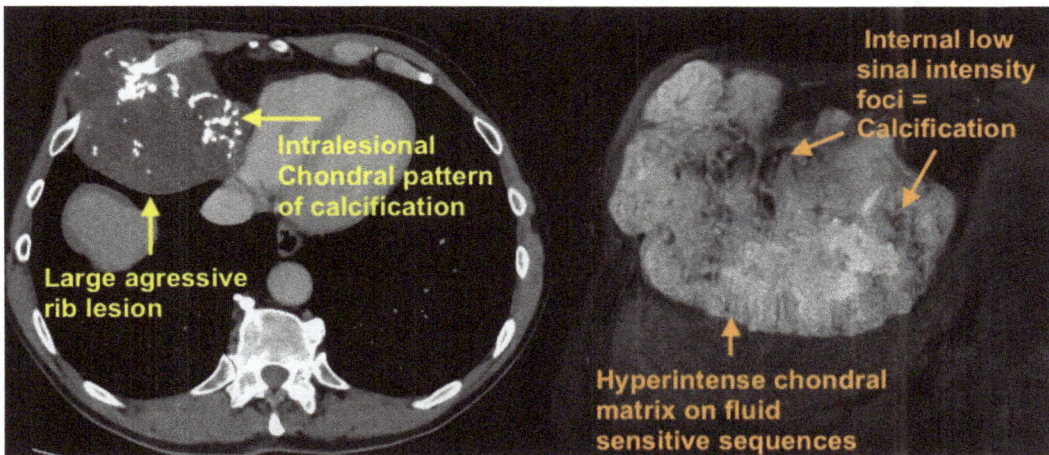

Figure 2.7.10 Imaging features of chondrosarcoma.

■ Typically, marrow oedema, soft tissue reactive change, reactive joint effusion, and thick/solid periosteal reaction are typically seen

■ Heterogeneous enhancement of the tumour following contrast as well as the reactive soft tissue

Chondrosarcoma (Figure 2.7.10)

■ Malignant cartilage-producing tumour

■ Second most common primary malignant bone tumour

■ Seen in the 4th–5th decades of life

- Presents with pain, swelling, and pathological fracture in one-quarter of cases
- Typically seen in long bones (femur, humerus, tibia) with a predilection for the metaphysis followed by the diaphysis
- May arise from a pre-existing cartilage mass such as an enchondroma or osteochondroma

CT/Radiographs

On CT and in radiographs, chondrosarcomas appear as lytic, destructive tumours with amorphous, irregular, calcified chondroid matrices that show characteristic "rings and arcs" or "popcorn" calcification.

MRI

On MRI, chondrosarcomas show a lobular growth pattern with intermediate T1W and high T2W/STIR signal. Imaging features are similar to those of chondroma except that they are >4 cm in size and there is endosteal scalloping.

Ewing Sarcoma (Figure 2.7.11)

- Second most common malignant primary bone tumour in children after osteosarcoma
- Three-quarters of patients are under age 20
- Male > female
- Typically a single-site disease; multiple lesions seen in a small number of cases
- Permeative lesion usually in the diaphysis of long bones: Femur, humerus, pelvic bones, and ribs
- Arises from the medullary cavity
- Aggressive with a wide zone of transition
- Extraosseous mass almost always present
- Onion-skinned periosteal reaction seen on CT and radiographs

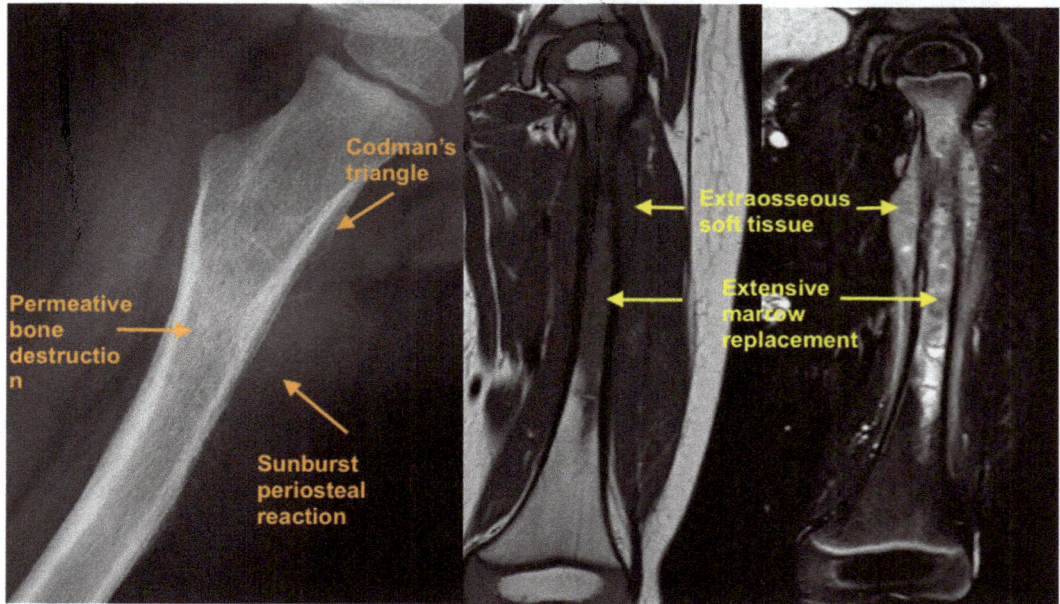

Figure 2.7.11 Imaging features of Ewing sarcoma.

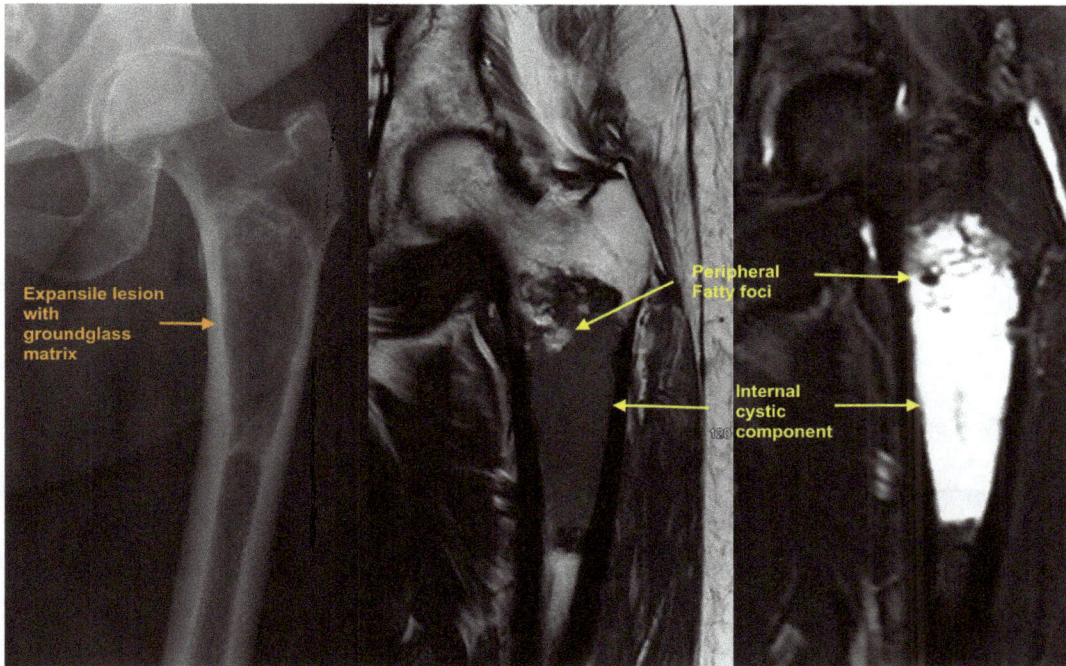

Figure 2.7.12   Imaging features of fibrous dysplasia.

MRI

- Non-specific

- Intermediate T1W and intermediate/high PDW/T2W/STIR signal

- Enhancement of solid tumour can allow overestimation of tumour burden

- Skip metastases are commonly seen; whole-body MRI is advised for staging T1W and STIR sequences

PAGET'S DISEASE (FIGURE 2.7.12)

- Male > female (3:2)

- Excessive and abnormal remodelling of the bone

- Three overlapping phases exist:
  - Phase 1: Lytic (incipient-active) due to the predominant osteolysis
  - Phase 2: Mixed (active) with osteoblastic activity on a background of osteolysis
  - Phase 3: Blastic (inactive), where osteoblastic activity subsides

- Any bone can be involved, although there is a predilection for the axial skeleton, with pelvis, spine, and skull the most common

- Monostotic disease is more common; however, in the presence of polyostotic disease, there is a predilection for the right side of the body and lower limb

CT/Radiograph

- Spine: Picture frame vertebra, vertical trabecular thickening, squaring of vertebra

- Pelvis: Cortical thickening and sclerosis, expansion of the pubic rami and ischium

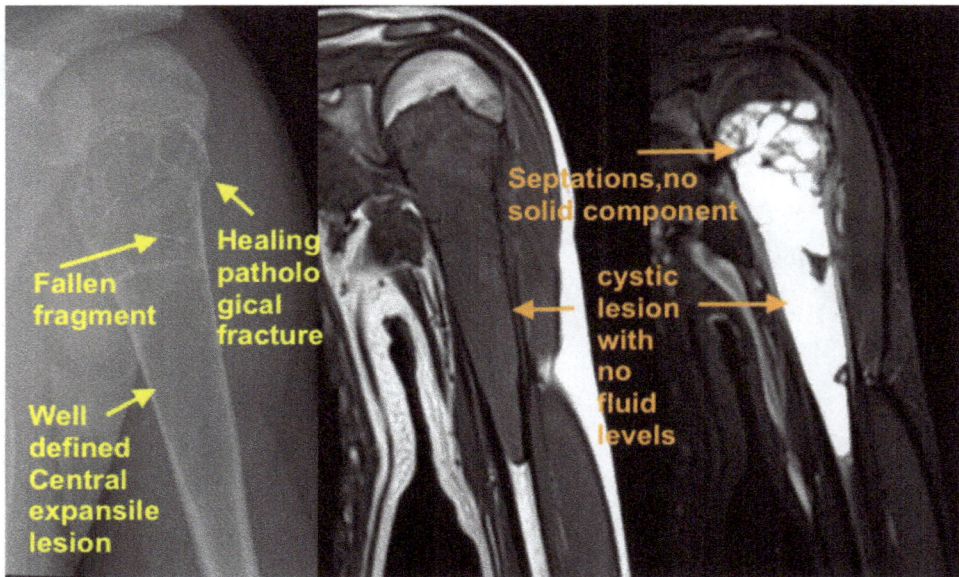

Figure 2.7.13 Imaging features of simple bone cyst.

- Skull: Cotton wool appearance (mixed lytic and sclerotic lesions), osteoporosis circumscripta (large lytic lesions)

MRI

- Marrow signal is variable and normal in most cases
- Early/active phase: Heterogeneously reduced T1W signal and increased T2W/STIR FS signal
- "Flame-shaped/blade of grass" hyperintense area seen on T2W/STIR FS signal
- Late phase: Reduced marrow signal on all pulse sequences

SIMPLE BONE CYST (FIGURE 2.7.13)

- Also known as a unicameral bone cyst
- Benign lytic lesion
- Usually, solitary
- Typically seen between ages 5 and 15
- Male > female (2.5:1)
- Begins within the physeal growth plate and extends into the diaphysis
- Centrally located within a long bone, commonly the proximal humerus
- Asymptomatic, unless there is a pathological fracture
- "Falling fragment" sign: Fracture fragments seen sunken at the bottom of the fluid-filled lesion

MRI

- Homogeneous fluid content
  - Low/intermediate T1W signal
  - Hyperintense T2W/STIR signal
- Signal characteristics are different in the presence of a fracture

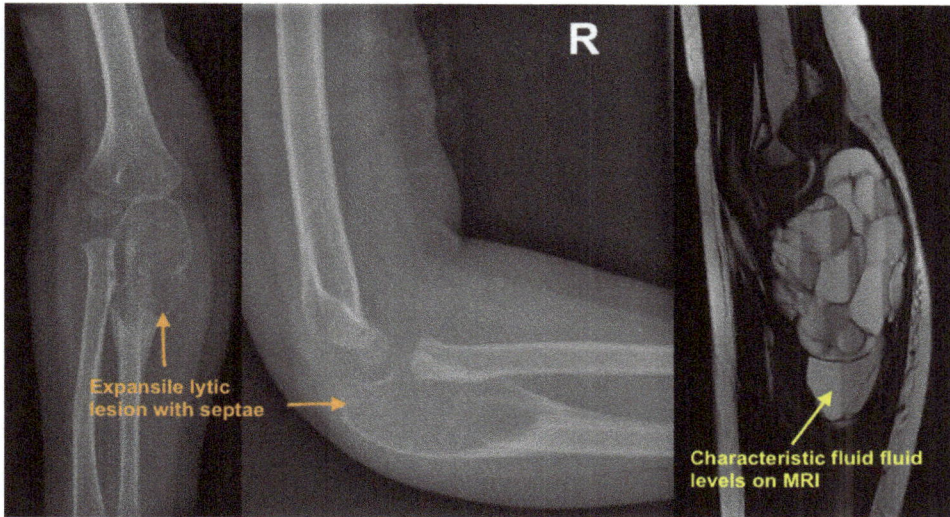

Figure 2.7.14   Imaging features of aneurysmal bone cyst.

ANEURYSMAL BONE CYST (FIGURE 2.7.14)

- Benign lytic lesion
- Primary aneurysmal bone cyst (ABC) accounts for 70% of cases
- Secondary ABC accounts for the remainder and arises in pre-existing benign or malignant tumours
- Present in the 2nd decade of life, typically <age 30
- Presents with pain and swelling

CT/Radiograph

- Expansile lytic lesion
- Thin sclerotic margin (eggshell)
- Eccentrically located in the metaphysis of a long bone adjacent to the unfused physeal growth plate

MRI

- Heterogeneous intermediate/high T1W signal
- Heterogeneous increased T2W/STIR PD signal
- No peri-lesional oedema

GIANT CELL TUMOUR (FIGURE 2.7.15)

- Locally aggressive lytic tumour
- >Age 30
- Closed epiphysis
- Lesion is invariably subarticular and eccentrically located
- Well-defined, narrow zone of transition
- Non-sclerotic margin
- Usually seen within the distal femur or proximal tibia

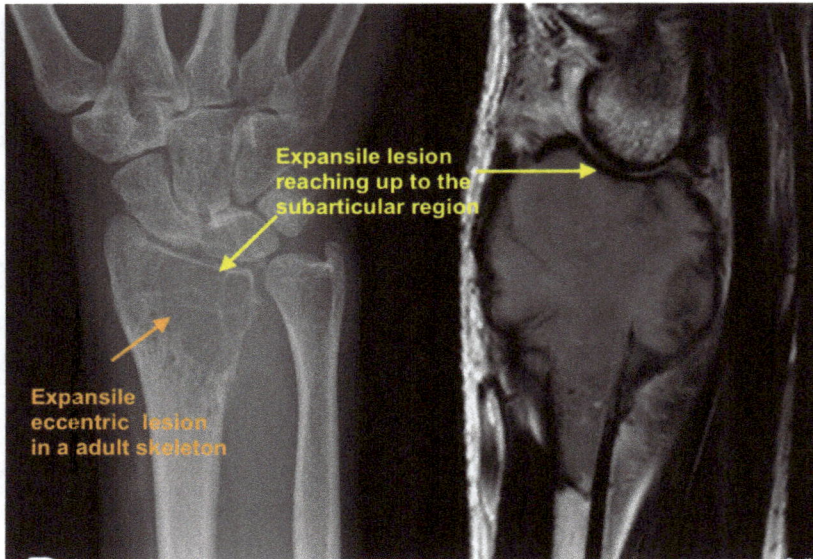

Figure 2.7.15   Imaging features of giant cell tumour.

MRI

- Intermediate T1W signal
- Heterogeneously high STIR signal
- T1W/PDW hyperintensity suggests haemorrhage
- Marked low SI foci on T2W GRE due to the presence of hemosiderin

CT/Radiograph

- CXR advised to look for lung metastasis
- In the event of recurrence or a pathological fracture, CT thorax is suggested

NON-OSSIFYING FIBROMA/FIBROUS CORTICAL DEFECT (FIGURE 2.7.16)

- Common benign lucent lesions
- Non-ossifying fibroma >2 cm
- Fibrous cortical defect <2 cm
- <Age 30
- Asymptomatic and usually an incidental finding
- Eccentric metaphyseal bone lesion located near the physis and commonly seen around the knee and distal tibia
- Found along the long axis of the bone

CT/Radiograph

- Lucent lesion with a thin, sclerotic rim that is often scalloped and slightly expansile
- With increasing age, the lesion migrates away from the physis
- Becomes sclerotic as healing occurs and "disappears" as it ossifies

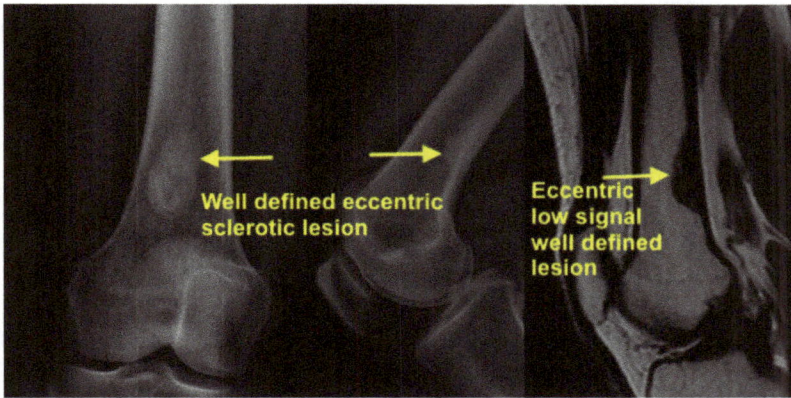

Figure 2.7.16   Imaging features of non-ossifying fibroma.

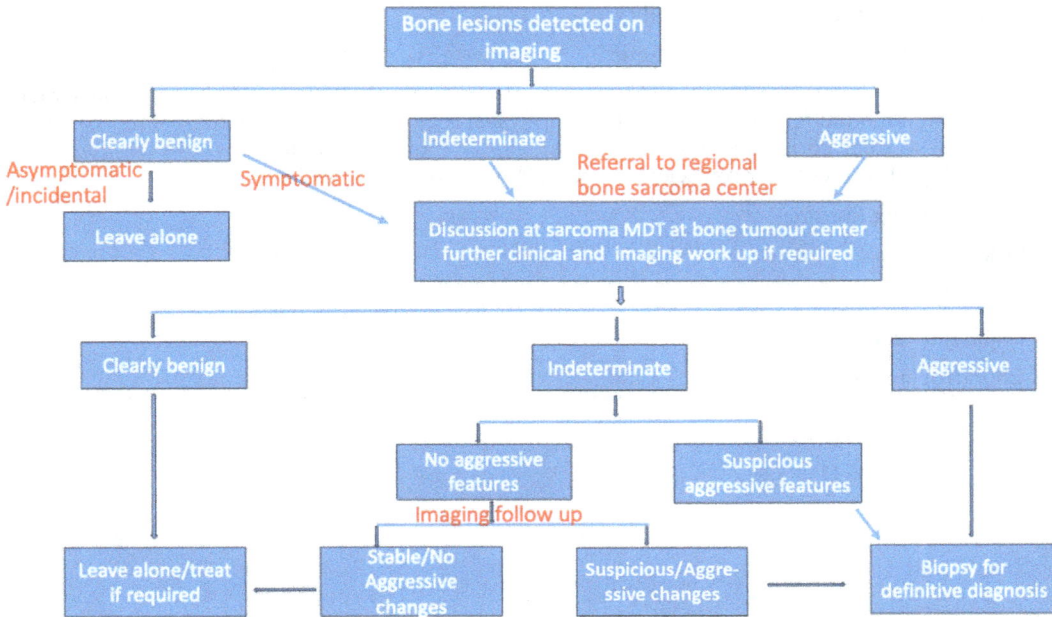

Chart 2.7.1   Referral pathway and approach to a bone lesion.

CONCLUSION

Characterisation of bone lesions requires a systematic approach, assessment of multiple parameters, and a combination of imaging modalities such as radiographs, CT, and MRI (usually without the benefit of gadolinium-based contrast medium). Imaging characteristics of the lesion in conjunction with the age of the patient and the tumour location can help the radiologist devise an appropriate list of differential diagnoses, if not the single correct diagnosis. Follow Chart 2.7.1 for a sample referral pathway.

SUGGESTED READING

■ Butt SH, Muthukumar T, Tyler P. Radiological Imaging of Primary Benign and Malignant Bone Tumours. In *Radionuclide and Hybrid Bone Imaging* (pp. 195–257). Berlin, Heidelberg: Springer; 2012 Sep 18.

SBA QUESTIONS

1) A 10-year-old presented with 3 months history of pain in the distal femur. A radiograph was performed. Which of the following parameters help in assessing the aggressiveness of the lesion?

    A. Age of the patient

    B. Location of the lesion in the bone

    C. Type of periosteal reaction

    D. Tumour matrix

    E. Distance from the joint

2) A bone lesion was identified on imaging incidentally during a CT scan. After imaging workup, it was not possible to conclusively say if the lesion was aggressive or non-aggressive. What should be the next step?

    A. Perform an image-guided biopsy for confirmation of diagnosis

    B. Discharge as it is an incidental lesion

    C. Refer to regional bone tumour centre for further evaluation and management

    D. Follow-up imaging to look for stability

    E. Get an opinion from a senior colleague

3) A 12-year-old presents with a 12-month history of pain in the thigh. Radiograph demonstrates thickened sclerotic posteromedial femoral cortex in the diaphyseal region. MRI shows extensive marrow oedema, and CT shows a thick cortex with solid periosteal response and a lucent focus within the thickened cortex measuring 11 mm with central sclerotic focus. What is your diagnosis?

    A. Non-ossifying fibroma

    B. Osteosarcoma

    C. Osteoblastoma

    D. Osteoid osteoma

    E. Chondroblastoma

Answers: (1) C, (2) C, (3) D

Chapter 2.8
Haematological Disorders

Kirran Khalid and Phillipa Tyler

LEARNING OBJECTIVES

■ To become familiar with the imaging appearances of red and yellow marrow

■ To understand the process and patterns of normal red-to-yellow marrow conversion

■ To appreciate common haematological conditions that result in yellow-to-red marrow reconversion

■ To recognise imaging features that allow differentiation between normal adult marrow, normal variants, non-neoplastic haematopoietic disorders, and malignant marrow disease

■ To utilise non-routine advanced MRI techniques such as Dixon chemical shift imaging as a diagnostic tool for marrow abnormalities

---

This is one of the most important chapters, not just for FRCR 2B purposes but also for marrow pathologies you might encounter during daily practice and MDTs. We recommend referring to it at least twice before the exam to maximise the understanding.

Haematological disorders encompass a wide range of conditions that affect not only the blood but also the bone marrow, one of the largest organs in the human body, accounting for approximately 4% of total body weight. It forms a gelatinous tissue consisting of haematopoietic stem cells, adipose cells, and stroma and is contained within a bony trabecular network in the medullary space consisting of osseous components, vessels, vascular sinuses, nerves, retinaculum cells, and lymphoid tissue.

MARROW PHYSIOLOGY

At birth, the bone marrow is composed almost entirely of haematopoietically active red marrow (appearing macroscopically red due to the presence of haemoglobin). It functions to produce blood cells, supplemented by **extra-medullary haematopoiesis (EMH) occurring in the liver and spleen**.

During childhood, the red blood cell life span increases and EMH ceases, with physiological conversion of red marrow into haematopoietically inactive yellow marrow (appearing yellow due to the presence of fat and carotenoids).

■ **Marrow conversion in the skeleton:** Red-to-yellow marrow conversion follows a predictable pattern, commencing peripherally in the appendicular skeleton and then extending towards the central axial skeleton, demonstrating a centripetal pattern in the phalanges of the hands and feet.

■ **Marrow conversion in an individual bone:** Within the long bones, red-to-yellow marrow conversion first occurs in the epiphysis—usually within 6 months of the radiological appearance of the secondary ossification centre—followed by the diaphysis and then extends towards the distal metaphysis followed by the proximal metaphysis.

■ **Vertebral marrow conversion:** Normal variant is typically seen in those under age 20, where yellow marrow is seen along the superior and inferior margins of the basi-vertebral veins. Triangular areas of yellow marrow adjacent to endplates at the anterior and posterior vertebral corners can also be seen.

■ **Adult red marrow retention sites:** Usually by age 25, red marrow is retained in the axial skeleton, skull, vertebral bodies, sternum, ribs, pelvis, and proximal humerus and femur:

• Most of the adult red marrow is located within the spine (Figure 2.8.1).

• Prominent residual red marrow in the long bones of adults is typically found in the medial proximal humeral metaphysis, the medial femoral neck, the medial proximal femoral metaphysis, the posterior distal femoral metaphysis, and the posterior proximal tibial metaphysis.

DOI: 10.1201/9781003500247-17

Several patterns of prominent yellow marrow distribution in adults are recognised and should not be mistaken for pathology.

Proximal Femur

■ Prominent yellow marrow in the proximal femoral epiphysis and trochanters (typically in patients under 50) and inferior to the medial femoral head

■ Multiple focal areas of prominent intertrochanteric yellow marrow that may coalesce (commonly in middle-aged patients)

■ Uniformly diffuse fatty marrow within the proximal femur (typically in patients over 50)

Adult Pelvis

■ Focal fatty marrow often found adjacent to the sacroiliac joints (commonly seen in patients over 40)

■ Acetabula (more commonly seen in patients under 40

■ Symphysis pubis

■ Diffuse fatty marrow in the sacrum and coccyx

IMAGING CHARACTERISTICS OF PHYSIOLOGICAL ADULT BONE MARROW

■ Conventional radiography is poor at differentiating between normal adult marrow distribution (Table 2.8.1) and red marrow reconversion.

■ MRI is the most sensitive imaging modality for evaluating bone marrow and can differentiate between red and yellow marrow due to differences in their fat and water content.

■ Non-fat suppressed, non-contrast T1-weighted turbo spin echo (T1W TSE) sequences are useful in the differentiation between yellow and red marrow, marrow oedema, and marrow infiltration.

Reporting Pearls

Imaging characteristics of marrow on non-fat-suppressed, non-contrast T1-weighted turbo spin echo (T1W TSE) sequence:

■ Both red and yellow marrow are hyperintense to skeletal muscle and intervertebral discs (Figure 2.8.1).

■ Red marrow should be a similar SI to the spinal cord and conus.

■ Marrow oedema returns a similar SI to red marrow on T1 but is usually less well-defined and unlike red marrow is markedly high signal on fat-suppressed fluid-sensitive sequences (Figure 2.8.2).

■ Marrow infiltration is typically isointense or hypointense to skeletal muscle, usually with well-defined margins.

IMAGING CHARACTERISTICS OF MARROW ON OTHER MRI SEQUENCES

Reassuring imaging features supporting the presence of non-pathological red marrow include:

■ A diaphyseal location

Table 2.8.1 Normal Cellular Composition of the Adult Bone Marrow

	Haematopoietic Cells	Fat Cells
Red marrow	60%	40%, consisting of • 40% water • 40% fat • 20% protein
Yellow marrow	5%	95%, consisting of • 80% fat • 15% water • 5% protein

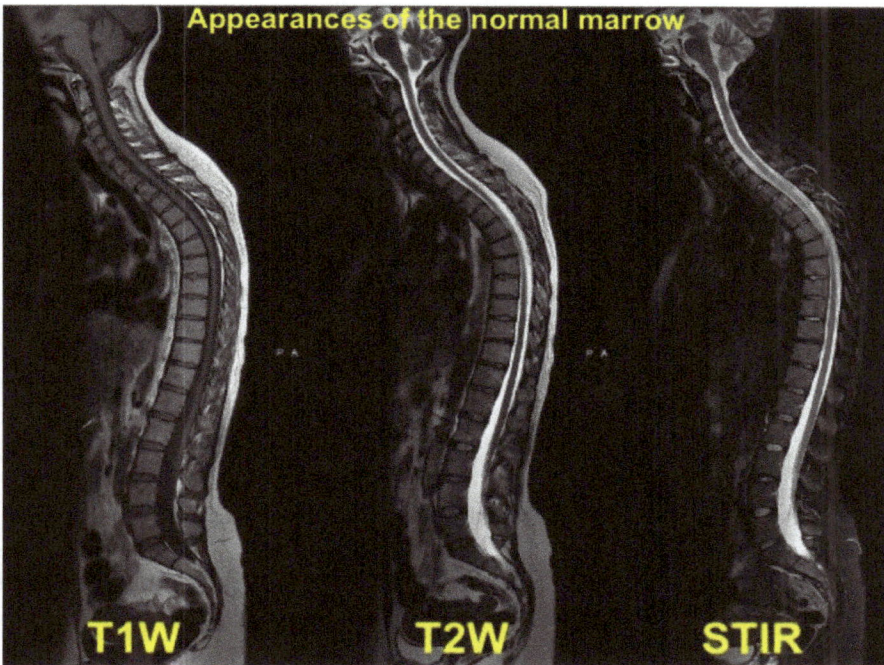

Figure 2.8.1 MRI appearances of normal marrow on T1W, T2W, and STIR whole-spine images.

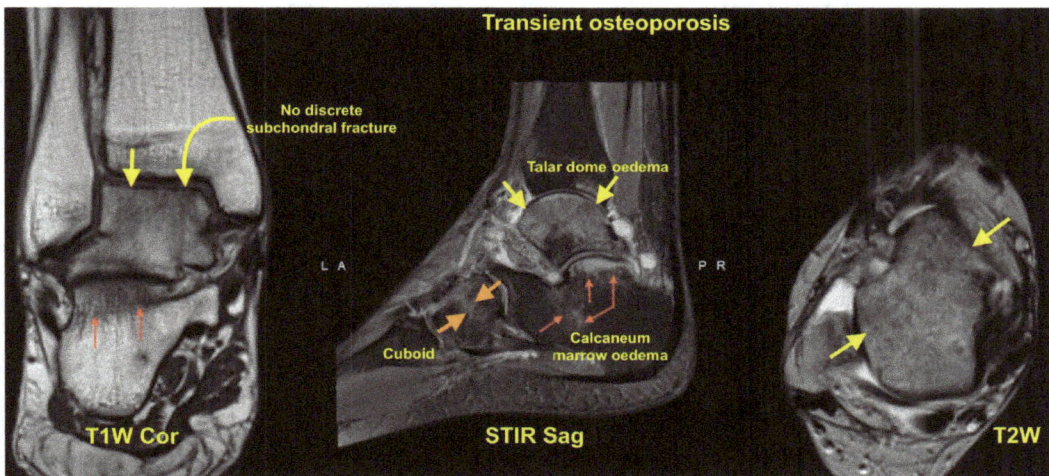

Figure 2.8.2 Multifocal marrow oedema syndromes in ankle: Transient osteoporosis (where no subchondral insufficiency fracture is visible on T1W image) versus true subchondral insufficiency fracture (not shown here). Worth investigating with serum vitamin D and DEXA in such cases.

- Hyperintense (bright) to skeletal muscle on T1W TSE sequences
- Absence of an associated soft tissue mass
- Absence of cortical destruction
- Table 2.8.2 describes typical marrow appearance on imaging

Table 2.8.2 Differential Marrow Appearance on MRI Sequences

T2-weighted fast spin echo (T2W FSE) sequences	Less apparent differentiation between red and yellow marrow since there is less difference between the SI of water and fat
Chemical fat saturation sequences (such as SPIR or SPAIR)	Suppression of SI from fat can be achieved to differentiate between physiological and pathological marrow
STIR sequences	Used to null fat SI by selecting an appropriate inversion time
Fat-suppressed proton density-weighted fast spin echo, STIR, and SPIR/SPAIR sequences	Yellow marrow is low signal and red marrow is intermediate to high signal, being mildly hyperintense relative to skeletal muscle On the contrary, marrow oedema and marrow infiltration are typically high signal on fat suppressed fluid sensitive sequences
Gradient echo sequences	Low signal; red marrow being markedly low signal

Red Marrow Reconversion

Primary non-conversion of red-to-yellow marrow or reconversion of yellow-to-red marrow in adulthood occurs in response to a variety of stresses endured by the body when the demand for red blood cells exceeds the production capacity of the existing marrow.

Causes of Red Marrow Reconversion

- Congenital
- Anaemia
- Malignancy
- High-level aerobic athletics
- Menstruation

- Chronic illnesses (cyanotic heart disease, chronic pulmonary disease and liver or kidney failure)
- Marrow replacement disorders
- Infection
- Smoking
- Obesity

The pattern of reconversion of yellow-to-red marrow occurs from the axial to the appendicular skeleton, in the opposite direction to that of red-yellow marrow conversion.

- In cases of severely increased haematopoietic requirement, epiphyseal red marrow conversion, marrow cavity expansion and extra-medullary haematopoiesis (EMH) may occur.

- The resulting red marrow hyperplasia is often patchy; the marrow heterogeneity may be the result of multiple focal areas of red marrow or islands of yellow marrow.

- It is prudent to correlate these appearances on T1W, T2W, and STIR sequences, with chemical shift imaging being particularly useful in cases of focal red marrow mimicking possible marrow replacement; focal red marrow demonstrates a significant drop in signal intensity on the out-of-phase sequence.

REPORTING PEARLS

Red marrow reconversion sites appear as areas of non-specific, slightly decreased SI on T1W TSE with corresponding slightly increased SI on STIR sequences (Figures 2.8.3 and 2.8.4), and either a patchy or more homogeneous distribution; potentially mimicking disease progression and/or metastatic disease.

- Reassuring features are a pelvic and proximal femoral location and bilateral symmetry, the latter demonstrated on whole-body MRI.

- Dixon out-of-phase imaging is useful in cases which are indeterminate on T1 and STIR.

Focal Nodular Marrow Hyperplasia (Figure 2.8.5)

Focal nodular marrow hyperplasia (FNMH) occurs in response to the body's increased oxygen demand in situations such as smoking, long distance running or excessive sporting activity, chronic anaemia, administration of haematopoietic growth factor, malignancy, and chronic illness.

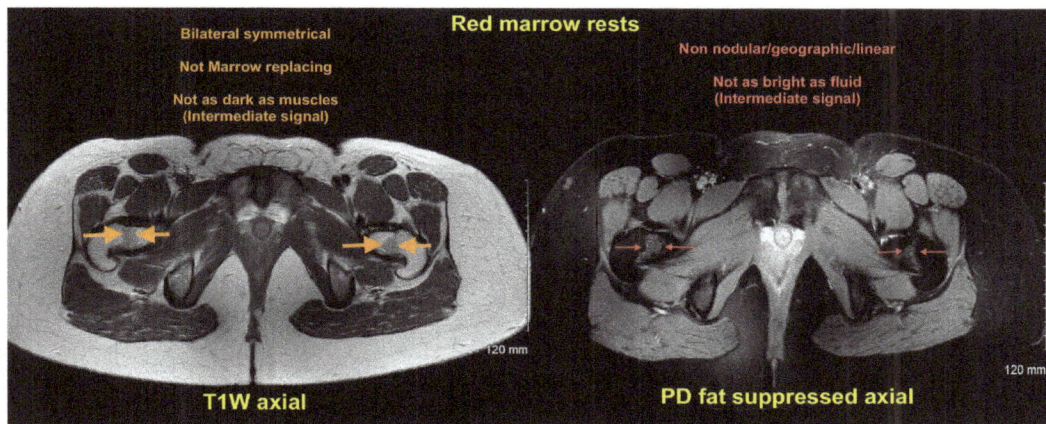

Figure 2.8.3 Normal red marrow in geographic distribution in both proximal femur (axial images).

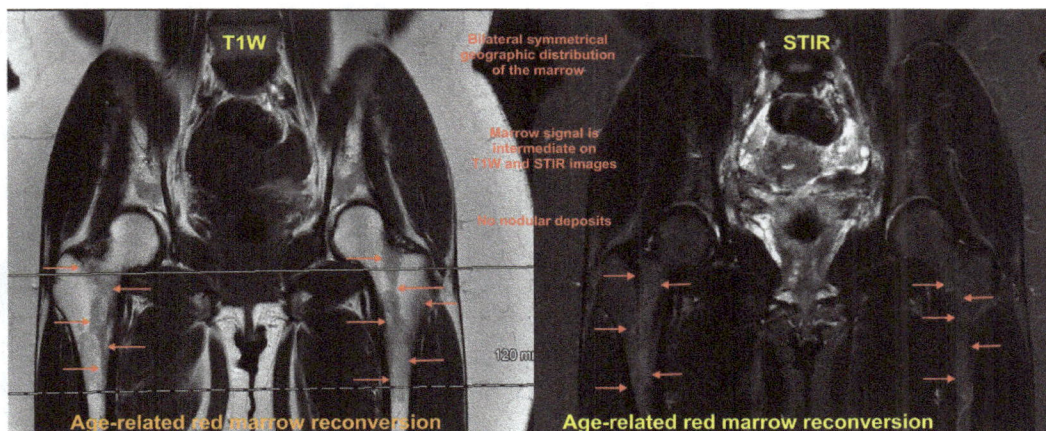

Figure 2.8.4 Normal red marrow in geographic distribution in both proximal femur (coronal images).

- The appearances on MRI represent geographic areas of red marrow.
- They are typically oval, less than 2 cm in size, with somewhat poorly defined margins (likely due to incomplete marrow conversion). They are frequently found in the appendicular skeleton, in the femoral and humeral metaphyses, and near the vertebral endplates (metaphyseal equivalent).

MRI Characteristics

- Hypointense (darker) on T1W TSE compared with surrounding marrow
- More importantly, hyperintense (brighter) or at least isointense to skeletal muscle on T1W FSE
- Lower signal on T2W FSE than surrounding marrow
- Variable signal on STIR
- "Bull's eye" sign; central fatty focus usually within an area of focal red marrow (not diagnostic)

143

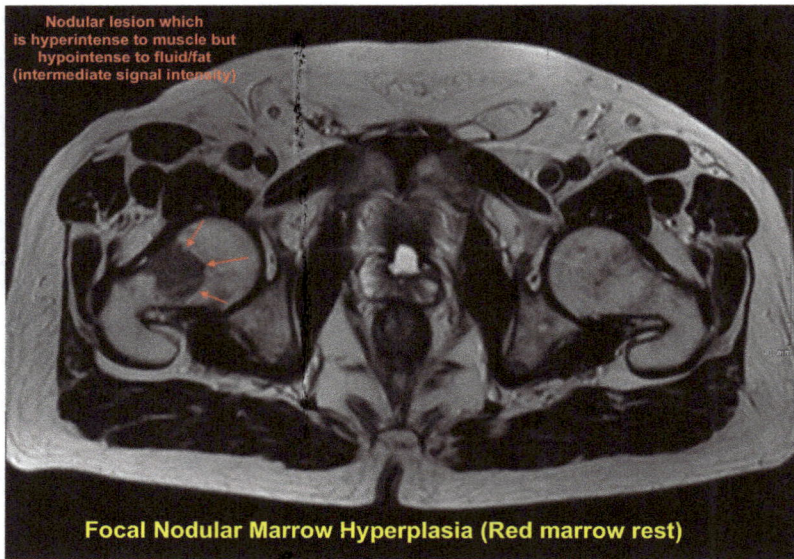

Figure 2.8.5 MRI appearances of a focal nodular marrow hyperplasia (red marrow rest). It can mimic solitary metastatic deposit.

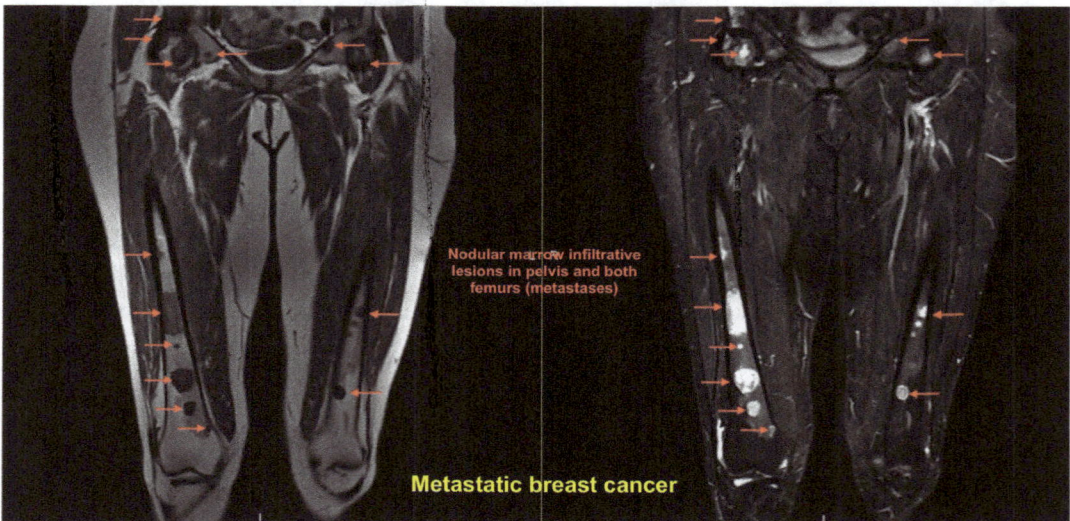

Figure 2.8.6 Multifocal metastatic disease in a known breast cancer patient.

Differential Diagnoses

FNMH can mimic bone metastases, leading to potentially unnecessary follow-up and even bone biopsy.

- Osteoblastic metastases are typically low signal on T1W and corresponding high signal on T2W/STIR images (Figure 2.8.6), and there may be a "halo sign," exhibiting a high T2W/STIR SI rim of oedema around a low signal lesion.

- In atypical haemangioma, a "polka dot" pattern is observed on CT and axial T2W FSE images secondary to thickened trabecula.

- Benign notochordal cell tumours: Mild medullary sclerosis on CT, always markedly hyperintense on T2W FSE sequences, with MRI SI characteristics comparable to the nucleus pulposus. Occur in the sacrum and coccyx, spine, and clivus.

As a rule of thumb, a SI drop of >20% on DIXON imaging using a 1.5T MRI scanner is a reliable cut-off value, indicating the presence of microscopic intralesional fat, and therefore excluding marrow infiltration or replacement.

Anaemia

Anaemia is the most common blood disorder and is a result of inadequate or defective red blood cell production, increased red blood cell breakdown, blood loss, or chronic disease, and can be hereditary or acquired.

- When red marrow replaces yellow marrow in the reverse pattern to that seen in the normal red-to-yellow marrow conversion, this is termed reconversion.

- Bone marrow reconversion occurs secondary to increased haematopoietic demand and can be physiological due to obesity or smoking, can occur in high-endurance athletes, and occurs following treatment with granulocyte colony-stimulating factor.

- Alternatively, reconversion can be pathological, such as in severe chronic anaemias, diabetes, and chronic respiratory disease.

Areas of marrow reconversion will retain the same signal characteristics as red marrow.

- Hypointense to normal marrow fat on T1W
- Mildly hyperintense to skeletal muscle, allowing differentiation from marrow infiltration

HAEMOGLOBINOPATHIES

Haemoglobinopathies are inherited disorders secondary to defective haemoglobin synthesis which produce severe anaemia, compensatory red marrow reconversion, and extramedullary haematopoiesis. The most common haemaglobinopathies are thalassaemia and sickle cell disease (SCD).

Thalassaemia

Thalassaemia is an inherited autosomal recessive disorder of haemoglobin synthesis.

- The genetic defect reduces globin chain synthesis, causing formation of abnormal haemoglobin molecules.

- Alpha-thalassaemia most commonly arises in West African populations and their descendants, whereas beta-thalassaemia is most prevalent in people living in or descended from Mediterranean countries, with 15% of the population carrying the beta-thalassaemia gene.

- Resultant abnormal haemoglobin molecules secondary to the defective synthesis of alpha- or beta-globin chains results in microcytic hypochromic anaemia, hepatosplenomegaly, medullary marrow expansion, and EMH.

- Medullary marrow expansion is a result of reduced bone density, cortical resorption, initial medullary trabecular thinning with subsequent trabecular coarsening (which can be seen as "cob-webbing" on pelvic radiographs).

- Imaging features of medullary marrow expansion in the spine are initially seen as increased vertebral body height, later progressing to multiple vertebral compression fractures.

- In the skull, medullary marrow expansion widens the diploic spaces, affecting the frontal region first and sparing the occiput. A "hair-on-end" appearance may be seen radiographically. On MRI, diffuse low marrow signal is observed on all pulse sequences.

- EMH masses are usually found in the paraspinal location, with MRI signal comparable with that of haematopoietically active red marrow (Figure 2.8.8). Inactive EMH masses may return a fat SI. Mild contrast enhancement can be seen in EMH masses containing haematopoietically active red marrow.

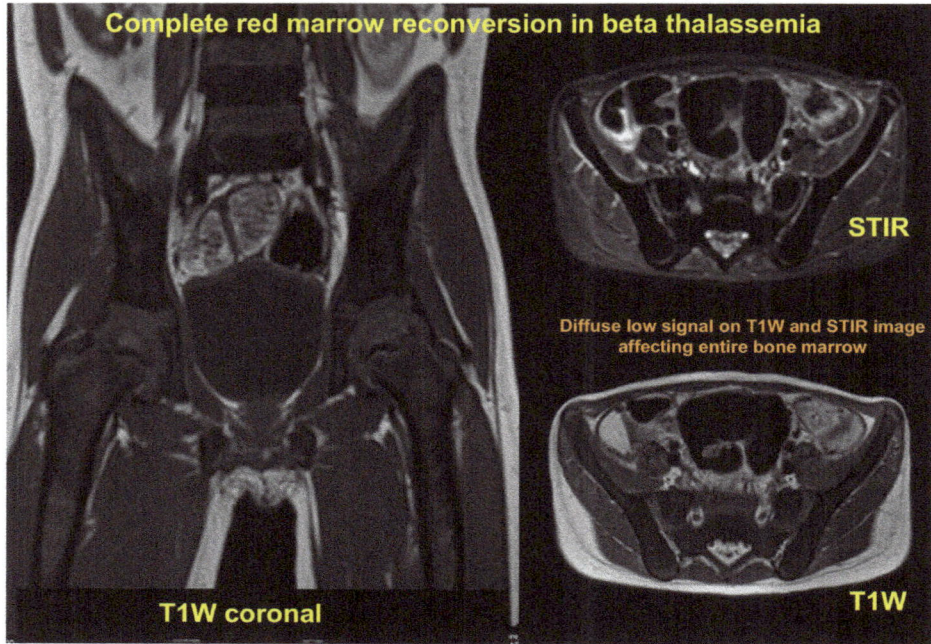

Figure 2.8.7 Diffuse marrow changes in a patient with beta-thalassemia.

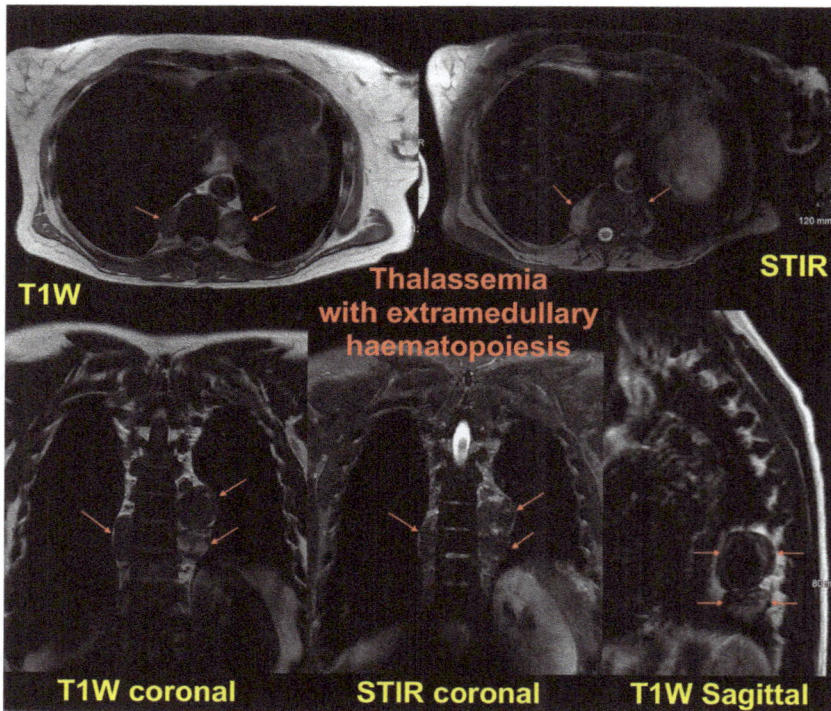

Figure 2.8.8 Patient with thalassemia-related diffuse red marrow proliferation and extramedullary haematopoiesis.

Paraspinal EMH masses are typically seen in the following locations:

- Anterior paraspinal soft tissues

- Posterior ribs (differentials for this location include neurogenic lesions which enhance much more avidly when compared with EMH masses)

- Mediastinum (differentials for this location include lymphoma and Castleman's disease)

- Pre-sacral space (patients are usually asymptomatic and the abnormality is seen as irregular soft tissue thickening. Differentials for a mass in this location include chordoma, lymphoma, extra-adrenal myelo-lipoma, radiation change, and sarcoma)

Marrow signal and osseous changes are secondary to:

- The disease itself

- Result of multiple transfusions

- Iron chelation treatment

Hyper-transfusion treatment aims to keep haemoglobin levels at or above 10 mg/dL and reduce the extent of marrow expansion.

- The resulting iron overload from repeated blood transfusions causes raised serum ferritin and iron deposition in the central and peripheral skeleton, seen as areas of very low signal marrow as well as susceptibility artefact on MRI, with a signal lower than skeletal muscle on all pulse sequences.

- Iron chelation removes the excess iron resulting from multiple transfusions.

- Iron deposition can affect the synovium and articular cartilage, resulting in loss of joint space, subchondral flattening, sclerosis and cyst formation, as well as osteophyte formation and chondrocalcinosis.

REPORTING PEARLS

- In untreated (un-transfused) thalassaemic patients, predominantly red marrow is present in the vertebral bodies, pelvis, and femora.

- In hyper-transfused but un-chelated patients, iron deposition is seen in the same distribution as red marrow.

- In hyper-transfused and chelated patients, iron deposition is typically seen in the spine and pelvis as well as foci of red marrow in the femora on a background of predominantly yellow marrow. As red marrow recedes with age, so does the iron deposition.

Sickle Cell Disease

SCD is an autosomal recessive haemolytic anaemia owing to a point mutation in the beta-globin chain that replaces glutamic acid with valine, resulting in an abnormally shaped haemoglobin molecule termed sickle cell haemoglobin (HbS).

- The highest incidence of SCD is in individuals of African descent but can also be found in those of Middle Eastern and Eastern Mediterranean origin.

- SCD results in a delay or absence of normal age-related red-to-yellow marrow conversion. Marrow hyperplasia can occur secondary to anaemia and results in medullary cavity expansion, cortical thinning and trabecular coarsening.

- MRI demonstrates diffuse intermediate signal on T1W TSE sequences.

- Persisting red marrow is typically found in the ankles, wrists, long bones, and axial skeleton.

- Vaso-occlusion predisposes to bone infarction and osteomyelitis.

- In infants and young children, bone infarcts often occur in the diaphyses of the tubular bones of the hands and feet.

- In adolescents and adults, bone infarction more commonly involves the metaphyses and epiphyses of long bones.

- On MRI, acute bone infarcts manifest as medullary oedema on T2W FSE and STIR sequences, periostitis, focal lytic lesions, adjacent soft tissue inflammation, and often growth arrest of the affected bone.

- Imaging features are difficult to differentiate from osteomyelitis. Infarcts heal with medullary sclerosis and myelofibrosis, resulting in a low signal on all MRI sequence and increased density on radiographs.

Acute osteomyelitis has a delayed presentation on radiographs, causing a lamellated periosteal response, with bone destruction and formation of a sequestrum and involucrum.

- MRI is more sensitive to early osteomyelitis and demonstrates ill-defined marrow oedema, periostitis, and soft tissue oedema.

- Geographic regions of marrow enhancement are typical of osteomyelitis on post-contrast MRI, while serpiginous peripheral enhancement is seen in acute bone infarction.

- Osteopenia occurs in SCD and predisposes to fractures, with spinal involvement typically resulting in "H-shaped vertebrae" (Figure 2.8.9).

Avascular necrosis (AVN) is common in SCD (Figures 2.8.10 through 2.8.12) and is secondary to vasocclusion caused by sickling red blood cells in the marrow that lead to blood stasis and cell sequestration and result in ischaemia and tissue hypoxia.

- Bone infarcts are observed in the medullary cavity and epiphysis (Figure 2.8.10), with the latter being in the subchondral location.

- Typically, the humeral and femoral heads are involved and eventual collapse of the normal spherical contour. More frequently, there is bilateral involvement, typically more extensive than AVN of other aetiologies.

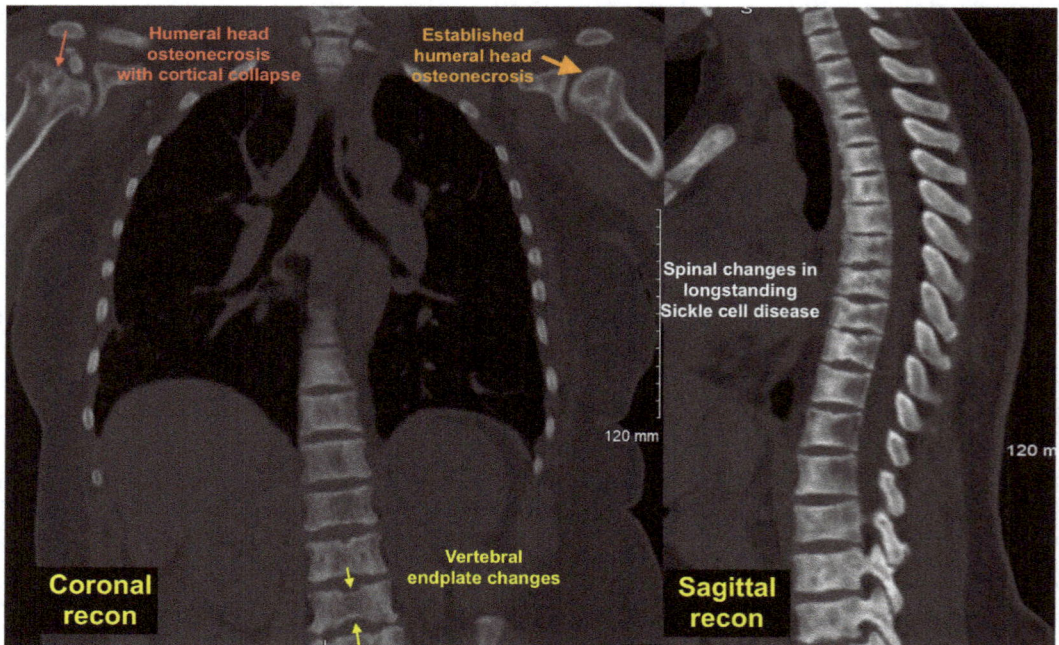

Figure 2.8.9 Humeral head osteonecrosis and H-shaped vertebral appearances following endplate infarcts in sickle cell disease.

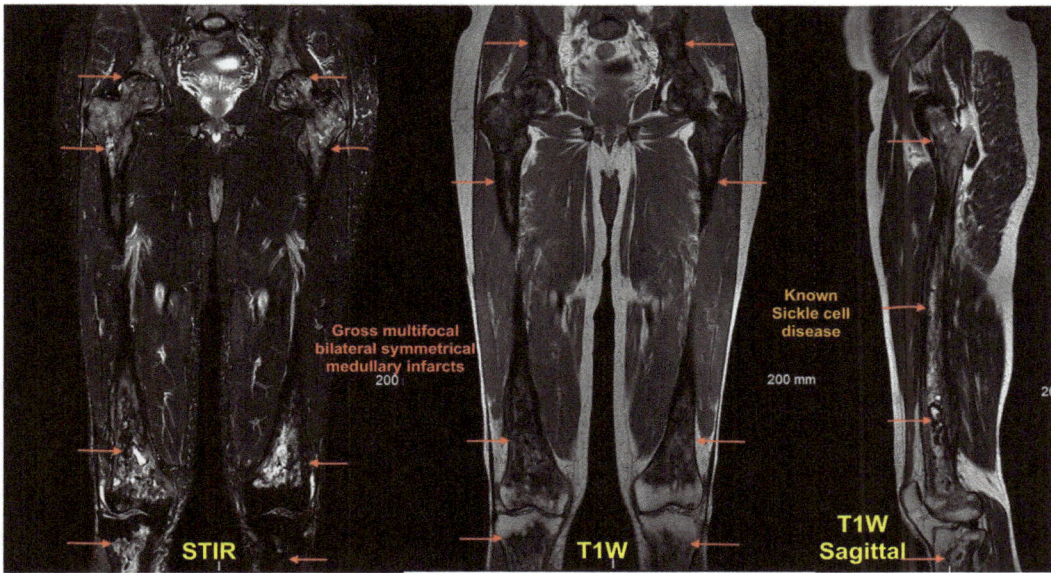

Figure 2.8.10 Diffuse medullary and subchondral infarcts in both lower limbs in a patient with sickle cell disease.

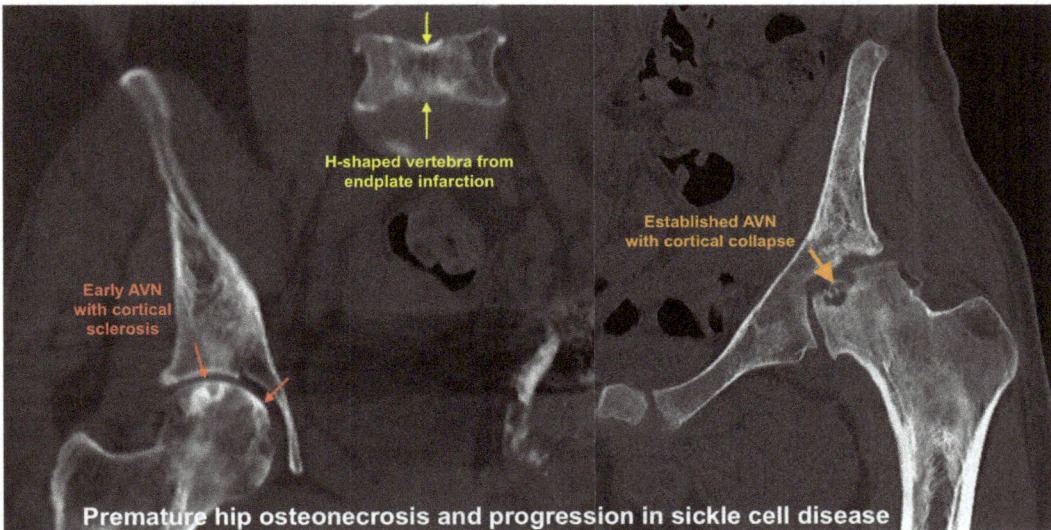

Figure 2.8.11 Osteonecrosis in vertebral endplates and both femoral heads: Right: early; Left: established.

- MRI is the investigation of choice. Infarction exhibits an area of bone marrow oedema with increased T2W signal in the acute phase and a fibrotic/sclerotic pattern observed as low signal on all pulse sequences in the chronic phase.

- With the passage of time, a low T1W signal serpiginous rim develops. "Double line sign" is observed on T2W images as a low signal peripheral border and a high signal inner border.

- Medullary AVN is far more common than acute osteomyelitis.

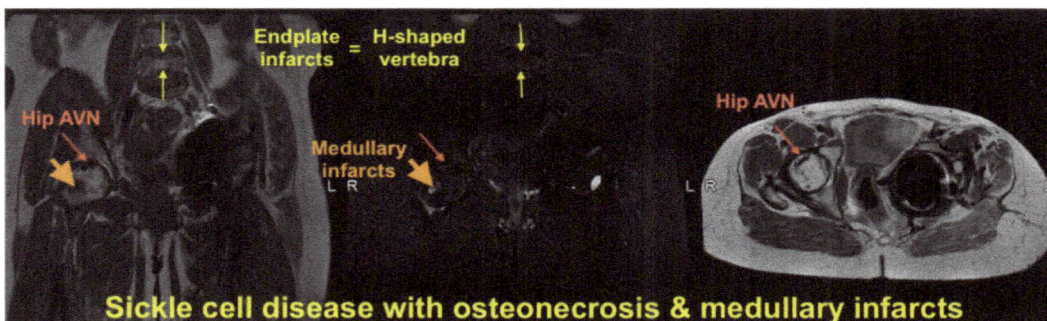

Figure 2.8.12 Sickle cell disease-related infarcts in different stages. See premature osteoarthritis in the left hip leading to early hip replacement.

MYELODYSPLASTIC SYNDROMES

Myelodysplastic syndromes (MDS) are a group of stem cell disorders in which abnormal or ineffective production of red blood cells, platelets, and white blood cells results in a variety of symptoms including chronic anaemia, bruising, bleeding, and frequent infections.

- MDS can be idiopathic, or it can follow previous chemotherapy, radiotherapy, or heavy metal or toxin exposure.

- On MRI, MDS demonstrates red marrow reconversion with a nodular, patchy, or diffusely decreased signal on T1W TSE sequences due to increased bone marrow cellularity, increased SI on T2W FSE, and a variably increased SI on STIR sequences.

- Repeated blood transfusions to treat the anaemia can result in iron overload and require iron chelators, with similar secondary MRI appearances to those occurring in hyper-transfused and chelated thalassaemic patients.

Aplastic Anaemia

Aplastic anaemia is a T-lymphocyte-mediated immune imbalance, which targets the haematopoietic system.

- Hypocellular or acellular bone marrow results in a pancytopenia affecting all cell lines. Aplastic anaemia is idiopathic in 50% of cases but can also be related to viral infections, hepatitis, and exposure to toxins and some drugs.

- Fatty marrow replacement results in a generalised increased marrow signal on T1W TSE sequences, and a low signal on STIR.

- MRI may be beneficial in guiding a bone marrow biopsy and prove useful in monitoring treatment response.

Systemic Mastocytosis

Systemic mastocytosis (SM) is a multi-organ system haematological condition with marrow involvement occurring in virtually all patients. Symptoms are secondary to the effects of mast cell derived mediators.

- SM is categorised into indolent, smouldering, and advanced subtype. Increased incidence of osteoporosis—more commonly seen in men—leads to an increased risk of vertebral compression fractures, which are mostly seen in the indolent subtype.

- Differential diagnoses include osteoblastic metastases and osteopoikilosis.

Variable MRI patterns are usually seen with smouldering and advanced subtypes:

- Normal appearance

- Activated marrow pattern—diffuse reduction of T1W signal and diffuse high signal on STIR

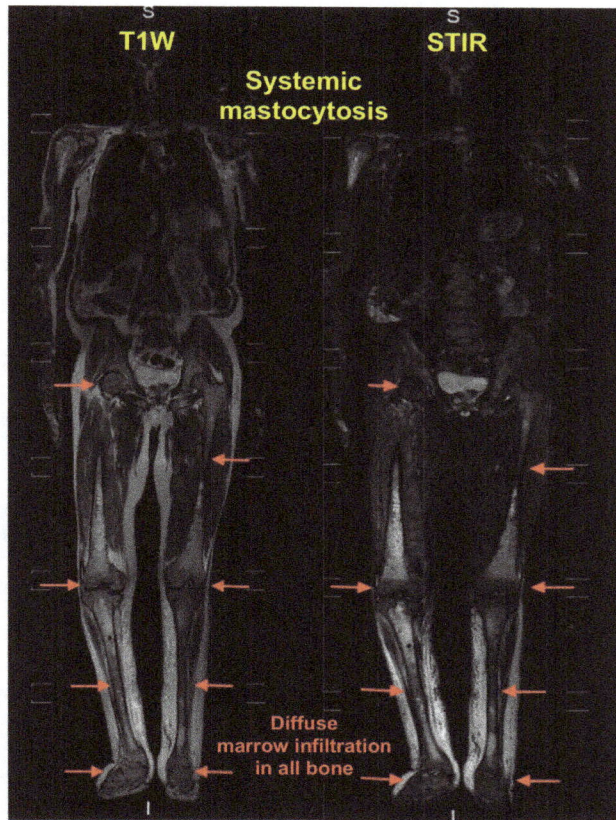

Figure 2.8.13 Marrow appearance of systemic mastocytosis.

■ Diffuse sclerotic marrow pattern commonly affects the axial skeleton, with reduction of both T1W and STIR signal (Figure 2.8.13)

■ Small-spotted sclerotic marrow pattern may be seen with tiny focal areas of reduced signal on T1W and STIR sequences, corresponding to osteoblastic foci demonstrated on radiography and CT

■ Osteolytic lesions may be seen and are sharply demarcated, low signal on T1W and high signal on STIR. Disease severity may be lower with this pattern of marrow involvement

Serous Atrophy of Bone Marrow (SABM)

SABM, also known as gelatinous bone marrow transformation, is a potentially reversible condition characterised by atrophy of fat cells within the marrow, loss of haematopoietic cells, and deposition of gelatinous substances including mucopolysaccharides within the marrow space.

■ Associated with cachexia, anorexia nervosa, anaemia, heart failure, hypoalbuninaemia, electrolyte imbalance, alcohol toxicity, and malignancy.

■ Typically seen in patients under age 30.

■ Increased risk of lower limb fractures.

■ MRI signal characteristics demonstrate reduced signal of the bone marrow and subcutaneous fat on T1W TSE sequence, giving an appearance similar to that of a fat suppressed sequence.

■ Increased marrow signal occurring on fluid-sensitive sequences gives the appearance of "failed fat suppression" due to the depletion of medullary fat.

151

- These MRI appearances are termed the "flip-flop" effect and are due to relative increase in water-to-fat content in the marrow cavity. Marrow changes may be focal or diffuse and can reduce the sensitivity of MRI in diagnosing occult fractures.

Lymphoma

Primary bone lymphoma (PBL) is one of the rarest intraosseous neoplasms of malignant lymphoid cells, typically without nodal or extra nodal involvement.

- PBL makes up ~3% of all malignant primary bone tumours and 1% of all lymphomas.

- Patients present between the 2nd–8th decades of life, with an average age of 50 years

- A biphasic age distribution maybe seen with an earlier peak at ~ age 20.

- PBL lesions may be lytic (~70% of cases), blastic (~28%), or mixed (~2%).

- Multifocal lesions have a worse prognosis than single sites of disease.

- MRI is the modality of choice and PBL presents as an extensive poorly defined lesion frequently in a long bone metadiaphysis with a large extra-osseous soft tissue component.

- PBL is rarely seen confined to the periosteum or cortex.

- Synovitis can occur at an adjacent joint, usually the knee, and bone lesions can cross joints to involve opposing bones.

- Lesions usually exhibit a low signal T1W and demonstrate variable signal on T2W (Figure 2.8.14), sometimes resulting in a "mosaic" pattern.

- Lesions show post-gadolinium enhancement in non-necrotic region.

- Lack of bone destruction and the presence of regional lymphadenopathy are characteristic, although pathological fractures occur in up to 25% of cases.

- Marrow signal abnormality can persist for years despite successful treatment.

- Differentials include secondary bone lymphoma, (SBL) which is lymphoma originating in an extraosseous site extending to bone or evidence of systemic disease.

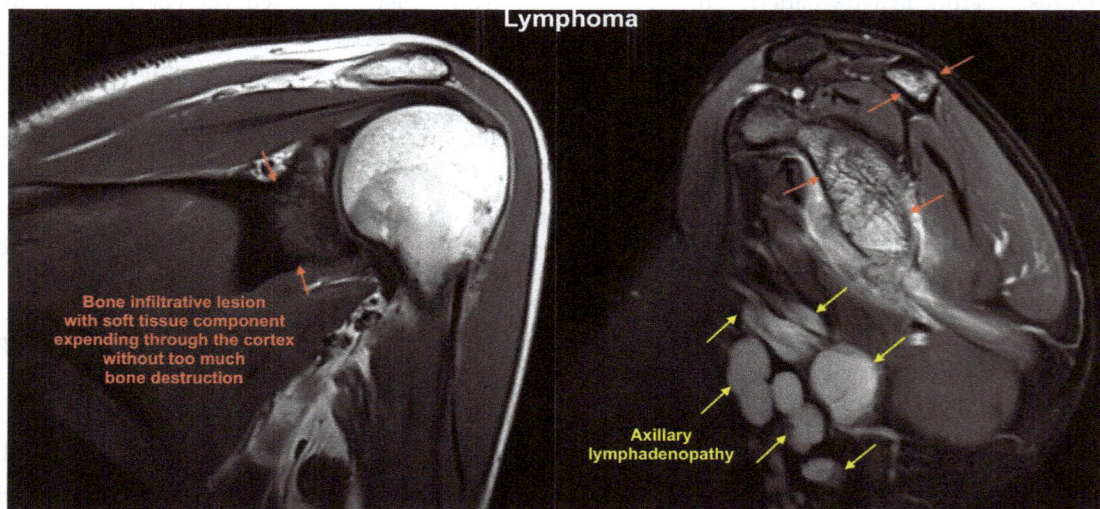

Figure 2.8.14 MRI features of lymphoma.

Leukaemia

Leukaemia, another haematological malignancy, demonstrates similar diffuse low T1W signal hypointense or isointense relative to intervertebral discs and skeletal muscle (comparable to lymphoma), increased T2W signal and diffuse enhancement of the abnormal marrow following intravenous contrast, *without* the typical extra-osseous soft tissue component seen in lymphoma (Figure 2.8.15).

- Acute leukaemia is the most common malignancy of childhood, whereas chronic leukaemia predominates adult patients.

- Radiographs may be normal, but osteopenia is a frequent finding.

- Radiographs demonstrate lucent metaphyseal bands, which are 2–15 mm wide, typically seen at sites of rapid growth, such as the proximal humerus, distal radius, proximal and distal femur, and proximal tibia.

- Periosteal response can be seen in 2–50% of patients, commonly involving the tibial and fibular diaphysis, which is typically thin or lamellated, although aggressive appearances may be seen.

- Pathological fractures maybe the first sign of an underlying disease process, with ~ 6–12% reported at initial presentation with ALL (Figure 2.8.15). CT is useful in demonstrating the degree of cortical destruction and the extent of endosteal scalloping, if present.

- MRI is also useful in the assessment of fractures.

- Benign fractures exhibit low T1W signal owing to bone marrow oedema and haemorrhage with foci of normal intervening fatty marrow.

- On the other hand, the abnormal T1W SI in pathological fractures is secondary to tumour infiltration, resulting in a more uniform low signal, with no intervening normal fatty marrow and well-defined convex margins.

Multiple Myeloma (MM)

MM is the most common primary bone malignancy, accounting for ~1% of all malignant disease and ~ 10% of all haematological malignancies. Production of an abnormal paraprotein leads to a wide m-band on

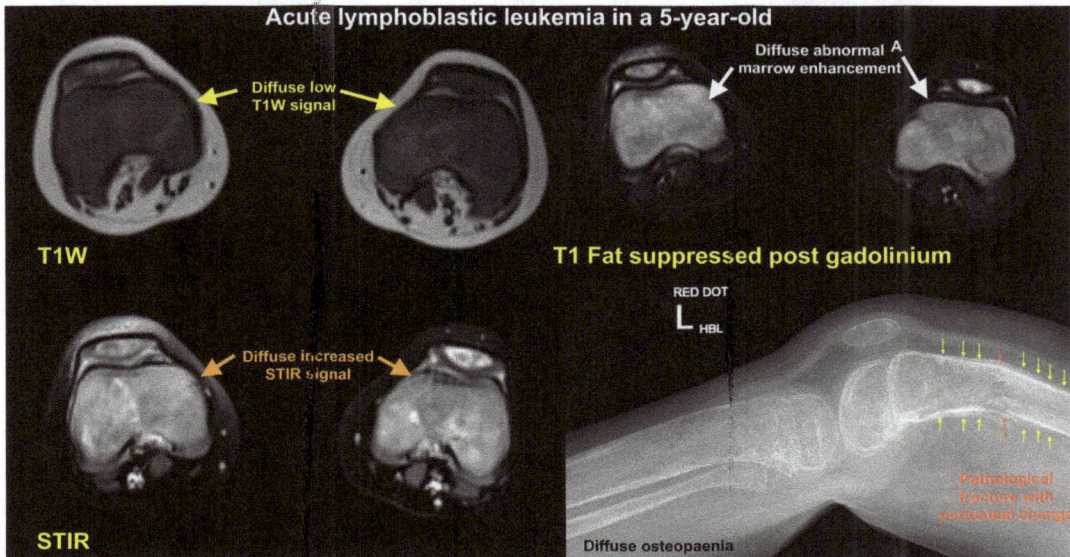

Figure 2.8.15 X-ray showing diffuse osteopaenia and a pathological fracture as well as diffuse marrow replacement with post-gadolinium enhancement in a child with acute lymphoblastic leukemia.

plasma electrophoresis, with a raised ESR and the production of light-chain immunoglobulins resulting in in Bence Jones proteinuria in over half the cases, contributing to diagnostic confidence.

■ 2:1 male predilection, with 75% of patients over the age of 50 (median age 65).

■ Up to 80% of MM patients develop skeletal involvement: the axial skeleton and proximal ends of the long bones being typically favoured. The combination of a good clinical history, MRI imaging features and specific laboratory results are prudent in diagnosis of MM.

■ At presentation, a normal marrow pattern on MRI may be seen in 50–75% of cases.

■ However, MM presents with a number of distinct bone marrow patterns (Figures 2.8.16 and 2.8.17):

• A focal pattern consists of localised areas of decreased T1W signal and corresponding increased FS T2W/STIR signal, which may easily be mistaken for metastatic disease. Occasionally, the lesions can be high signal on T1W proving difficult detection, and in such instances the lesion may only be conspicuous on T2W sequences.

• Diffuse pattern exhibits a globally reduced T1W signal, high signal on T2W-fat-suppressed and STIR images, as well diffuse enhancement following intravenous contrast. Haematopoietic marrow hyperplasia (non-malignant marrow abnormality) can mimic the diffuse pattern.

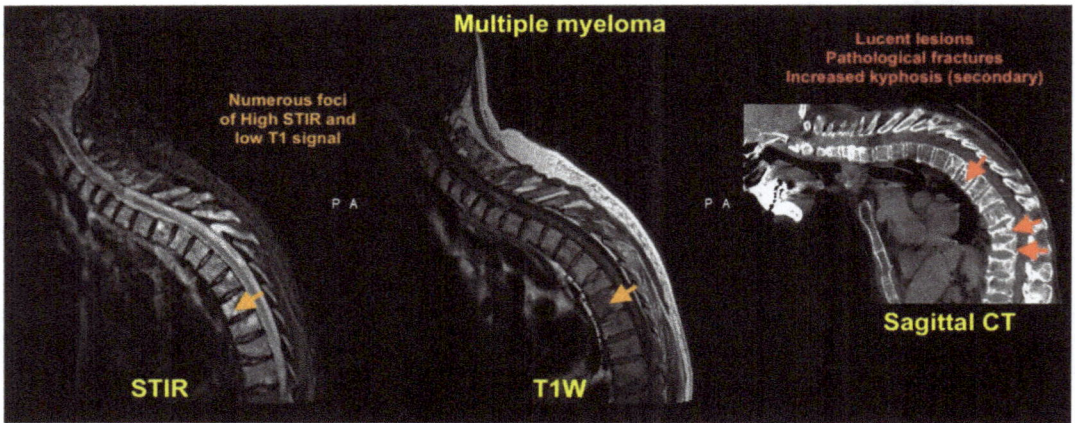

Figure 2.8.16 MRI features of multiple myeloma.

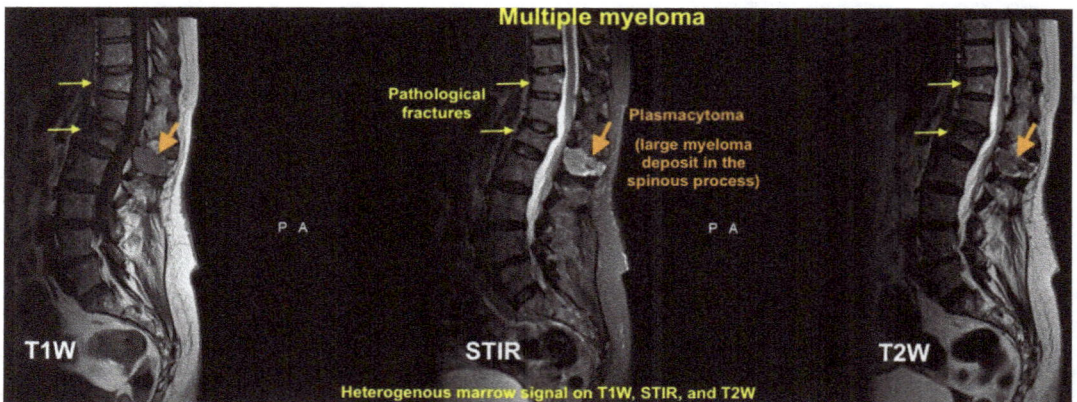

Figure 2.8.17 Multiple myeloma with spinous process plasmacytoma.

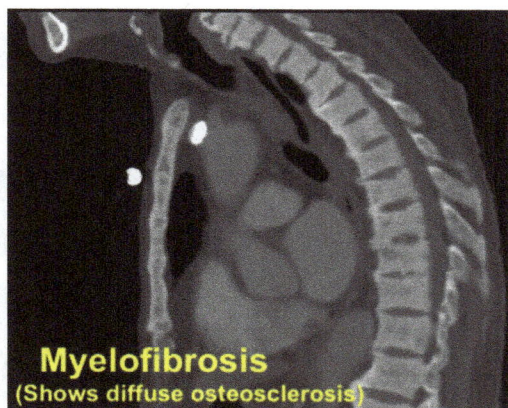

Figure 2.8.18 CT features of myelofibrosis.

- Focal and diffuse patterns manifest as a focal T1 low signal lesion (better demarcated on fat suppressed sequences) on a background of diffusely low signal marrow

- Variegated pattern consists of multiple tiny foci of low signal on T1W and corresponding high signal on T2W/STIR, a pattern invariably seen with early stage. Heterogeneous marrow secondary to advancing age may mimic the variegated pattern

Whole-body diffusion-weighted MRI is the gold standard modality in patients with asymptomatic myeloma and plasmacytoma (solitary myeloma).

Myelofibrosis

■ The bone marrow replaced with collagenous connective tissue causing progressive fibrosis.

■ The musculoskeletal manifestation of myelofibrosis is osteosclerosis (Figure 2.8.18), and this may exhibit a diffuse pattern or no bony architectural distortion.

■ Typical sites of disease include the axial skeleton, ribs, proximal humerus, and femur.

■ Radiologically one can see narrowing of the intramedullary cavity secondary to endosteal new bone formation.

■ Patchy lucencies may also be observed due to the presence of fibrous tissue.

■ Myelofibrosis can cause homogenously hypointense marrow signal (Figure 2.8.19).

■ A bone scan may produce a "superscan" appearance.

CONCLUSION

Within bone marrow, focal and diffuse abnormalities can mimic neoplastic disease, which may be identified on MRI. To avoid misdiagnosing normal marrow, changes due to physiological reconversion, and lesions associated with oedema-like marrow signal intensity as neoplastic pathology, radiologists should be cognisant of normal changes in the distribution of yellow and red marrow with age, the appearances of marrow reconversion and the commoner focal and multifocal non-neoplastic lesions that may be seen incidentally on MRI. Recognition of associated features such as EMH and post-treatment changes is necessary to avoid over-investigation of physiological and benign disease processes.

SUGGESTED READING

■ Saifuddin A, Tyler P, Hargunani R. *Musculoskeletal MRI*. CRC Press; 2016 Mar 23.

■ Helms CA, Major NM, Anderson MW, Kaplan P, Dussault R. *Musculoskeletal MRI e-Book*. Elsevier Health Sciences; 2008 Dec 9.

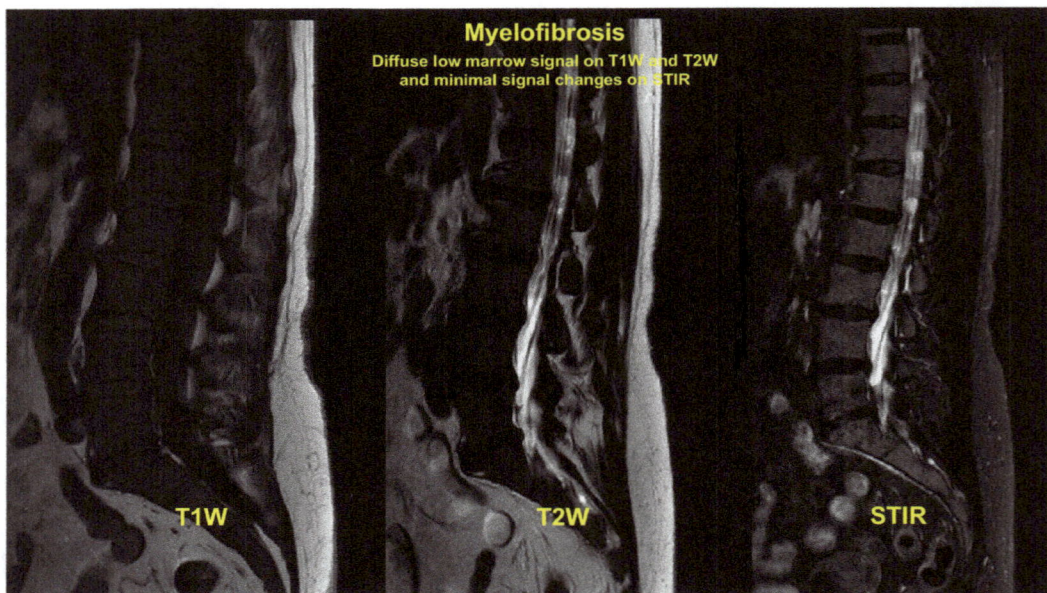

Figure 2.8.19 MRI features of myelofibrosis.

SBA QUESTIONS

1) Which of the following is NOT a presentation of myelomatous infiltrative disease?

   A. Monoclonal gammopathy of uncertain significance

   B. Multiple myeloma

   C. Plasmacytoma

   D. Smouldering myeloma

   E. Chloroma

2) A 10-year-old paediatric patient from an African immigrant family presented to A&E with swollen left calf and sepsis. X-rays of the left tibia and fibula revealed central lucency with surrounding sclerosis in the left tibia and adjacent solid periosteal reaction. MRI was performed to assess the area further. It revealed diffuse hypointense signal on T1W images through the entire tibia and fibula with a few serpiginous lines on T1W and STIR in the fibula as well as intramedullary collection on STIR with further diffuse intermediate signal on STIR in visualised bones. What is the most likely diagnosis?

   A. Alpha-thalassemia

   B. Beta-thalassemia

   C. Osteosarcoma

   D. Sickle cell disease

   E. Ewing sarcoma

3) What is the most specific organism responsible for such appearances?

   A. *Staphylococcus aureus*

   B. *Salmonella* species

   C. *Streptococcus pneumoniae*

   D. *Campylobactor jejuni*

   E. *Escherichia coli*

4) What is the most common organism responsible for such appearances?

   A. *Staphylococcus aureus*

   B. *Salmonella* species

   C. *Streptococcus pneumoniae*

   D. *Campylobactor jejuni*

   E. *Escherichia coli*

Answers: (1) E, (2) D, (3) B, (4) A

Chapter 2.9
Multisystemic Diseases with Musculoskeletal Manifestations

Siddharth Thaker, Anand Kirwadi, and Harun Gupta

LEARNING OBJECTIVES

■ To understand characteristic imaging features of a few selected multisystemic diseases

■ To learn the multifocal nature of the disease and highlight a few red flags which require further management promptly

■ To learn the different associations with multisystemic diseases and required follow-up

INTRODUCTION

In this chapter, we will understand various multisystemic diseases which are completely unrelated to each other. However, all pathologies present with characteristic imaging features. The candidates must know classical appearances following pathologies to score better. Many multisystemic diseases are the outcome of specific genetic mutations (genetic mutations are divided into germline—which can be inherited—or somatic—individual specific). Such diseases require clinical and imaging follow-up and genetic and familial counselling according to a the nationally agreed genetic framework.

SARCOIDOSIS

■ Multisystemic inflammatory disorder with non-caseating granuloma forming in various organs. It usually involves lungs, skin, lymph nodes, eyes, and the musculoskeletal and central nervous systems.

■ Occurs in patients younger than their 40s.

■ African American and Caucasians > Asians.

■ Presenting symptoms include low-grade fever, easy fatiguability, unintentional weight loss, general health decline, and evidence of lymphadenopathy.

■ Musculoskeletal involvement is uncommon (up to 13%).

■ Imaging is used to diagnose musculoskeletal manifestation in known disease and isolated musculoskeletal sarcoidosis with lung or systemic changes.

■ Chest X-ray is paramount for assessing for bilateral hilar lymphadenopathy and parenchymal infiltrates.

■ Small bone involvement on X-ray is usually bilateral and asymmetrical, affecting the middle and proximal phalanges (Figure 2.9.1). This occurs following years of soft tissue involvement and is characterised by a "moth-eaten" appearance of the cortex due to granulomatous lesions, a lace or grid pattern due to destruction of the Haversian system, and compensatory trabecular thickening.

■ Long bone involvement on X-rays: Variable appearances from bony lysis to osteosclerosis; focal lesion may mimic tumour. Look for adjacent tenosynovitis.

■ Axial skeletal involvement on CT: Great mimicker, appearances involve a lytic lesion with trabecular thickening (like haemangioma), solitary sclerotic vertebra (like ivory vertebra), vertebral and paravertebral lesions with uninvolved disc (mimicking TB), and diffuse sclerosis (like metastases).

■ MRI: Lytic lesions appear low signal on T1W and high signal on STIR; sclerotic lesions appear low signal on all sequences; treated lesions may show fibrous or fatty matrix.

■ Joint sarcoidosis or Lofgren's syndrome (tetrad—fever, arthralgia, erythema nodosum, and hilar lymphadenopathy): Knees and ankles are most commonly involved. Acute sarcoid arthritis mimics rheumatoid or infective arthritis and chronic sarcoid arthropathy.

DOI: 10.1201/9781003500247-18

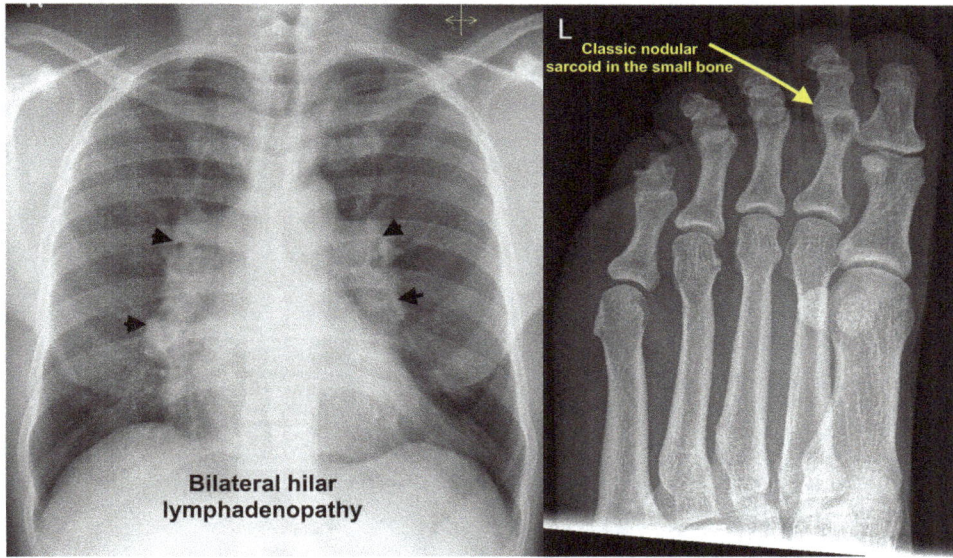

Figure 2.9.1 Classic hilar lymphadenopathy in pulmonary sarcoidosis with small bone involvement.

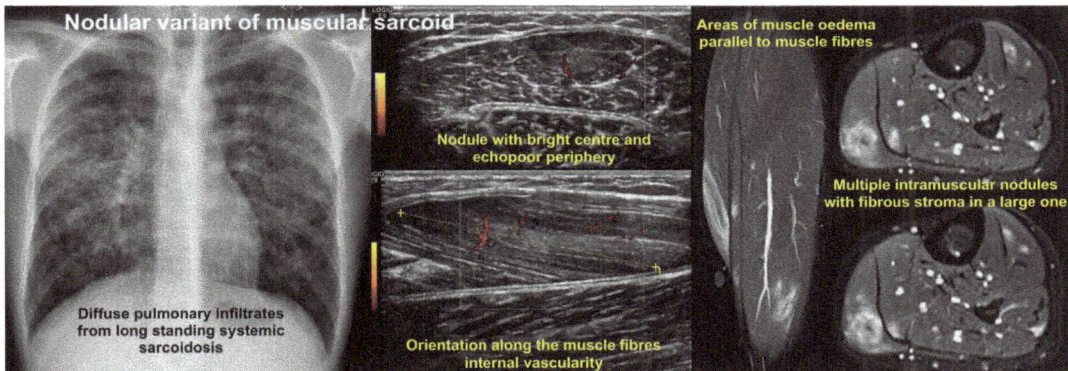

Figure 2.9.2 Pulmonary changes in long-standing sarcoidosis with ultrasound and MRI appearances of nodular variant of muscular sarcoid.

- Muscle sarcoidosis or acute sarcoid myositis mimics muscular dystrophies and inflammatory myopathies and shows diffuse muscle oedema on MRI (steroid-induced myopathy is a differential).

- Chronic sarcoid myopathy is common in postmenopausal women; MRI shows normal or bilateral muscle atrophy and fatty infiltration.

- In nodular sarcoid myopathy, US shows echogenic centre and echopoor periphery compared with muscle; star appearance, internal vascularity on Doppler imaging, sometimes mimic sarcoma and requires biopsy. MRI is the most sensitive; fusiform nodules along the muscle fibres and myotendinous junction show differential signal intensity and contrast enhancement depending upon the age (Figure 2.9.2).

- Cutaneous sarcoid: Erythema nodosum, red and tender nodule at any subcutaneous bony prominence; mimics sarcoma, requires biopsy sometimes to prove.

- Sarcoid tenosynovitis: Preferential involvement of wrists, fingers, and ankles. US is the imaging technique of choice, extensor tendons > flexor tendons, associated with soft tissue nodules around.

HEREDITARY MULTIPLE EXOSTOSES

- Also known as diaphyseal aclasis: Autosomal dominant transmission.

- Characteristic findings: Multiple osteochondromas with secondary bony deformities, present as multiple, painless, hard lumps involving the long bones and around joints with secondary changes. Usually osteochondromas point AWAY from the adjacent joints. (Differential diagnosis: Trevor's disease, characterised by epiphyseal osteochondroma, pointing TOWARDS the joint causing its widening.)

- Genetic mutation: EXT gene.

- Diagnosis is usually in the first decade of life; lesions can be sessile or pedunculated, and bilateral is more common than unilateral.

- Calvarium is usually spared. The most common bones affected are the distal femur, proximal tibia, ankle, wrists and hands, humerus, ribs, and pelvis.

- X-rays (Figure 2.9.3) are the imaging technique of choice. Forearms show pseudo-Madelung deformity, or "bayonet hands," due to ulnar shortening and curve. Distal femurs show Erlenmeyer flask deformities

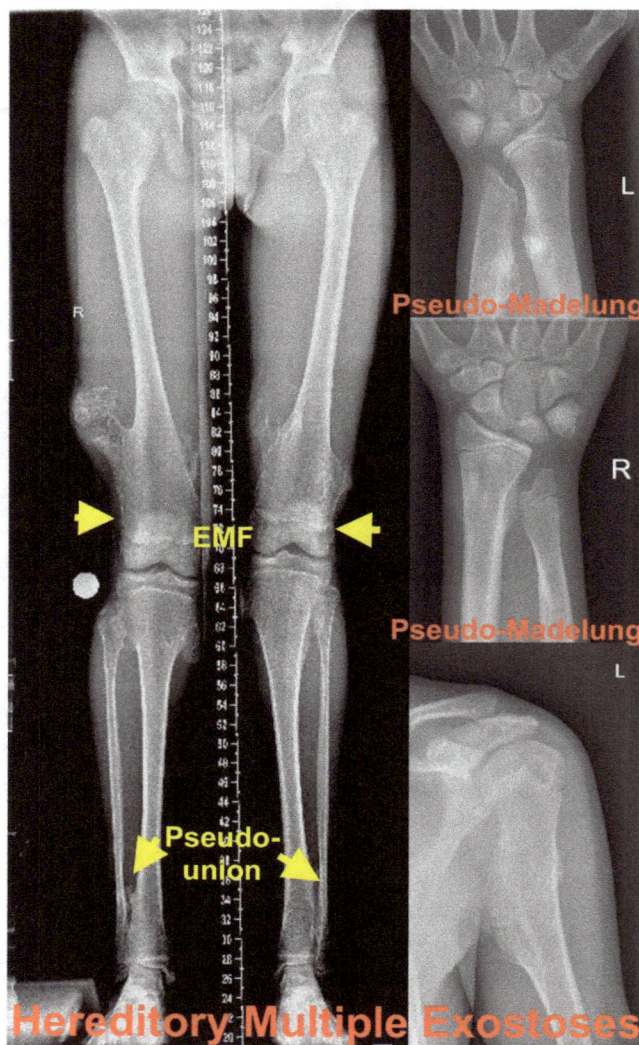

Figure 2.9.3 Pathognomonic features of hereditary multiple exostoses.

due to widening of the distal metadiaphysis. The proximal femur and hip show coxa valga due to vertical orientation of the femoral necks. Limb length shows discrepancies.

- Complications include bone deformities, fractures, vascular and neural impingement, pseudoaneurysm, secondary bursa formation, nerve entrapment (especially radial and peroneal), pseudo-unions, and most importantly malignant transformation of the cartilage cap.

- Malignant transformation of the cartilage cap usually manifests as chondrosarcoma, with cartilage cap thickness > 2 cm on an MRI. A large soft tissue mass with untraceable rarefied cortex in previous traceable bony contours of the lesion in an adult is highly suggestive of malignancy and requires bone tumour centre referral as a 2-week wait.

Ollier's Disease and Maffucci Syndrome

- Most common enchondromatosis subtypes.

- Associated with IDH1 and IDH2 mutations.

- Ollier's disease: Multiple enchondroma especially in the long bones and small bones of hands and feet.

- Maffucci syndrome: Multiple enchondroma + soft tissue haemangioma.

- Both diagnosed in the first decade of life.

- Malignancy risk: Maffucci syndrome is rarer than Ollier's disease. Chondrosarcoma from bony lesions and angiosarcoma from soft tissue lesions. Also susceptible to extraskeletal malignancies like gliomas, mesenchymal ovarian tumours, and intraabdominal solid organ tumours.

- Enchondromas on X-rays: Stippled or punctate cartilage matrix within elongated radiolucent lesions with a thin rim of radiodense bone, cause expansile remodelling, thinning of cortices, and endosteal scalloping (Figure 2.9.4). Maffucci syndrome additionally presents multiple small round soft tissue calcifications due to phleboliths (Figure 2.9.5).

- Cortical destruction, bone expansion, permeative bone destruction, and aggressive periosteal reaction, especially in skeletally mature patient suggest malignant transformation into chondrosarcoma.

- CT detects matrix mineralisation, lesion margins, endosteal scalloping, associated soft tissue mass in chondrosarcoma; also used for surgical planning.

- On MRI, there are lobular areas of low to intermediate signal on T1W with corresponding increased signal on fluid-sensitive images. Mass forming areas outside the bone and associated pathological fractures are concerning features (Figure 2.9.6).

- PET-CT is used to assess malignant transformation.

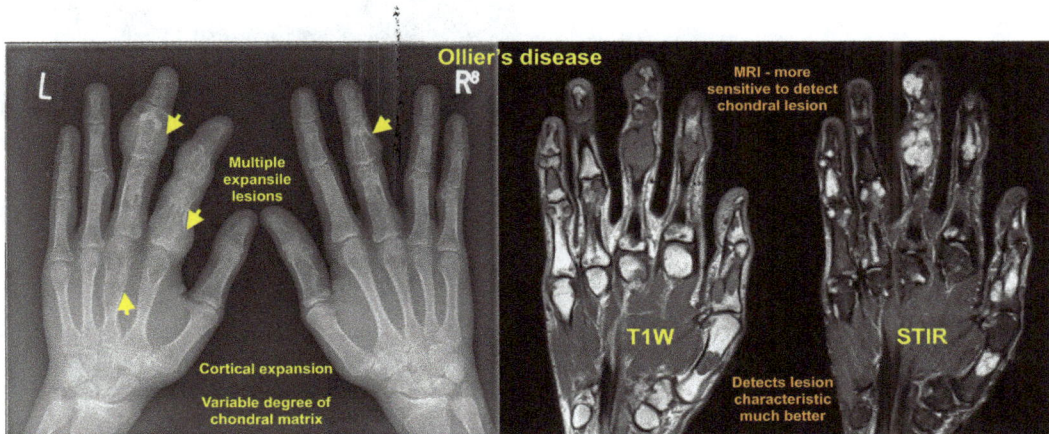

Figure 2.9.4 Classic radiographic and MRI appearances of Ollier's disease.

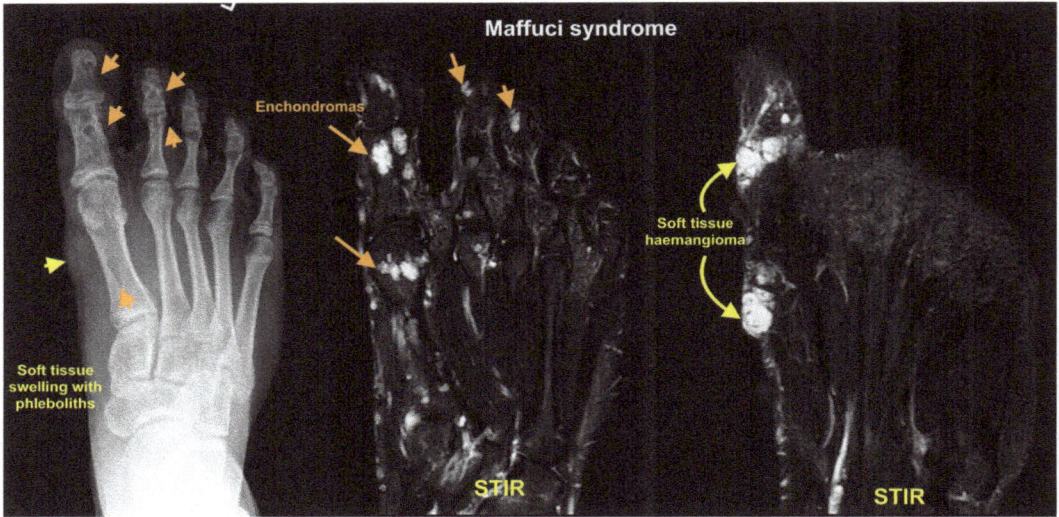

Figure 2.9.5 Classic imaging appearances of Maffucci syndrome (enchondroma + soft tissue haemangioma on MRI). (Image courtesy of Dr Ganesh Hegde, RNOH, Stanmore, UK.)

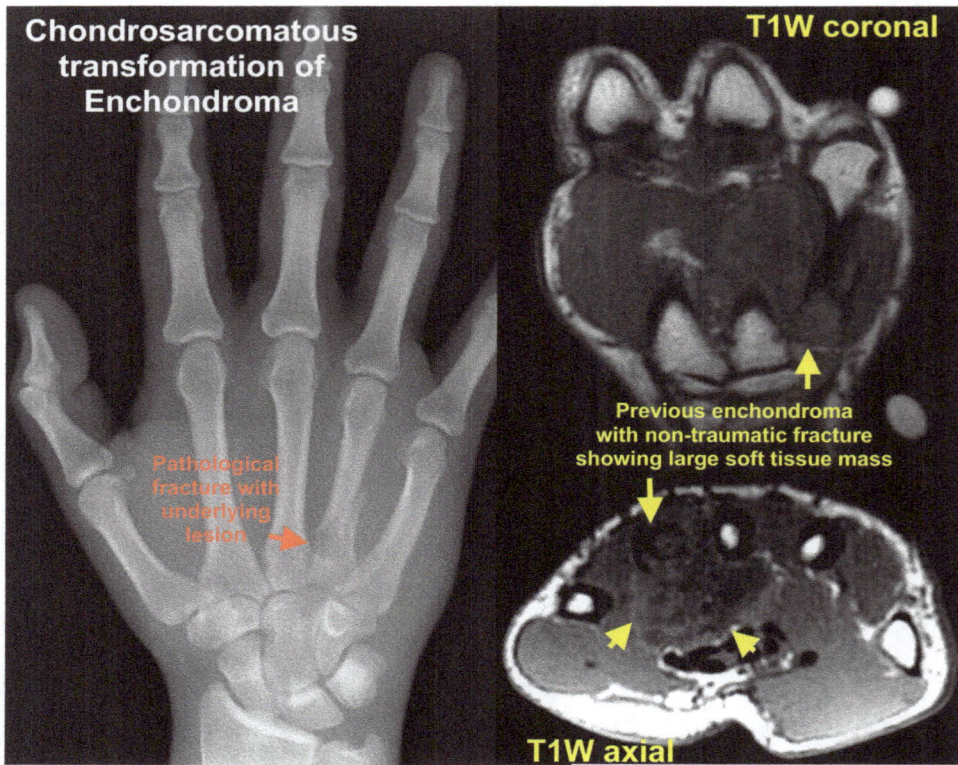

Figure 2.9.6 Chondrosarcomatous transformation of a digital enchondroma with pathological fracture and soft tissue mass.

McCune–Albright Syndrome

- Triad: Polyostotic fibrous dysplasia (FD), cutaneous pigmentation (known as café au lait spots), and hyperfunctioning endocrinopathy (hyperthyroidism, Cushing syndrome, precocious puberty, and diabetes).

- Associated with sporadic GNAS gene mutation.

- Polyostotic FD involves femur, tibia, pelvis, ribs, craniofascial bones, and spine.

- X-ray appearance: Intramedullary expansile lesion with ground glass matrix and no periosteal reaction classical of fibrous dysplasia; variety of lesion matrices including ground glass, sclerotic, and mixed, shows "rind sign" and fusiform rib enlargement.

- CT demonstrates features of FD in more detail than X-rays; better assesses craniofascial FDs and detects neural compromise; also assesses bone deformities and fractures (Figure 2.9.7).

- MRI: Not particularly useful apart from craniofascial lesions; FDs show low to intermediate T1W signal corresponding to high STIR signal and avid contrast enhancement.

- Benign transformation: Myxoid or aneurysmal bone cyst-like changes on MRI.

- Malignant transformation: Soft tissue mass, cortical destruction, aggressive periosteal reaction, pathological fracture.

- Intraductal papillary mucinous neoplasm and breast fibroadenoma are also associated.

Mazabraud Syndrome

- Syndromic association of fibrous dysplasia and intramuscular myxoma (strong link with GNAS1 mutation).

- Intramuscular myxomas can be multiple and are usually located in vicinity to fibrous dysplasia of the bone.

- Imaging features (Figure 2.9.8) are classical of intramuscular myxoma (see Chapter 2.6) and fibrous dysplasia, as mentioned earlier.

- Pelvis and lower limb (thighs) are more commonly involved.

- Fibrous dysplasia precedes for years before development of myxoma.

- Treatment depends upon symptoms caused by bone and soft tissue lesion.

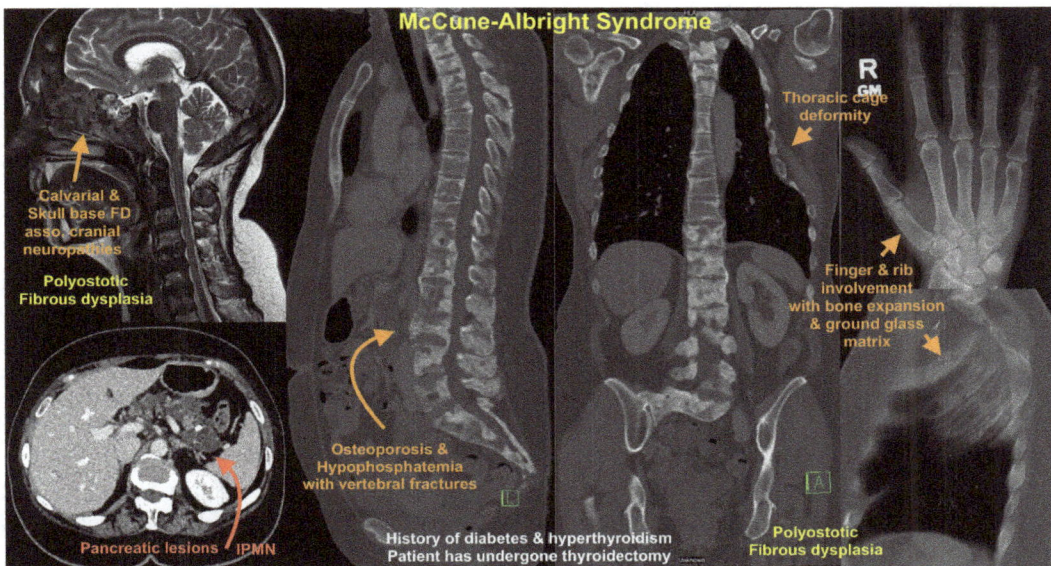

Figure 2.9.7 Imaging features in McCune–Albright syndrome.

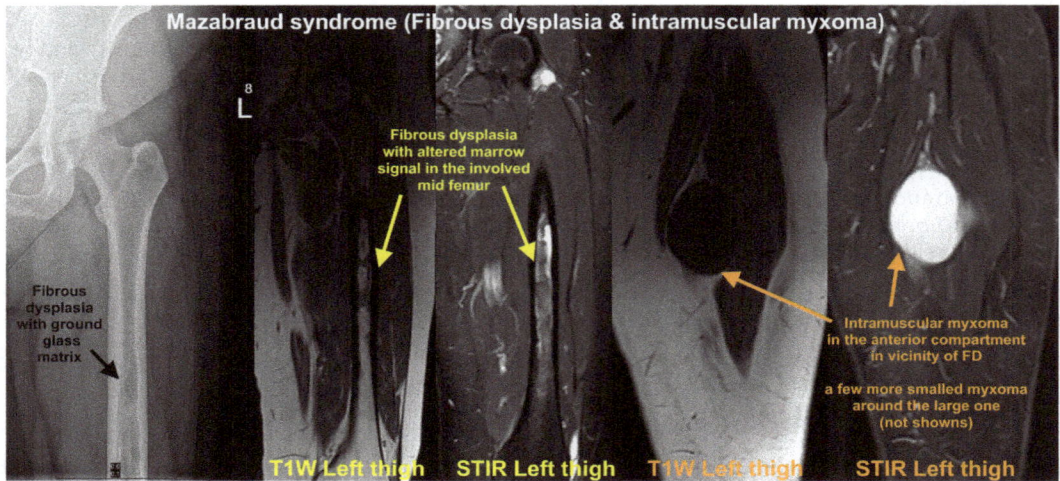

Figure 2.9.8 Imaging features of Mazabraud syndrome on X-ray (fibrous dysplasia) and MRI (intramuscular myxoma).

Gardener Syndrome

- One of the polyposis syndromes associated with APC genes.

- Frequently presents to sarcoma MDTs due to its association with various soft tissue tumours.

- Common associated tumours are GI tract polyps, epidermal inclusion cysts and fibromatoses (see Chapter 2.6 for imaging appearances), desmoid tumours of anterior abdominal wall and mesentery, breast fibroadenomas, osteomas in the mandible and skull, dentigerous cysts, ampullary, and thyroid carcinomas.

NEUROFIBROMATOSIS TYPE 1

- One of the most common neurocutaneous syndromes or phacomatoses; associated with NF1 gene and autosomal dominant transmission

- Criteria-based multidisciplinary team diagnosis

- Characteristic cutaneous findings: Café au lait spots (>6, highly predictive of NF1), cutaneous neurofibroma, and axillary and inguinal freckling

- Plexiform neurofibroma: Superficial or deep nerve sheath tumours along the length of the entire neural structure involved, cause mass effect and infiltration, appear as confluent multinodular fusiform masses along the neural axis, and show target sign and mass effect on T2W or fluid-sensitive images on MRI (Figure 2.9.9)

- Central CNS manifestations: Optic pathway glioma, sphenoid dysplasia (bare orbit sign), FASIs, dural ectasia, nerve sheath tumours, and meningocele

- Neural crest tumours: Pheochromocytoma and catecholamine-secreting tumours

- Thoracic and abdominal manifestations: Interstitial lung disease, cyst and bulla formation, pneumothorax, pulmonary hypertension, neurofibroma, gastrointestinal stromal tumours, and secondary bowel obstruction

- Musculoskeletal manifestations: Scoliosis (most common abnormality, often involves lower cervical and upper thoracic spine), associated with vertebral scalloping, foraminal widening, transverse process, rib remodelling, and dural ectasia

- Appendicular bone remodelling: Tibia and fibula are most commonly involved; anterolateral tibial bowing, fracture, and pseudoarthrosis are most common manifestations

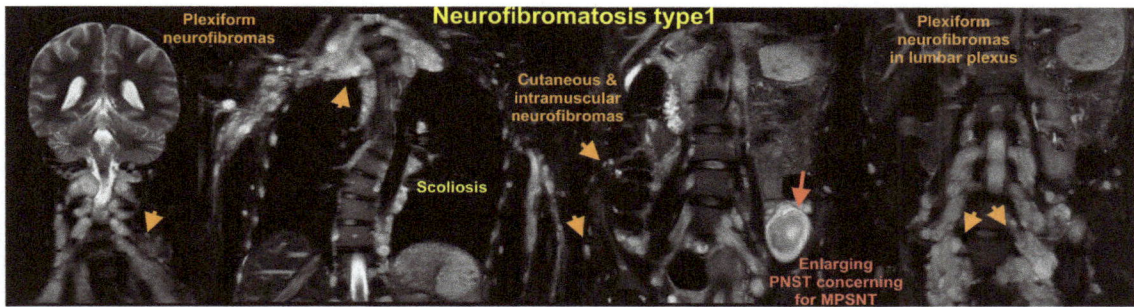

Figure 2.9.9 Plexiform cutaneous and intramuscular neurofibroma, scoliosis, and enlarging PNST in neurofibromatosis type 1.

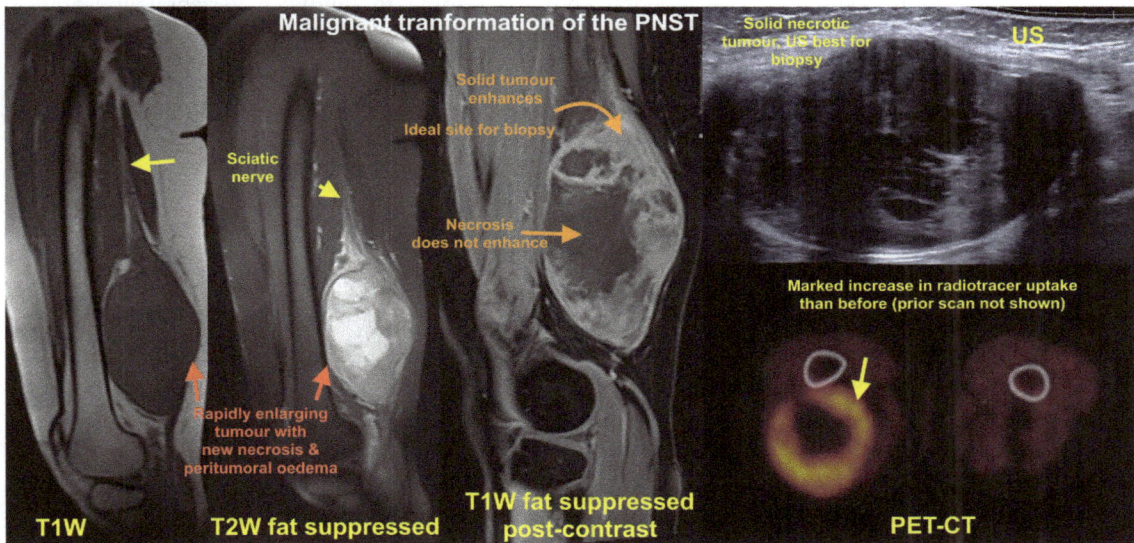

Figure 2.9.10 Ultrasound, MRI, and PET-CT appearances of the malignant transformation of the PNST in a neurofibromatosis type 1 patient.

Neurofibroma in diagnosed and undiagnosed cases of NF1 are one of the most common presentations to sarcoma MDTs.

- Ultrasound and image-guided biopsies are used to diagnosed PNST/neurofibroma in NF1.

  - Ultrasound: Well-defined, solid, echopoor mass with internal vascularity, contiguous with peripheral nerves, smaller nerves around cutaneous or intramuscular neurofibromas may not be visible.

- MRI shows characteristic features as described (target sign).

  - Signs of malignant transformation of PNST into MPNST: Sudden and rapid enlargement, peritumoral oedema, change in the internal signal characteristics and enhancement pattern, sudden increased radiotracer uptake compared to prior scans, and associated new neurological deficits (Figure 2.9.10). MPNST is the most feared complication and reason for surveillance.

  - Usually, annual clinical and imaging follow-up is recommended in NF1.

  - Whole-body MRI is used for imaging follow-up.

  - More focused MRI is performed if any PNST shows suspicious features, often with contrast.

  - Suspected MPNSTs require PET-CT and biopsies.

OSTEOPETROSIS

- Also known as marble bone disease or Albers–Schonberg disease

- Autosomal recessive and Autosomal dominant transmission (Rarer: X-link recessive)

- Abnormal osteoclasts functions leading to osteosclerosis of variable patterns

- X-ray is the most common modality and shows four distinct patterns:

  - Diffuse sclerosis involving skull, spine, pelvis, and appendicular bones (most common presentation)

  - Enlargement and expansion of long bone metaphyses (Erlenmeyer flask deformity, also seen in hereditary multiple exostoses, Gaucher's disease, and achondroplasia)

  - "Bone-within-a-bone" appearance: Mostly involves vertebrae, pelvis, long bones, and phalanges (Figure 2.9.11) (*Differential diagnoses*: Sickle cell anaemia, thalassemia, rickets, acromegaly, and Gaucher's disease)

  - Sclerosis and thickening of the vertebral endplate leading to sandwich vertebral appearances (Figure 2.9.11)

Hypertrophic Pulmonary Osteoarthropathy

- A syndrome presenting with diffuse metadiaphyseal pain affecting both forearms and lower legs, associated with solid, non-aggressive periosteal reaction affecting both distal forearms and lower legs without underlying bone lesions, and specifically in the setting of lung parenchymal diseases.

- Clubbing of nails is also associated.

- Common lung diseases causing HPOA include bronchiectasis, lung abscess, bronchogenic cancers, lymphoma, and parenchymal metastases.

- Similar bony features in GI tract and liver diseases are termed hypertrophic osteoarthropathy.

- Differentials include chronic venous insufficiency, thyroid acropachy, shin splints, hypervitaminosis A, thyroid acropachy, and normal variant.

- X-rays: Unilateral or bilateral long bone metaphyseal or metadiaphyseal smooth periosteal reaction without underlying tumour; can mimic osteomyelitis in presentation (Figure 2.9.12).

- MRI: Diffuse periosteal reaction with marrow signal abnormality (Low signal on T1W corresponding to high STIR/T2W-FS signal), non-specific, reviewing MRI in the clinical context is most important.

- Bone scan: Symmetrical tracer uptake on metadiaphyseal surface (tram-track sign).

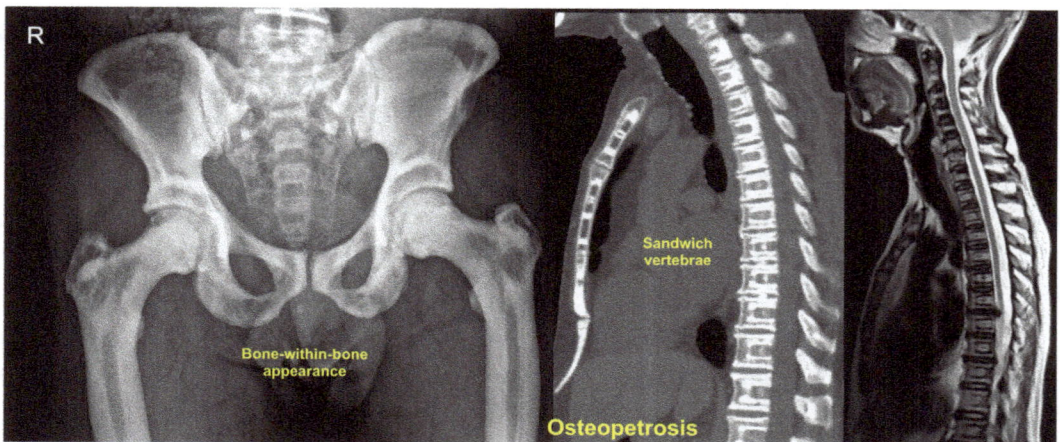

Figure 2.9.11 Characteristic imaging appearances of autosomal dominant osteopetrosis type 2.

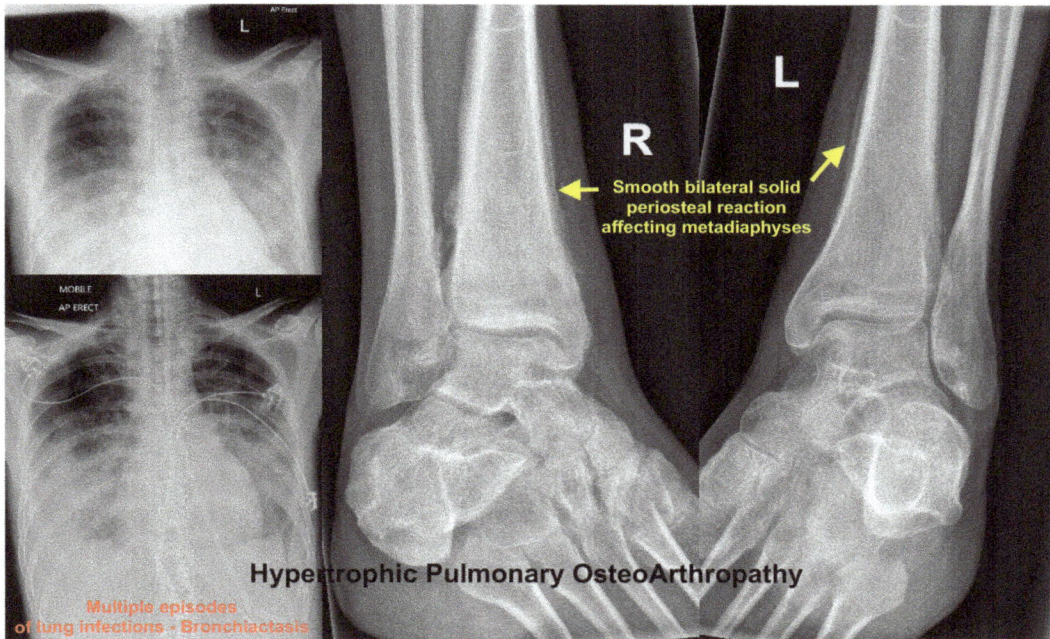

Figure 2.9.12 Chest X-rays showing pulmonary infiltrates in multiple admissions and typical radiographic features of hypertrophic pulmonary osteoarthropathy.

CONCLUSION

Various multisystemic diseases have characteristic musculoskeletal manifestations on imaging. Although uncommon, practising musculoskeletal radiologists should be familiar with such imaging appearances to direct patient care in appropriate direction. More importantly, the patient should be referred to appropriate genetic or familial counselling if genetic association of the diagnosed syndrome is possible.

SUGGESTED READING

- https://www.nhs.uk/conditions/neurofibromatosis-type-1/treatment/

SBA QUESTIONS

1) An 85-year-old female with known osteoporosis presented to A&E with acute pain, limb shorting, and inability to weight bear on the right side. She confirmed Zolendronate therapy for osteoporosis in the last few years and denies a significant fall. X-rays of the pelvis and right femur were performed to rule out fracture. Which of the following is least likely to be a bisphosphonate-related fracture?

   A. Displaced right proximal femur fracture in the subtrochanteric region

   B. Small area of cortical thickening in the left proximal femur in the subcortical region

   C. Sclerotic line in the midshaft of the right femur

   D. Sclerotic line in the medial neck of the left femur

   E. None of the above

2) A 66-year-old Asian male presented to A&E with a foul-smelling ulcer at the plantar surface of the posterior calcaneal tuberosity. He has a history of long-standing, poorly controlled type II diabetes mellitus. Foot and ankle X-rays were performed at the A&E to assess for suspected osteomyelitis. Which of the following imaging appearances is NOT consistent with features of pedal changes of diabetic foot?

A. Non-visualisation of distal and middle phalanges of 2nd and 3rd toes

B. Air foci in the pedal soft tissue in the region of posterior calcaneal tuberosity

C. Lack of cortex at the posterior calcaneal tuberosity

D. Vascular calcification in the small vessels of the foot

E. Thickening and punctate calcification around the distal Achilles tendon at the calcaneal insertion

3) Which of following MRI appearances is most likely to represent an osteoporotic compression fracture?

A. A linear hypointense signal in the middle of the posterior cortex with fatty marrow around it on T1W image

B. A linear hypointense signal just above the inferior endplate without any retropulsed fracture fragment on T1W image

C. A linear hypointense signal in the middle of the vertebra with absence of fatty marrow around and bulging posterior vertebral wall on T1W image

D. A linear hypointense signal through fused vertebral body and posterior elements on T1W image with cord oedema on STIR image

E. All of the above

Answers: (1) D, (2) E, (3) B

BONUS QUESTIONS

1) A 42-year-old female presented with a painless slow-growing lump in the left anterior thigh. She described activity-related discomfort locally. The MRI showed a well-capsulated solid lesion that appeared hyperintense on T1W and STIR images in the rectus femoris. It showed avid enhancement on post-gadolinium images. There was an abnormal marrow signal (hypointense on T1W and hyperintense on STIR) area in the adjacent femur midshaft. It showed ground glass appearances on the X-ray but no cortical expansion or pathological fracture. What is the most likely diagnosis?

A. Ollier's disease

B. Maffucci syndrome

C. Mazabraud syndrome

D. Gardener syndrome

E. Hereditary multiple exostosis

2) A 28-year-old semi-professional footballer presented with numbness in the first webspace of the right foot. The plain radiographs through the right ankle showed a small osteophyte arising from the tibial plafond, and the MRI showed scarring in the anterior joint capsule, a small ganglion near the tarsal tunnel, and mild ankle joint effusion. Which anatomical structure is the most likely cause of the patient's symptoms?

A. Lateral cutaneous branch of the sural nerve

B. Medial plantar calcaneal nerve

C. Superficial peroneal nerve

D. Deep peroneal nerve

E. Dorsalis pedis artery

3) A 63-year-old gentleman presented with atraumatic left shoulder pain. The MRI showed mild glenohumeral joint effusion and cartilage loss in the posterior glenoid. Additionally, there was a small posterosuperior labral tear with a paralabral cyst and muscle oedema affecting only the infraspinatus muscle on STIR images. What is the most likely location of the paralabral cyst?

   A. Supraspinatus notch

   B. The spine of the scapula

   C. Spinoglenoid notch

   D. Biceps-labral junction

   E. Posterior IGHL labro-ligamentous complex

4) A 24-year-old female presented with right knee pain, swelling, and episodes of locking. The radiograph showed moderate joint effusion. The MRI showed early erosions and numerous intra-articular bodies which appear hypointense on T1W, PD-weighted, and STIR images. A few of the nodules show susceptibility artefacts on gradient echo (GRE) images. What is the most likely diagnosis?

   A. Primary synovial chondromatosis

   B. Nodular tenosynovial giant cell tumour

   C. Diffuse tenosynovial giant cell tumour

   D. Rheumatoid arthritis

   E. Haemophilic arthropathy

Bonus Question Answers: (1) C, (2) D, (3) C, (4) E

Chapter 2.10
Endocrine Bone Disorders

Joseph KT, Madhavi K, and Ankit Tandon

LEARNING OBJECTIVES

- Know heterogenous endocrine conditions and their effects on the musculoskeletal system

- Appreciate imaging appearances of metabolic disorders and their mimics

- Understand relevant imaging recommendations once certain pathologies are diagnosed

---

This is one of the most important chapters focusing on commonly asked pathologies as single best answers (SBA), long cases and table viva during FRCR examinations. All such cases require methodical approach focusing on bone density and combination of imaging findings in the appropriate biochemical context. This is a long chapter with a lot of information, concepts, and points to remember. Therefore, we have provided "Key Points to Remember" at the beginning of each topic that may be helpful during exam revisions.

CONDITIONS CAUSING INCREASED BONE DENSITY

- Paget's disease

- Renal osteodystrophy

- Fluorosis

- Acromegaly

PAGET'S DISEASE

Key Points to Remember

- Radiographs are generally sufficient to diagnose Paget's disease given its characteristic features observable in each stage.

- The most frequent presentation occurs during the mixed phase.

- Familiarity with imaging patterns on CT and MRI is crucial for avoiding misdiagnosis, as these findings can occur incidentally.

- MRI is warranted in cases where there is suspicion of neoplastic transformation or neurological compression.

Introduction

Paget's disease, also known as osteitis deformans, is a metabolic bone disorder of unknown etiology that predominantly affects adults. It is characterised by excessive bone resorption followed by the formation of structurally aberrant bone. The polyostotic form is the most common, affecting approximately 66% of patients, followed by the monostotic form. While most individuals are asymptomatic, those exhibiting symptoms may present with pain, deformities, fractures, or neuromuscular symptoms, depending on the distribution of the disease and the bones involved.

- The disease progresses through three primary phases: Predominant osteoclastic activity in the lytic phase, concomitant osteoclastic activity and osteoblastic activity in the mixed phase, and marked osteoblastic activity in the blastic phase.

- These phases are reflected through elevated serum and urine hydroxyproline levels, indicative of increased resorption, and elevated serum alkaline phosphatase signifies osteoblastic activation.

DOI: 10.1201/9781003500247-19

- These biochemical markers are useful for monitoring disease activity and evaluating therapeutic efficacy. Imaging modalities further elucidate the pathological stages of the condition.

Imaging Features

Radiographs

- Radiographs are the mainstay in the diagnosis.

- In long bones, the lytic phase is characterised by a distinctive wedge-shaped area of radiolucency in the metaphysis with a lack of sclerosis, which may resemble a flame or a blade of grass (Figure 2.10.1). This advancing osteolytic wedge typically initiates in the subchondral bone of the epiphysis and extends peripherally into both the metaphysis and the diaphysis.

- In the later stages of the lytic phase, one may observe subperiosteal cortical thickening along with accentuation and coarsening of the trabecular pattern, often accompanied by an enlargement of the bone contours.

- In the skull, the progression of osteolysis is manifested as significant areas of radiolucency, particularly within the frontal and occipital bones, often referred to as osteoporosis circumscripta (Figure 2.10.2). These cranial lesions are notably pronounced in the inner calvarial tables and frequently cross suture lines.

   The mixed phase of Paget's disease shows features of both the lytic and blastic phases. Most patients are diagnosed during the mixed phase, marked by decreased osteoclastic activity and increased osteoblastic activity.

- This phase is defined by all **four** cardinal features of the disease: **advancing osteolysis, coarsening and thickening of bone trabeculae along the lines of stress, cortical thickening, and bone expansion**.

- Thickening and sclerosis of the iliopectineal and ischiopubic lines are often noticed. Changes around the acetabulum can lead to acetabular protrusion. In the spine, the mixed phase of Paget's disease is marked by cortical thickening along all four margins of the vertebral body cortex, creating a distinctive picture-frame appearance (Figure 2.10.3).

- In the skull, abnormal bone deposition presents a characteristic cotton-wool appearance, featuring globular to fluffy foci of varying density (Figure 2.10.2).

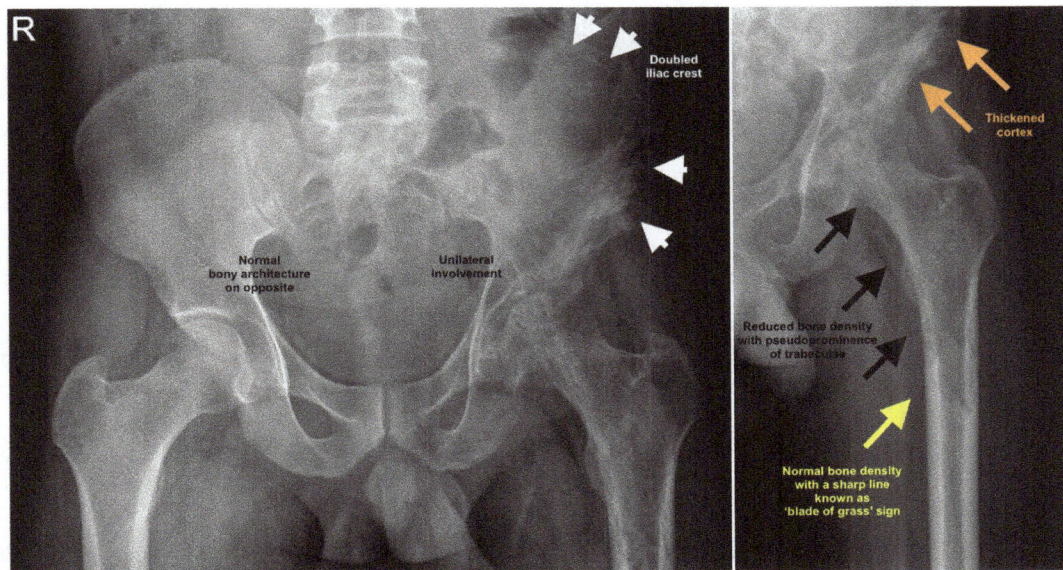

Figure 2.10.1 X-rays showing classical features of Paget's disease in the left hemipelvis and blade of grass sign.

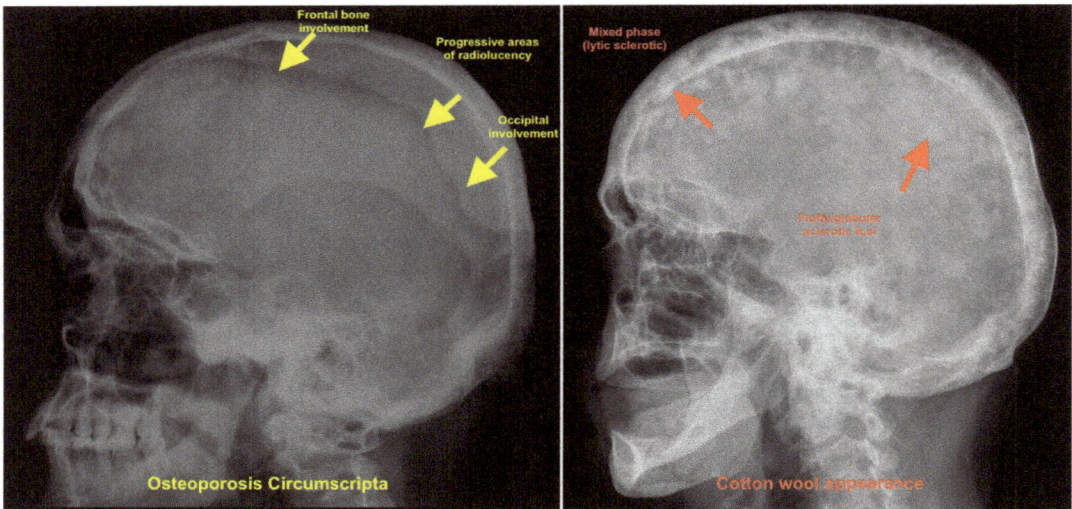

Figure 2.10.2 X-ray features of lytic and mixed phases of the Paget's disease in the skull.

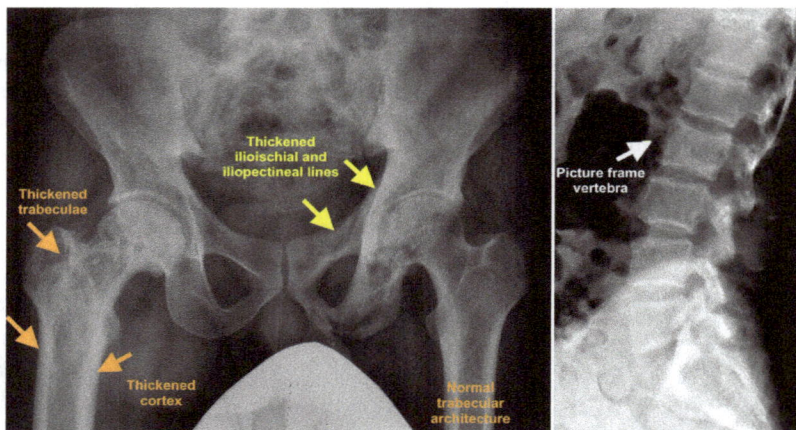

Figure 2.10.3 X-ray features of polyostotic Paget's disease in the pelvis and picture frame vertebra in the spine.

The blastic or late inactive phase is marked by decreased osteoblastic activity, resulting in osteosclerosis.

- In the pelvis and long bones, key features include coarsening of the trabecular structure and cortex thickening, which causes bone enlargement.

- Due to the excessive deposition of abnormal bone, these bones become weak and are more susceptible to transverse fatigue fractures, commonly known as "banana fractures."

- The occurrence of multiple fractures and abnormal bone repair can lead to progressive bowing deformities. In the spine, osteosclerosis gives the vertebrae an "ivory vertebra" appearance and results in the enlargement of the vertebral body, with or without involvement of the posterior elements.

- The presence of enlarged vertebrae helps differentiate Paget's disease from other causes of diffuse vertebral sclerosis.

The findings on CT are similar to those observed in radiographs, with lytic areas appearing as attenuated trabeculae. The thickening of trabecular structures and the sclerosis seen in the mixed and blastic phases are better visualised through CT. Familiarity with these CT findings is essential to mitigate the risk of misdiagnosis, as incidental findings may occur.

On MRI, Paget's disease may present with a range of marrow appearances that vary according to the disease stage.

- Osteolysis is depicted as high signal intensity on T2-weighted images and low signal intensity on T1-weighted images.

- Heterogeneous marrow signals due to bone oedema-like signals and thickened trabeculae are a common appearance in the mixed phase, often mimicking osteomyelitis (Figure 2.10.4).

- The trabecular thickening and sclerosis in the blastic phase appear as low signal intensity across all imaging sequences.

- **A considerable characteristic feature of the disease is that fatty marrow is generally preserved**, even in advanced stages, unless complications such as fractures or sarcomatous transformation occur.

- The emergence of new aggressive lytic areas, cortical disruptions, soft tissue masses, or mass-like marrow replacement indicates sarcomatous transformation.

- MRI is instrumental in evaluating spinal cord compression or cranial nerves. The irregular bone formation along the inner margins of the cranial vault can compress nearby nerves and brain tissue, leading to neurological symptoms.

Imaging Recommendations

- Incidental lesions should be correlated with laboratory markers to evaluate disease activity.

- Cross-sectional imaging is recommended when there is a suspicion of malignant transformation or neurological deficits. Once proven, staging CT is recommended.

Mimics of Vertebral Paget's Disease

- Osteomyelitis typically presents with localised bone destruction and the presence of a sequestrum, while Paget's disease is characterised by bone enlargement and thickening.

- Vertebral haemangioma: The key feature of haemangioma is the significant thickening of the vertical trabeculae. Unlike in haemangiomas, Paget's disease commonly involves thickening all four cortices of the vertebral body and involving the posterior spinal elements.

- Osteoblastic metastasis or lymphoma: bone expansion and cortical thickening are absent. Paget's disease may occasionally show diffuse sclerosis of an entire vertebral body.

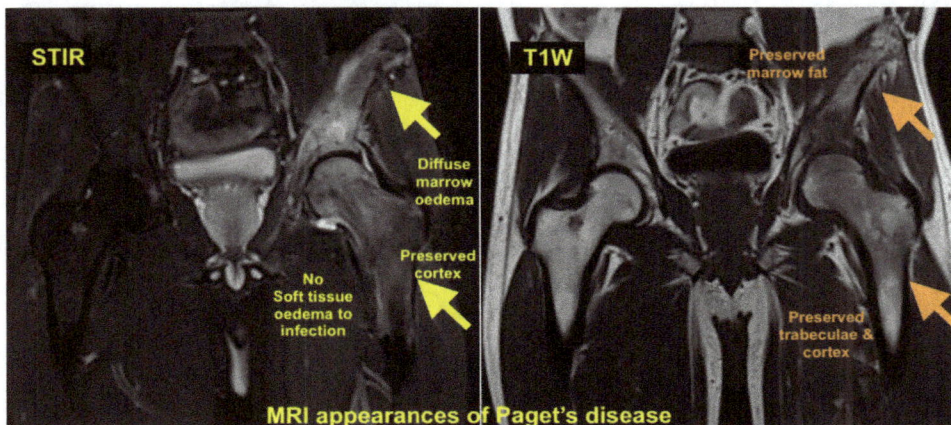

Figure 2.10.4 MRI features of Paget's disease mimicking acute osteomyelitis. Note preserved fat signal on T1W image.

Renal Osteodystrophy
Key Points to Remember

- Secondary hyperparathyroidism, osteoporosis, osteosclerosis, and osteomalacia are common musculoskeletal manifestations of this condition.

- Often involved bones are axial skeleton, especially the sacroiliac joints and the hands.

- A thorough understanding of renal osteodystrophy is essential for radiologists, particularly in cases that overlap or have similarities with other metabolic musculoskeletal disorders.

Introduction

Renal osteodystrophy refers to a constellation of findings observed in the setting of chronic renal insufficiency secondary to both vitamin D deficiency causing osteomalacia and secondary hyperparathyroidism as a response to low serum calcium levels.

- In chronic renal failure, elevated serum phosphate depresses serum calcium levels, leading to hyperplasia of the parathyroid glands and increased levels of parathyroid hormone.

- Despite the increased radiodensity/osteosclerosis, the bone is structurally weak and prone to stress fractures.

- Axial skeleton involvement is common.

Imaging Features

- Deposition of bone in the subchondral areas of the vertebral bodies leads to the formation of dense bands along the superior and inferior margins, giving rise to the appearance known as a rugger-jersey spine (Figure 2.10.5).

- Additional findings associated with secondary hyperparathyroidism may aid in establishing a secure diagnosis, including osteomalacia, osteopenia, brown tumours, as well as soft tissue and vascular calcifications.

- Insufficiency fractures are a common complication.

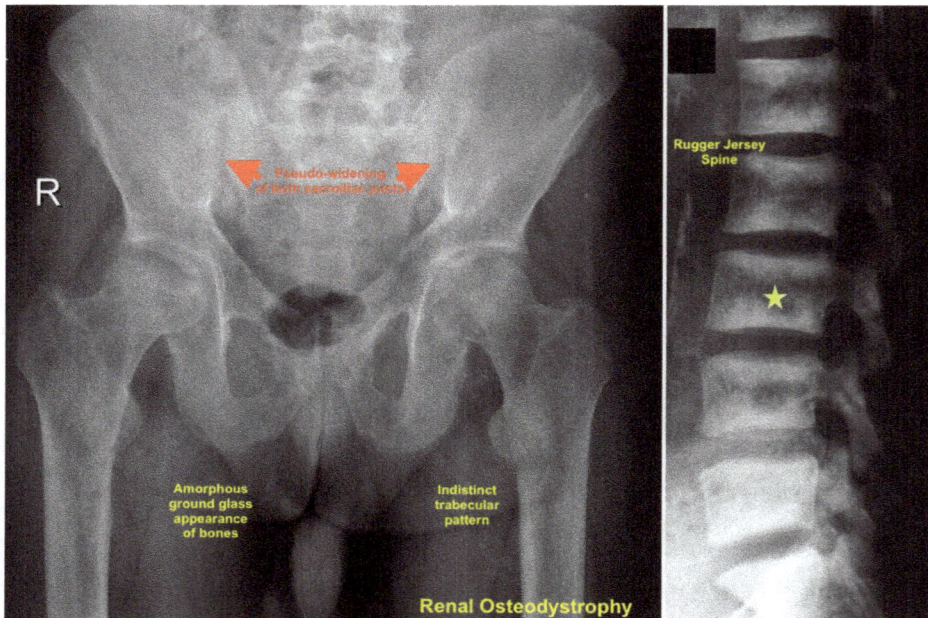

Figure 2.10.5   Pelvic and spinal features of renal osteodystrophy on X-rays.

- Other complications seen in patients on long-term dialysis include deposition of amyloid, arthritis, and osteonecrosis.

Imaging Recommendations If Newly Diagnosed

- Imaging evaluation should include the search for evidence of either primary or secondary hyperparathyroidism resorption of the bones, bone tumours, and soft tissue calcifications.

- Ultrasound of the abdomen to assess the kidneys.

- Neck ultrasound or nuclear scan for parathyroid lesions.

- To correlate with serum calcium and phosphorous.

Fluorosis
Key Points to Remember

- Common in endemic regions.

- Diffuse osteosclerosis with additional findings of periostitis and ligament calcifications are key imaging features of skeletal fluorosis.

Introduction

Skeletal fluorosis is a chronic metabolic bone disease due to prolonged ingestion, or rarely, inhalation of fluoride ions in regions where high fluoride levels are naturally present. The condition is often asymptomatic and may be discovered incidentally during a radiological examination. Its symptoms can vary widely and may include general weakness, diffuse skeletal pain, limited mobility, and neurological deficiencies, along with elevated levels of fluoride in the serum and urine.

Imaging

- The key imaging features are diffuse osteosclerosis with flowing osteophytes and thickening and ossification of the ligamentum flavum and the posterior longitudinal ligament.

- Thickening and ossification are also seen at the entheseal attachments of the ligaments, tendons, muscles, and interosseous membrane calcification (Figure 2.10.6).

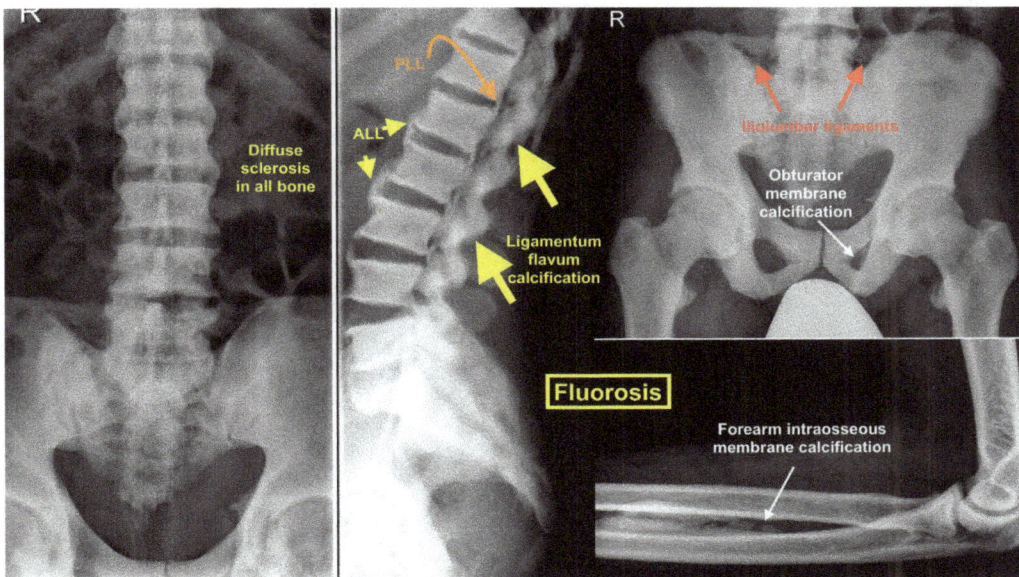

Figure 2.10.6 X-ray features of fluorosis.

- Diffuse periosteitis is another feature of skeletal fluorosis.

Imaging Recommendations If Newly Diagnosed

- Forearm radiographs for characteristic interosseous membrane ossification.

- Check for the endemic history, dental fluorosis, and elevated serum and urine fluoride levels.

Mimics
Fused Spine

- Diffuse idiopathic skeletal hyperostosis: Ligamentous ossification and enthesopathy are common manifestations of diffuse idiopathic skeletal hyperostosis; however, bone density is usually normal in this condition (Figure 2.10.7).

- Diffuse osteosclerosis: Osteopetrosis, myelofibrosis, renal osteodystrophy, osteoblastic metastatic disease, hypervitaminosis D, and plasma cell dyscrasias. None of these cause periostitis or mineralisation at tendons/ligaments.

- Diffuse periostitis: Hypervitaminosis A, hypertrophic osteoarthropathy, venous stasis (limited to lower limbs), and thyroid arthropathy (limited to hands); however, these do not cause diffuse osteosclerosis.

ACROMEGALY
Key Points to Remember

- Characteristic radiographic features help in early diagnosis.

- Soft tissue changes may develop earlier than bone alterations and therefore must be carefully looked for.

- Early manifestations include widened joint spaces of the hand and foot and increased intervertebral disc spaces.

- Radiologists must be aware of the possible manifestation of acromegaly as nerve enlargements and entrapments.

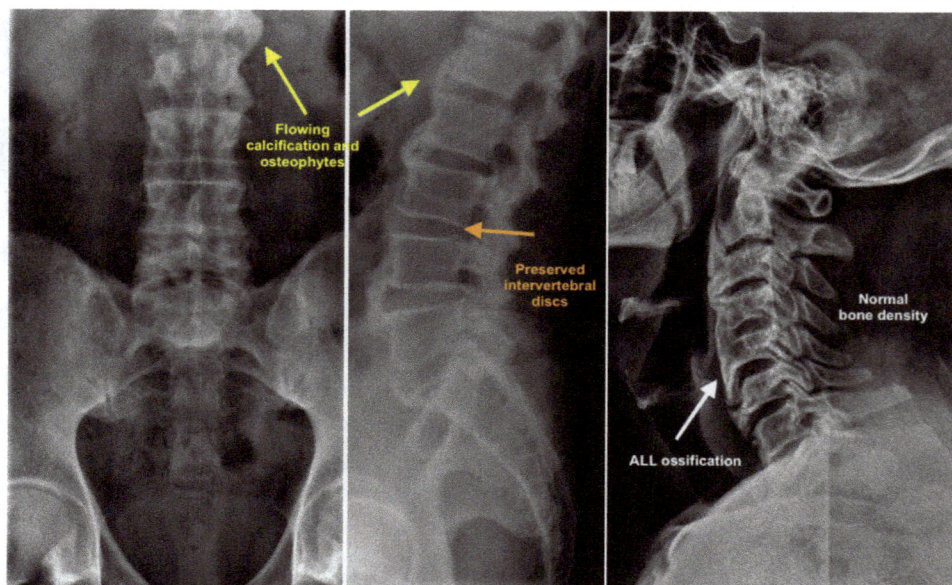

Figure 2.10.7 X-ray features of diffuse idiopathic skeletal hyperostosis.

Introduction

Acromegaly is characterised by the excessive secretion of growth hormone from a pituitary adenoma and, less commonly, hyperplasia of eosinophilic cells. Growth hormone (GH) leads to various systemic effects and progressive physical changes.

- The hallmark clinical features of acromegaly include a prominent forehead, mandibular hyperplasia, a thickened tongue, broadening of the extremities, and thickening of soft tissues.

- If GH production occurs before the closure of long bone growth centres, it can lead to gigantism.

- Other symptoms can include bitemporal hemianopsia and chronic headaches, both resulting from the progressive growth of the adenoma.

The skeletal effects of growth hormones are significant, as they stimulate the proliferation of chondrocytes, fibroblasts, and osteocytes, which results in new bone formation and irregular thickening of the bone cortex. Musculotendinous insertions may develop bony excrescences and spurs, increasing ectopic bone formation.

Imaging

- Soft tissue changes are predominantly observed in the hands and feet, with a heel pad thickness exceeding 20 mm suggestive of acromegaly, although this measurement alone is not definitive.

- In the skull, key features include an enlarged sella turcica, thickened skull bones, prominent occipital protuberances, frontal bossing, prognathism, and an enlarged mandible. Sinus overgrowth in the frontal and maxillary regions may lead to malocclusion.

- Spinal manifestations can include platyspondyly, increased disc heights, a widened atlanto-dental interval, and excessive osteophyte formation.

- In the hands, features include widened phalangeal shafts and metacarpals, spade-shaped ungual tufts, enlarged sesamoids, and bony protuberances (Figure 2.10.8).

- Early degenerative arthritis, carpal tunnel syndrome, and foraminal and spinal canal stenosis are common complications.

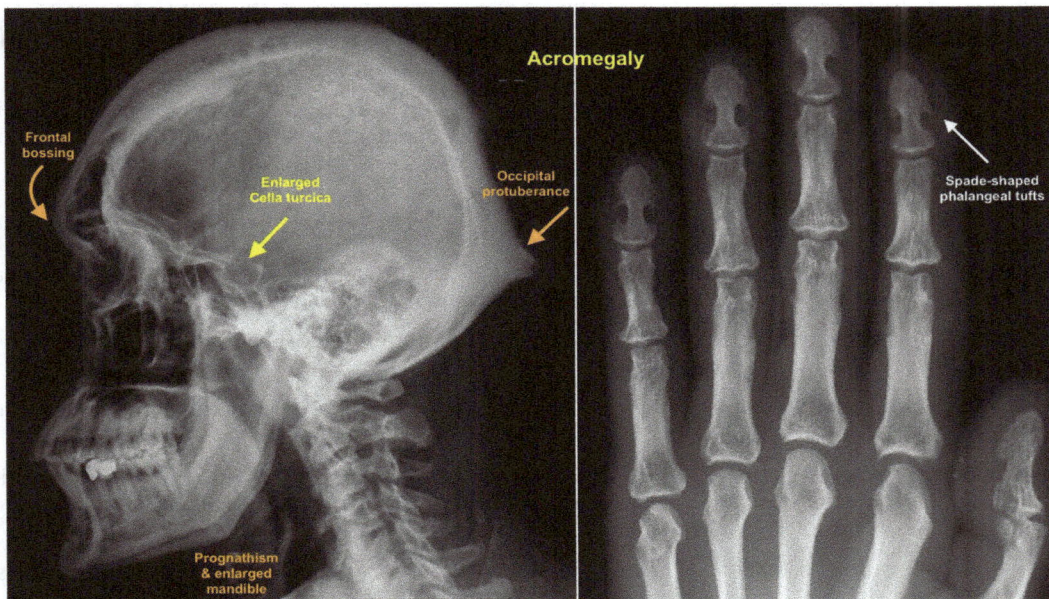

Figure 2.10.8   Features of acromegaly on skull and hand X-rays.

Imaging Recommendations If Newly Diagnosed

- MRI brain with gadolinium: A pituitary protocol to assess pituitary adenoma.
- Check for elevated basal growth hormone and insulin-like growth factor-1 levels.

CONDITIONS CAUSING REDUCED BONE DENSITY

- Osteoporosis
- Rickets and osteomalacia
- Oncogenic osteomalacia
- Scurvy
- Alkaptonuria d/d DISH
- Osteogenesis imperfecta

OSTEOPOROSIS
Key Points to Remember

- Conventional radiography remains the mainstay in the diagnosis.
- Key imaging features are reduced density, cortical thinning, and endosteal resorption.
- Thorough knowledge is essential to differentiate between benign osteoporotic fractures and malignant vertebral fractures to ensure appropriate clinical management.

Introduction

Osteoporosis is the most common metabolic bone disorder, characterised by decreased bone density while maintaining normal bone structure. It occurs when bone formation is insufficient or when bone resorption exceeds bone formation.

- Osteoporosis may be localised, as seen in disuse osteoporosis, or generalised throughout the body. Osteoporosis is either primary, where no cause is identified, or secondary due to several causes including nutritional deficiencies and infective, inflammatory, and neoplastic disorders.
- The imaging characteristics of osteoporosis can vary depending on the rate of its progression. Osteoporosis leads to significant morbidity and mortality, mainly due to fragility fractures. The three most common fracture sites are the forearm, hip, and spine.

Imaging Features
Radiographs

- Conventional radiography remains the most commonly used imaging technique; however, it usually detects pathological changes only after about 30% of bone mass has been lost.
- Key features associated with osteoporosis include cortical thinning, endosteal resorption, and a decrease in the amount of trabecular bone.
- An early sign of the disease in the spine is the verticalisation of trabecular structures, which occurs due to the loss of horizontal trabeculae.
- As osteoporosis progresses, the integrity of the vertical trabecular structure is compromised, leading to the collapse of the endplate, reduced height and further thinning of the cortices and, in later stages, thinned-out cortices result in an "empty box" appearance (Figure 2.10.9).
- The hallmark feature of osteoporosis is the occurrence of fractures, which may present as vertical insufficiency fractures in the sacrum and compression fractures in the vertebrae. Severe osteoporosis can mask nondisplaced fractures in conventional radiographs, making diagnosis difficult where MRI would be problem solving (Figure 2.10.10).

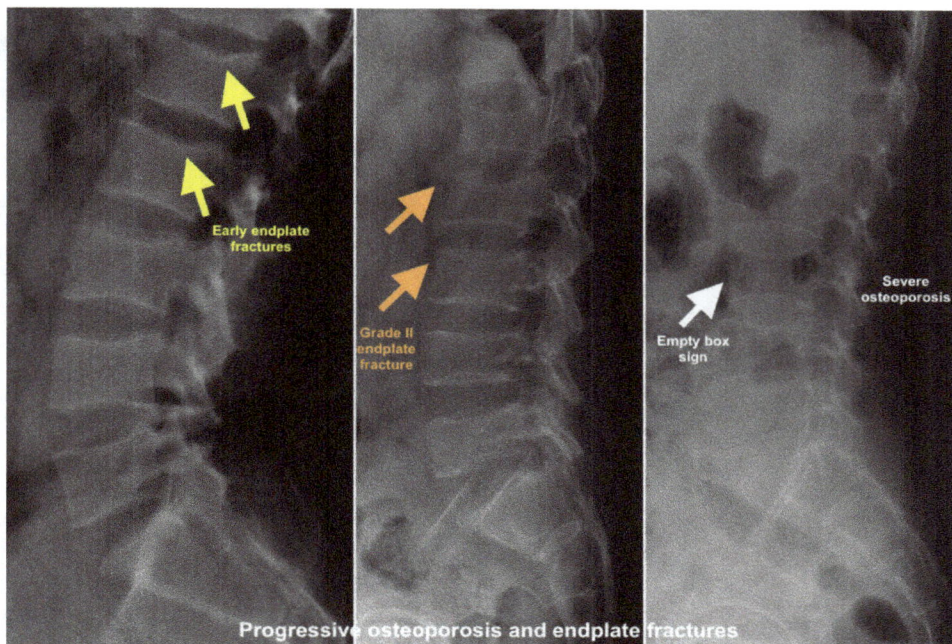

Figure 2.10.9   Osteoporosis and endplate fractures on spinal X-rays.

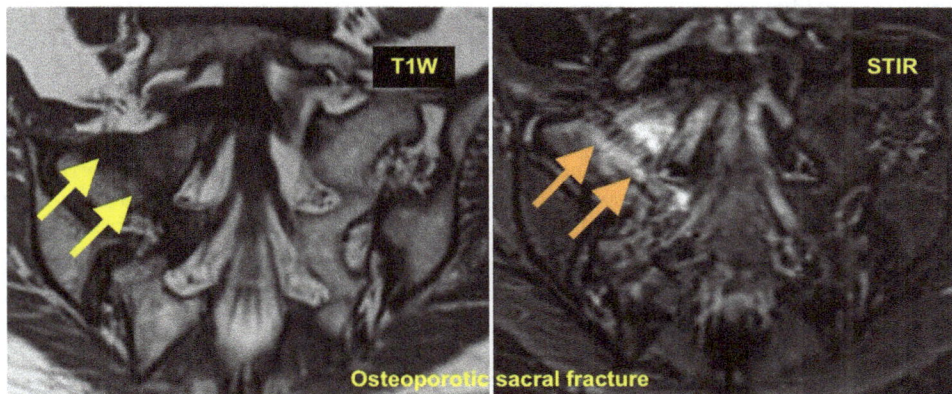

Figure 2.10.10   Right sacral alar osteoporotic fracture on MRI.

- In cases of severe pain with normal radiographs, CT or MRI is beneficial for proper diagnosis. It is crucial to differentiate between benign osteoporotic fractures and malignant vertebral fractures to ensure appropriate clinical management. Plain X-rays, CT, and radionuclide bone scans have not always reliably distinguished between benign and malignant causes, but MRI usually can (Figure 2.10.11, Table 2.10.2).

Imaging Recommendations If Newly Diagnosed

- Additional cross-section imaging is suggested to identify fractures and causes of severe pain in cases with severe osteoporosis on conventional radiographs.

- MRI is recommended if any suspicion of malignancy.

- Suggest bone mineral density assessment to assess the risk of fractures.

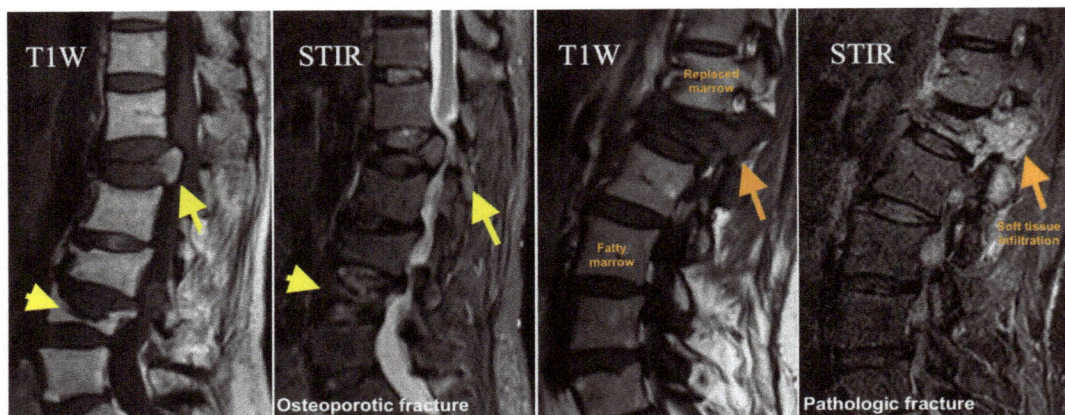

Figure 2.10.11 MRI features of osteoporotic versus metastatic fractures.

> ## OSTEOMALACIA/RICKETS
> ### Key Points to Remember
>
> - Osteomalacia has reduced bone density with or without Looser zones.
> - Key radiographic features of rickets include a widened growth plate, along with cupping and fraying of the metaphysis.
> - Important to identify associated osteopetrotic rickets and oncogenic osteomalacia since the treatment differs.

Introduction

Incomplete mineralisation resulting from a deficiency in calcium salts within the osteoid leads to the development of osteomalacia in adults and rickets in children. Various factors contribute to this condition, including gastrointestinal absorption issues and renal tubular dysfunction; however, the primary abnormalities are predominantly associated with calcium, phosphorus, and vitamin D metabolism.

- Osteomalacia that is associated with paraneoplastic disorders is known as oncogenic osteomalacia or tumour-induced osteomalacia. This condition is characterised by elevated serum levels of FGF23 and low phosphorus levels.
- Nuclear scans [^{68}Ga-DOTATATE, OctreoScan] are highly sensitive in identifying paraneoplastic lesions, which can be in soft tissue or bone (Figure 2.10.12).
- Rickets can be classified into two types based on the main mineral deficiency: calcipenic and phosphopenic.
- Rachitic manifestations are most pronounced at the sites of the greatest growth, such as the knee (distal femur and proximal tibia), distal tibia, proximal humerus, distal radius and ulna, and the anterior ends of the middle ribs.
- These findings are noted on the metaphyseal side of the growth plate because unmineralised osteoid accumulates in this area. The failure of mineralisation results in disorganised chondrocyte growth, and hypophosphatemia hinders the apoptosis of hypertrophic chondrocytes. This leads to excessively long cartilage cell columns, which contributes to the radiographic findings of a widened growth plate, as well as cupping and fraying of the metaphyses.

Imaging

- Radiographic findings in osteomalacia are generally nonspecific and include reduced bone density, diminished cortical definition, and a coarsened trabecular pattern.

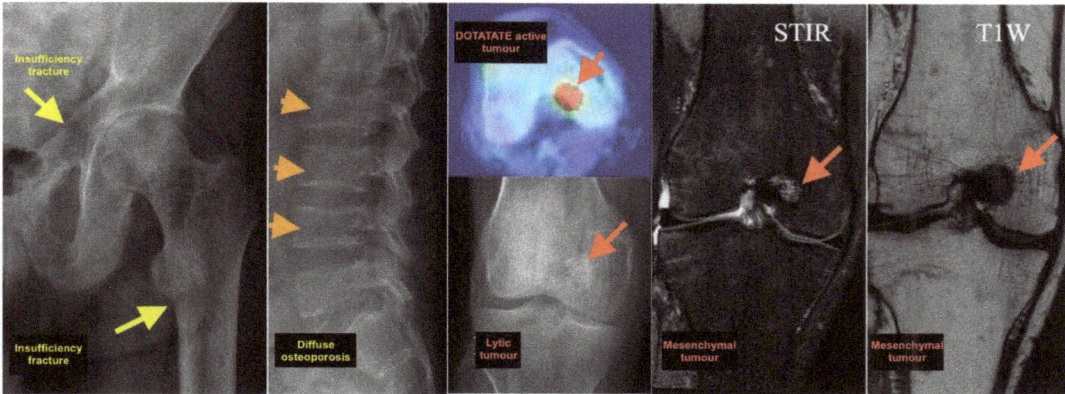

Figure 2.10.12 Oncogenic osteomalacia and insufficiency fractures caused by a mesenchymal tumour in the knee.

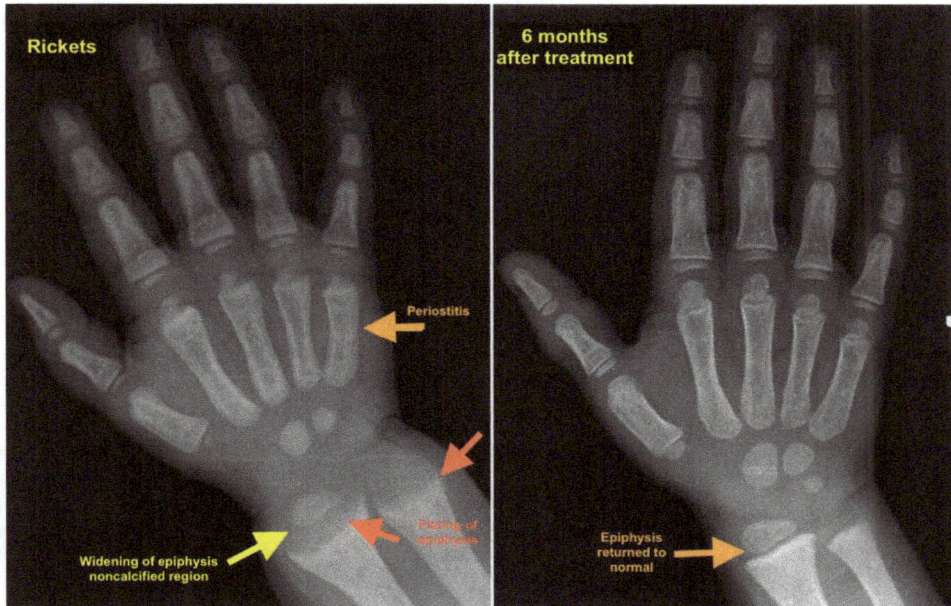

Figure 2.10.13 X-ray features of untreated and treated rickets.

- Commonly observed deformities encompass protrusio acetabuli, kyphoscoliosis, and an increased concavity of the endplates in the spinal region. Looser zones, or pseudo-fractures, represent insufficiency fractures characterised by linear radiolucent bands that are oriented perpendicularly to the long axis of the affected bone.

- These zones are most commonly identified in the pubic and ischial rami, medial femoral necks, ribs, scapulae, and long bones, typically located on a bowing deformity's concave (compressive) side.

- The radiographic findings associated with rickets include a widened growth plate, irregularities and osteopenia on the metaphyseal side of the growth plate, and flaring and fraying of the metaphysis (Figure 2.10.13).

- The key radiographic features in the healing phase are a widened growth plate, mild metaphyseal cupping, and sclerosis along the metaphyseal side. Other features include bowing deformities, fractures, rachitic rosary, bell-shaped thorax, widened sutures, a squared appearance of the skull, and basilar invagination.

Imaging Recommendations If Newly Diagnosed

- In newly diagnosed osteomalacia, further assessment with lab and nuclear scan is recommended to identify associated paraneoplastic disorders since the treatment differs.

SCURVY
Key Points to Remember

- Although relatively rare, this condition should be considered, especially in undernourished children. Early diagnosis and treatment are crucial, as symptoms may also present with nonclassical findings.

- The classic radiological features include a sclerotic epiphyseal rim, dense provisional metaphyseal calcification, metaphyseal spurs, and metaphyseal cupping.

Introduction

Scurvy is a nutritional deficiency of vitamin C (ascorbic acid). It primarily affects infants, typically between the ages of 6 and 24 months. Although rare in adults, scurvy can occur when there is a severe dietary vitamin C deficiency. A lack of vitamin C leads to abnormal collagen formation, resulting in vascular fragility and irregular bone matrix. Musculoskeletal manifestations occur in 80% of scurvy patients, with characteristic radiologic findings.

Imaging Features

- Radiographic features are most commonly seen at the site of rapidly growing areas such as the distal femur, proximal tibia, fibula, distal radius, ulna, proximal humerus, and distal ends of the ribs.

- Diffuse osteopenia that affects both cortical and trabecular bone is highly characteristic.

- Additionally, there is a decrease in and disorganisation of cartilage proliferation along the growth plates, resulting in an irregular appearance on the metaphyseal side. On this side, a dense band at the zone of provisional calcification, known as the Frankel line, signifies the sclerotic provisional calcification zone (Figure 2.10.14).

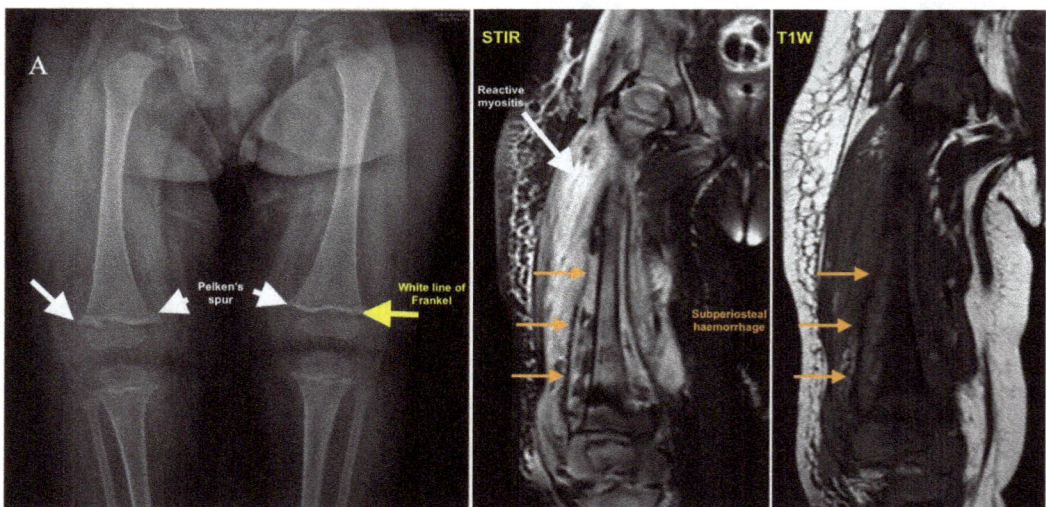

Figure 2.10.14 X-ray and MRI features of scurvy.

- The peripheral extension of this calcification zone results in a pointed contour of the metaphyses, commonly termed beaking. The fragility of the trabeculae in this area leads to subepiphyseal "corner" fractures.

- A distinct line adjacent to the Frankel line, known as the Trummerfeld zone, indicates the accumulation of haemorrhage in this region, which is prone to fracture.

- Subperiosteal haemorrhage leads to elevation of the periosteum and a periosteal reaction. In MR imaging, the bone marrow appears low signal on T1W and heterogenous high signal on T2W images, and edema-like signal in the STIR images with subperiosteal haemorrhage visible as periosteal elevation accompanied by increased T1 and T2 signal intensity beneath the periosteum (Figure 2.10.14).

Imaging Recommendations If Newly Diagnosed

- Check vitamin C levels and exclude imaging mimics, particularly hematological malignancies.

Mimics

- Non-accidental injury has only corner fractures, but the growth plate is normal.

- Oedema-like marrow signal on STIR images may mimic chronic non-bacterial osteitis [CNO]; however, the growth plate is normal in CNO.

- Diffuse low signal of marrow on T1W images may mimic haematological malignancies except that in malignancies, the pattern of bone marrow involvement is diffuse.

ALKAPTONURIA
Key Points to Remember

- Darkly stained diapers or discolouration of urine are the early clue to the diagnosis.

- Early marked arthritis in major joints such as knees, hips, and shoulders in a young patient is pathognomonic.

- Severe osteoporosis, multilevel intervertebral disc ossification, and narrowing of the disc spaces are the three most frequent radiographic findings.

Introduction

Alkaptonuria (AKU), also referred to as "black bone" or "black urine," is a rare metabolic disorder of autosomal recessive inheritance from a mutation in the homogentisic acid oxidase (HGO) enzyme, which is located on chromosome 3q. Due to the deficiency of HGO, there is an accumulation of homogentisic acid in both the blood and urine.

- Homogentisic acid gets deposited in the soft tissues, tendons, cartilages, large joints, and intervertebral discs often referred to as ochronosis.

- Ochronosis usually affects the thoracolumbar spine and typically spares the cervical spine and sacroiliac joints.

- Dark staining of diapers or dark discolouration of urine is an early indicator for diagnosis in infancy and childhood.

- The common clinical presentation is tendon tears or ochronotic arthritis in the 3rd or 4th decade of life; this delayed presentation is associated with a reduced renal clearance of homogentisic acid that occurs with ageing.

Imaging

- The key radiographic features of the condition include severe osteoporosis, multilevel intervertebral disc calcification accompanied by disc space narrowing, syndesmophyte formation, and early onset of significant osteoarthritis (Figure 2.10.15).

- Enthesopathy changes occur at the distal insertion sites of tendons and ligaments, which may present with soft tissue deposits that can be observed with or without calcification; ultrasound is particularly effective for visualising these changes.

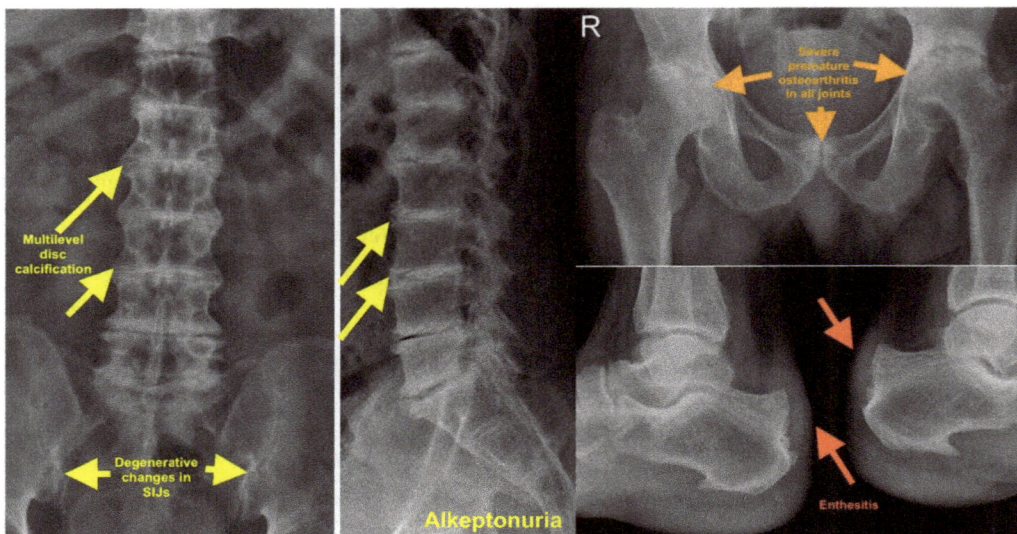

Figure 2.10.15 X-ray features of alkaptonuria/ochronosis.

- The tendons most commonly affected include the Achilles tendon, as well as the quadriceps and patellar tendons.

- MRI is typically reserved for evaluating complications such as tendon and ligament tears, as well as spinal canal and foramen stenosis resulting from severe disc extrusions.

Mimics

- **Diffuse idiopathic skeletal hyperostosis (DISH)**: Lack of intervertebral disc ossification and early marked osteoarthritis differentiates from alkaptonuria.

- **Ankylosing spondylitis**: The key differentiating feature is the lack of involvement of the sacroiliac joints and disc calcifications in alkaptonuria.

- **Intervertebral disc ossification**: It is seen in various conditions, including degenerative, metabolic, crystal, and chronic inflammatory arthropathies; however, very dense central (nucleus pulposus) calcification associated with osteopenia is noted in ochronosis where calcification begins in the lumbar spine and ascends.

OSTEOGENESIS IMPERFECTA
Key Points to Remember

- Conventional radiographs play an important role both in preoperative setting and in follow-up

- Key radiographic features are osteopenia, multiple fractures, and bone deformities

- Hyperplastic callus is seen in type V osteogenesis imperfecta

---

Introduction

Osteogenesis imperfecta (OI), commonly known as brittle bone disease, is a genetic disorder that affects connective tissues due to abnormalities in the synthesis or processing of type I collagen.

- There are multiple types of osteogenesis imperfecta.

- In general, type I is the most common type and is mild without associated deformity, while type II is the least common type and is fatal in the perinatal period. Type III is severely deforming, while type IV is deforming but less so than type III.

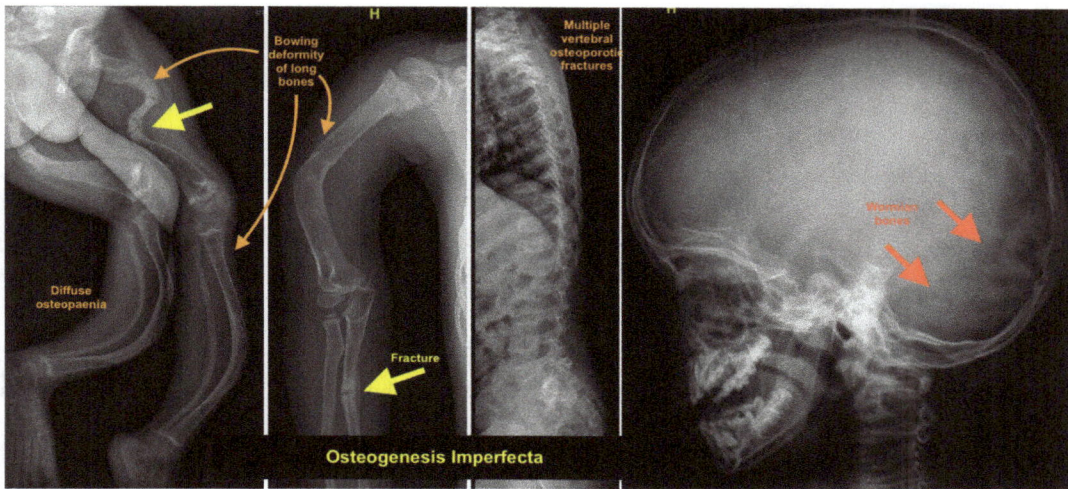

Figure 2.10.16 X-ray features of osteogenesis imperfecta.

- The hallmark features of OI include bone fragility and susceptibility to fractures, bone deformity, and diminished growth.

- The osteogenesis imperfecta (OI) diagnosis is based on clinical evaluation and can be confirmed through genetic testing. Nevertheless, imaging plays a crucial role in assessing fractures and deformities in both preoperative and follow-up settings.

Imaging

- Diffuse osteopenia is characterised by thinning of both trabecular and cortical bone and is a common feature in all forms of OI.

- Fractures frequently occur in the axial and appendicular skeletons, particularly affecting the diaphyses of long bones and compression fractures of the vertebrae.

- Hyperplastic callus and interosseous membrane ossification are typically seen in type V OI. Bone deformities arise due to excessive malleability and plasticity, with anterolateral deformity being the most common type. Additionally, wormian bones are often observed (Figure 2.10.16).

- In some forms of osteogenesis imperfecta, there may rarely be a prominent occipital region that resembles a "Darth Vader" appearance, or a flattening of the cranial vault accompanied by transverse infolding of the cranial base, referred to as a "tam o'shanter skull."

Imaging Recommendations If Newly Diagnosed

- Genetic analysis with mutations in the COL1A1 and COL1A2 genes

---

PARATHYROID AND THYROID ABNORMALITIES CAUSING REDUCED BONE DENSITY

- Hyperparathyroidism including tumoral calcinosis in secondary HPT
- Hypoparathyroidism/pseudohypoparathyroidism
- Hypothyroidism/hyperthyroidism

HYPERPARATHYROIDISM
Key Points to Remember

- Key imaging features are diffuse osteopenia and bone resorption.

- Thorough knowledge of bone resorption in the axial skeleton, especially the sacroiliac joints, is essential to avoiding misdiagnosis of spondyloarthritis.

- Brown tumours are more common in chronic renal insufficiency and secondary hyperparathyroidism.

Introduction

- Hyperparathyroidism is characterised by elevated parathyroid hormone (PTH) levels, which results in increased bone resorption. Primary hyperparathyroidism occurs when the parathyroid glands secrete PTH independently, bypassing the normal feedback inhibition exerted by serum calcium levels.

- The most common cause is parathyroid adenoma or carcinoma; it is rarely due to parathyroid hyperplasia.

- Secondary hyperparathyroidism is common as a response to low serum calcium levels, often due to chronic renal failure or renal insufficiency, which disrupts PTH metabolism and leads to hyperplasia of the parathyroid glands. This condition can also result from vitamin D deficiency and low dietary calcium.

Imaging

- The main imaging features include diffuse osteopenia and bone resorption. Subperiosteal bone resorption usually starts on the radial sides of the middle and index fingers' middle phalanges. It leads to acroosteolysis if resorption occurs at the distal phalanges. It can also occur in areas such as the ribs, lamina dura, humerus, femur, and upper medial tibia (Figure 2.10.17).

- Bone resorption may occur in trabecular, intracortical, endosteal, subchondral, and other regions. In the skull, it results in a "salt-and-pepper" appearance, complicating the distinction between the inner and outer tables.

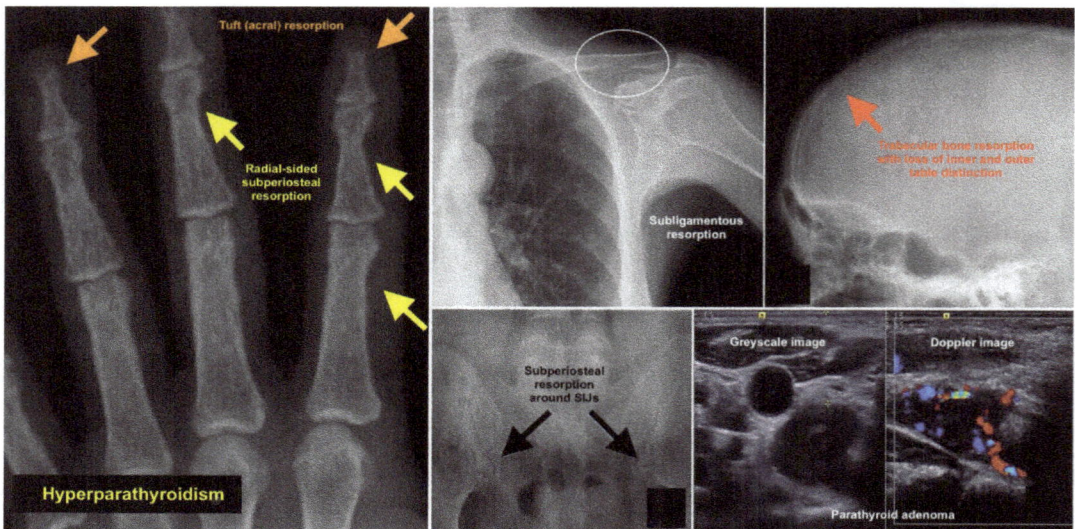

Figure 2.10.17 X-ray features of hyperparathyroidism caused by a parathyroid adenoma.

- Trabecular resorption causes a smudgy look, while intracortical resorption manifests as cortical tunnelling, common in hyperparathyroidism.

- Subchondral resorption can affect any joint, often beginning at the distal interphalangeal joints in the hands and potentially spreading to other joints. It can also occur especially at the iliac side of the sacroiliac joint and the clavicular side of the acromioclavicular joint and tends to affect both sides of the sternoclavicular joint (Figure 2.10.17).

- Subligamentous or subtendinous resorption can occur in various anatomical locations, most commonly in the calcaneus, clavicle, greater and lesser tuberosities of the humerus, greater and lesser trochanters of the femur, anterior inferior iliac spine, and ischial tuberosity.

- Brown tumours are lytic lesions resulting from PTH-induced osteoclast activation (Figure 2.10.18). These are often seen in secondary hyperparathyroidism. While typically solitary, these tumours can also be multifocal, increasing the risk of pathologic fractures.

- They are commonly found in the facial bones, ribs, pelvis, and femora and may significantly increase in size and decrease post-resection of parathyroid adenoma.

- Soft tissue and vascular calcifications and chondrocalcinosis are also commonly seen in secondary hyperparathyroidism.

Imaging Recommendations If Newly Diagnosed

- Check serum calcium, phosphorous, and PTH levels.

- Ultrasound neck to assess parathyroid lesions (Figure 2.10.17).

- Scintigraphy or 4D-CT to localise parathyroid adenoma.

OTHER PARATHYROID-ASSOCIATED METABOLIC BONE DISORDERS
Key Points to Remember

- Increased bone density, and intracranial and soft tissue calcifications are key imaging features in hypoparathyroidism and pseudohypoparathyroidism.

- Brachydactyly is a specific feature of pseudohypoparathyroidism.

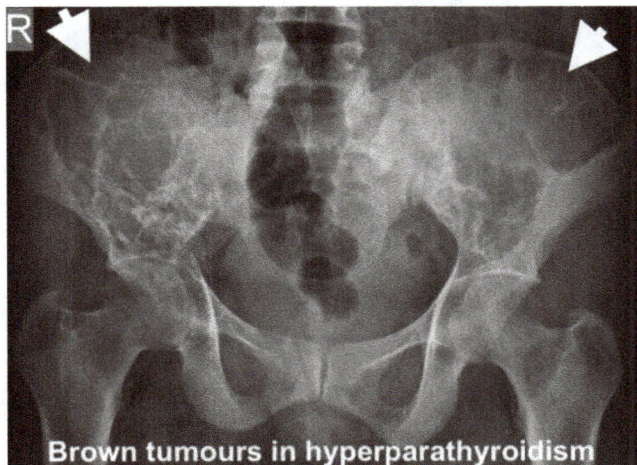

Figure 2.10.18 Brown tumours on pelvic X-ray.

Introduction

- Hypoparathyroidism and pseudohypoparathyroidism are two metabolic bone disorders associated with the parathyroid glands.

- Hypoparathyroidism is an acquired condition, primarily resulting from iatrogenic injury to the parathyroid glands during thyroid surgery or the removal of the parathyroid glands. Other causes may include autoimmune diseases or genetic factors like DiGeorge syndrome.

- The common clinical presentation is short stature, depression, and anxiety.

- On the other hand, pseudohypoparathyroidism is a congenital hereditary disorder in which the body does not respond properly to the parathyroid hormone (PTH), which affects phosphate excretion. This insensitivity to PTH can be due to several factors, including end-organ insensitivity, defective hormone production, or anti-enzymes in the serum or tissues.

- The clinical features of pseudohypoparathyroidism are short stature, obesity, intellectual disability, corneal or lenticular opacities, and brachydactyly.

- There is also a condition known as "pseudo-pseudohypoparathyroidism," characterised by physical appearances and imaging findings similar to those of pseudohypoparathyroidism but with normal blood marker levels.

Imaging

In hypoparathyroidism, the main imaging features include diffuse or localized increased bone density, thickening of the skull vault with narrowed diploic spaces, intracranial and soft tissue calcifications, and dense metaphyseal bands. In rare cases, there is ossification of the spinal ligaments (Figure 2.10.19). In pseudohypoparathyroidism, the key imaging features consist of short metacarpals, short metatarsals with coned epiphyses, short phalanges, and intracranial and soft tissue calcifications. If hypoparathyroidism or pseudohypoparathyroidism is newly diagnosed, check the serum calcium, phosphorous, and parathormone levels, and suggest CT brain in hypoparathyroidism to assess the intracranial calcifications additionally.

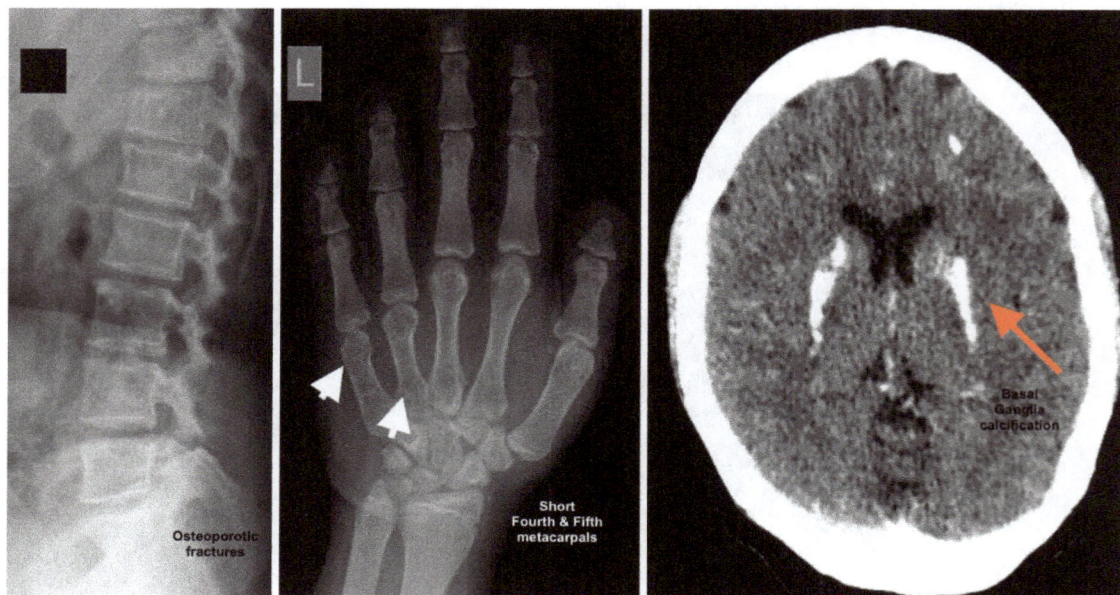

Figure 2.10.19 Imaging features of hypoparathyroidism.

THYROID-ASSOCIATED METABOLIC BONE DISORDERS
Key Points to Remember

- The characteristic skeletal manifestations in congenital hypothyroidism are delayed ossification, irregular and fragmented epiphysis

- Hyperthyroidism often presents with severe osteoporosis and features of thyroid acropachy in follow-up cases of Graves' disease

Introduction

- Hypothyroidism can be either congenital or acquired.

- Congenital hypothyroidism may result in significant skeletal abnormalities and delays in development. Conversely, acquired hypothyroidism typically manifests with mild skeletal abnormalities, if any. Acquired hypothyroidism can arise following surgical intervention, radioactive iodine therapy, or due to glandular atrophy.

- Additionally, it may be associated with acute or chronic thyroiditis, such as Hashimoto's disease, as well as infiltrative disorders like amyloidosis or lymphoma. Other contributing factors include certain medications, iodine deficiency, or a pituitary disorder leading to thyroid-stimulating hormone deficiency.

- Hyperthyroidism is predominantly caused by the excessive secretion of thyroid hormone from the thyroid gland, which can occur diffusely, as observed in Graves' disease, or focally in cases associated with single or multiple adenomas.

Imaging

- Congenital hypothyroidism often leads to delayed skeletal development in children. The key imaging features are absent, irregular, or fragmented distal femoral and proximal tibial epiphyses, resembling multiple epiphyseal dysplasia.

- Additionally, dental development may also be delayed.

- Hyperthyroidism often presents with osteoporosis.

- Thyroid acropachy, which is characterised by digital clubbing, periosteitis, and soft tissue edema, is associated with Graves' disease. This condition typically occurs after treatment when the patient reaches a euthyroid or hypothyroid state. The periosteitis is particularly pronounced along the radial borders of the metacarpals, metatarsals, and the diaphysis of the middle and proximal phalanges.

Imaging Recommendations If Newly Diagnosed

- Check the lab values: Serum T3, T4, and TSH levels.

- Ultrasound thyroid to assess thyroiditis and nodules.

CHARCOT'S NEURO-OSTEOARTHROPATHY
Teaching Points

- Plain radiographs may be normal in the early stages of Charcot's neuro-osteoarthropathy (CNO); hence, close-interval follow-up is recommended.

- MRI is recommended in a clinically suspected active CNO with a normal appearance of the plain radiographs to confirm or exclude the disease since offloading and immobilisation are the most important initial treatment.

- MRI is the imaging choice to assess the disease activity.

- The CNO has periarticular bone marrow oedema, whereas osteomyelitis is characterised by diffuse bone marrow oedema, typically at pressure points, often accompanied by a skin ulcer in these areas.

Table 2.10.1 Modified Eichenholtz Classification

Stage	Clinical Features	Radiographic Findings	Treatment
0 (Acute: Inflammatory)	Swelling, erythema & warmth	Normal	Patient education, serial radiographs to monitor progression, & protected weight-bearing
I (Acute Charcot: Developmental/ fragmentation)	Marked erythema, swelling & warmth	Osteopenia, fragmentation, joint subluxation or dislocation (Figure 2.10.20)	Protected weight-bearing with cast or brace should be used until radiographic resolution of fragmentation and presence of normal skin temperature
II (Subacute: Coalescence stage)	Decreased warmth, erythema & swelling	Absorption of debris, sclerosis, fusion of larger fragments	Total contact cast or brace, Charcot restraint orthotic walker, or clamshell ankle–foot orthosis
IV (Chronic: Remodelling)	Absence of warmth, erythema & swelling; deformities	Consolidation of deformity, joint arthrosis, fibrous ankyloses, rounding & smoothing of bone fragments	Plantigrade foot: Custom inlay shoes with rigid shank and rocker-bottom sole. Nonplantigrade foot or ulceration: Debridement, deformity correction, or fusion with internal fixation

Introduction

- CNO is a progressive destructive neuroarthropathy.

- It can be seen in any neurological condition/disorder causing sensory loss. The most common cause is diabetes, and the other causes include leprosy, spinal cord injury, alcoholism, and congenital insensitivity to pain.

- The etiopathogenesis is multifactorial, and the proposed mechanism consists of a neurotraumatic (loss of pain sensation and proprioception) and neurovascular (autonomic vascular reflex with hyperaemia) theory.

- The (modified) Eichenholtz classification, based on clinical and X-ray findings, is frequently used for clinical evaluation of a suspected Charcot foot (Table 2.10.1).

Imaging

- Radiographs: The ankle and foot views should include the AP, mortise, and lateral projections.

- The radiographs should ideally be taken while the patient is weight-bearing or standing. If a patient cannot stand, non-weight-bearing radiographs are an option, but they may not display more obvious malalignments when the patient is standing.

- Radiographs are adequate to establish the diagnosis and to stage and monitor the disease.

- The condition typically affects the midfoot and hindfoot, including structures such as the metatarsophalangeal, Lisfranc, talonavicular joints, and the medial column comprising the navicular, cuneiforms, and the 1st, 2nd, and 3rd metatarsals (Figure 2.10.20).

- It may also cause articular disease around the talus as well as avulsion of the calcaneal tuberosity. The severity of the deformities is best assessed on 3D CT scan images.

- **MRI:** MRI is the preferred imaging technique to establish an early diagnosis of Charcot's foot (Figure 2.10.21).

- MRI makes it possible to assess the effectiveness of off-loading therapy and the direction of the healing process (monitoring: active or inactive disease) (Figure 2.10.22).

- Another significant role of MRI is its ability to evaluate further complications of a Charcot's foot, particularly soft tissue infections and osteomyelitis (Figure 2.10.23).

- The CT or SPECT-CT is an alternative choice if MRI is unavailable or contraindicated. The level of evidence to establish diagnosis and assess disease activity is low. CT bone reconstruction is useful in surgical planning.

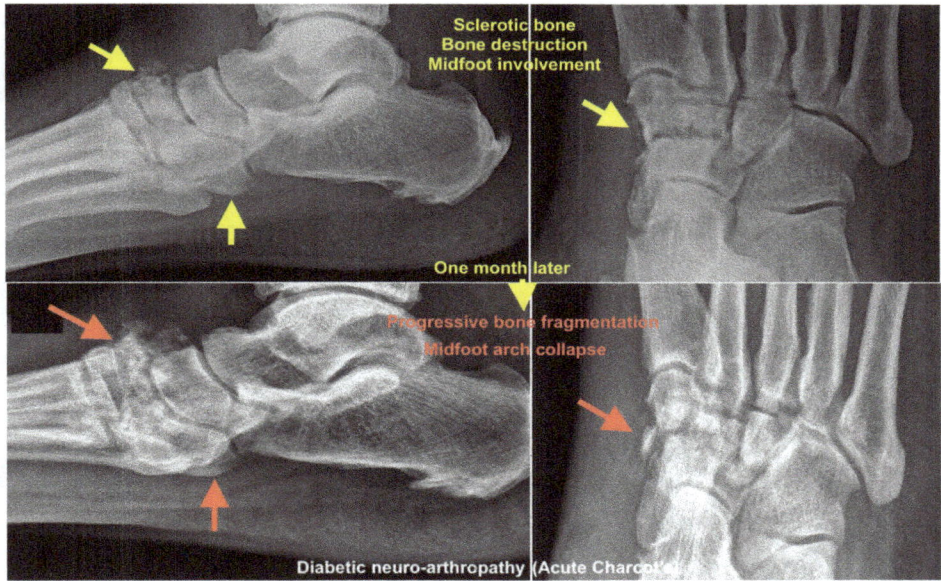

Figure 2.10.20   Progressive midfoot X-ray changes of diabetic (Charcot's) neuroarthropathy.

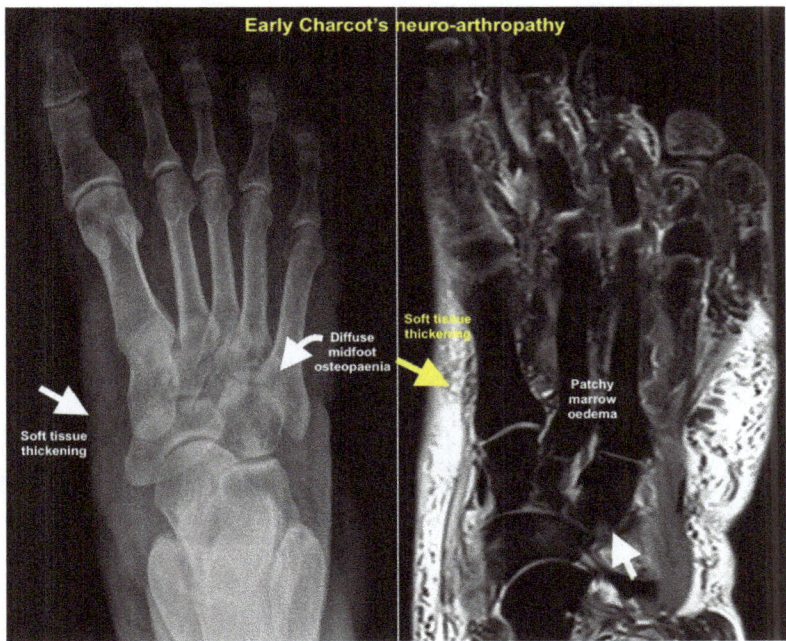

Figure 2.10.21   Imaging appearances of early diabetic neuroarthropathy.

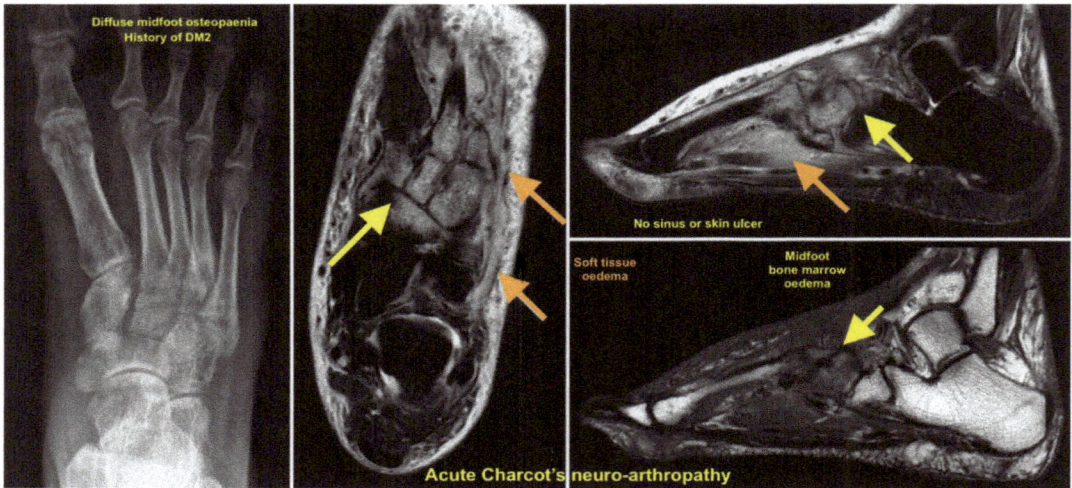

Figure 2.10.22 X-ray and MRI features of acute diabetic neuroarthropathy (Charcot's).

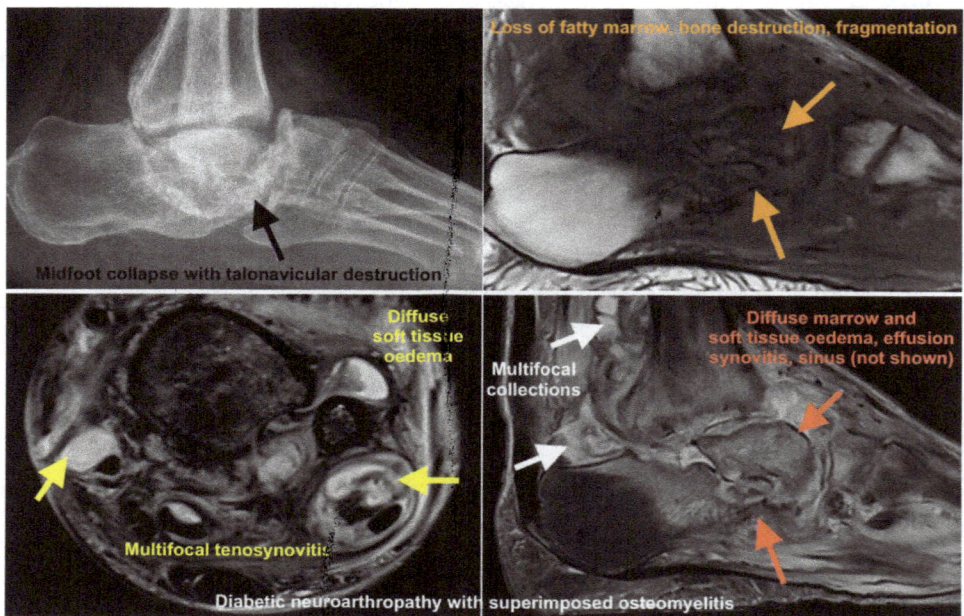

Figure 2.10.23 X-ray and MRI features of acute osteomyelitis superimposed on diabetic neuroarthropathy.

Imaging Recommendations If Newly Diagnosed

- MRI is indicated if there is suspicion of osteomyelitis on plain radiographs.
- MRI is the imaging choice to assess disease activity. Ultrasound may help if MRI is not available.

Table 2.10.2 Differences between Charcot's Neuroarthropathy and Osteomyelitis

	Charcot's Neuroarthropathy	Osteomyelitis
Location	Periarticular, multiple joints are affected	Single bone usually, the weight-bearing areas as affected (metatarsal heads, calcaneum, and cuboid).
Sinus tracts, skin ulcers	+/−	Often present
Collection/effusion	Present	Usually larger than CNO
Intra-articular bodies	Often present	Often absent since they will be resorbed by inflammation
Ghost sign (indistinct bone on T1 becomes evident post-Gd)	Absent	Present

SUGGESTED READING

- Chang CY, Rosenthal DI, Mitchell DM, Handa A, Kattapuram SV, Huang AJ. Imaging findings of metabolic bone disease. *Radiographics*. 2016;36(6):1871–1887. https://doi.org/10.1148/rg.2016160004. PMID: 27726750.

- Panwar J, Kandagaddala M, Bhat TA, Hsu C, Mitra P. The forgotten art of plain radiography in the evaluation of metabolic bone disease. *Indian J Musculoskelet Radiol*. 2020;2(1):3–19.

- Smith SE, Murphey MD, Motamedi K, Mulligan ME, Resnik CS, Gannon FH. From the archives of the AFIP. Radiologic spectrum of Paget disease of bone and its complications with pathologic correlation. *Radiographics*. 2002;22(5):1191–1216. https://doi.org/10.1148/radiographics.22.5.g02se281191. PMID: 12235348.

- Broski SM, Folpe AL, Wenger DE. Imaging features of phosphaturic mesenchymal tumors. *Skeletal Radiol*. 2019;48(1):119–127. https://doi.org/10.1007/s00256-018-3014-5. Epub 2018 Jul 9. PMID: 29987349.

- Gulko E, Collins LK, Murphy RC, Thornhill BA, Taragin BH. MRI findings in pediatric patients with scurvy. *Skeletal Radiol*. 2015;44(2):291–297. https://doi.org/10.1007/s00256-014-1962-y. Epub 2014 Aug 12. PMID: 25109378.

- Biswas S, Miller S, Cohen HL. Scurvy in a malnourished child: Atypical imaging findings. *J Radiol Case Rep*. 2022;16(9):11–15. https://doi.org/10.3941/jrcr.v16i9.4545. PMID: 36324605; PMCID: PMC9584558.

- Gazzotti S, Sassi R, Aparisi Gómez MP, Moroni A, Brizola E, Miceli M, Bazzocchi A. Imaging in osteogenesis imperfecta: Where we are and where we are going. *Eur J Med Genet*. 2024;68:104926. https://doi.org/10.1016/j.ejmg.2024.104926. Epub 2024 Feb 16. PMID: 38369057.

- Renaud A, Aucourt J, Weill J, Bigot J, Dieux A, Devisme L, Moraux A, Boutry N. Radiographic features of osteogenesis imperfecta. *Insights Imaging*. 2013;4(4):417–429. https://doi.org/10.1007/s13244-013-0258-4. Epub 2013 May 19. PMID: 23686748; PMCID: PMC3731461.

- Naik M, Khan SR, Owusu D, Alsafi A, Palazzo F, Jackson JE, Harvey CJ, Barwick TD. Contemporary multimodality imaging of primary hyperparathyroidism. *Radiographics*. 2022;42(3):841–860. https://doi.org/10.1148/rg.210170. Epub 2022 Apr 15. PMID: 35427174.

- Khan AA, Hanley DA, Rizzoli R, Bollerslev J, Young JE, Rejnmark L, Thakker R, D'Amour P, Paul T, Van Uum S, Shrayyef MZ, Goltzman D, Kaiser S, Cusano NE, Bouillon R, Mosekilde L, Kung AW, Rao SD, Bhadada SK, Clarke BL, Liu J, Duh Q, Lewiecki EM, Bandeira F, Eastell R, Marcocci C, Silverberg SJ, Udelsman R, Davison KS, Potts Jr JT, Brandi ML, Bilezikian JP. Primary hyperparathyroidism: Review and recommendations on evaluation, diagnosis, and management. A Canadian and international consensus. *Osteoporos Int*. 2017;28(1):1–19. https://doi.org/10.1007/s00198-016-3716-2. Epub 2016 Sep 9. PMID: 27613721; PMCID: PMC5206263.

- Bennett J, Suliburk JW, Morón FE. Osseous manifestations of primary hyperparathyroidism: Imaging findings. *Int J Endocrinol*. 2020;2020:3146535. https://doi.org/10.1155/2020/3146535. PMID: 32148487; PMCID: PMC7054819.

- Patidar PP, Philip, Rajeev; Toms, Ajit1; Gupta, Keshavkumar. Radiological manifestations of juvenile hypothyroidism. *Thyroid Research and Practice* 9(3):102–104, Sep–Dec 2012. | https://doi.org/10.4103/0973–0354.99660

- Wukich DK, Schaper NC, Gooday C, Bal A, Bem R, Chhabra A, Hastings M, Holmes C, Petrova NL, Santini Araujo MG, Senneville E, Raspovic KM. Guidelines on the diagnosis and treatment of active Charcot neuro-osteoarthropathy in persons with diabetes mellitus (IWGDF 2023). *Diabetes Metab Res Rev.* 2024 Mar;40(3):e3646. https://doi.org/10.1002/dmrr.3646. Epub 2023 May 23. PMID: 37218537.

- Yang C, Tandon A. A pictorial review of diabetic foot maifestations. *Med J Malayasia*.2013 Jun;68(3):279–89. PMID:23749027

SBA QUESTIONS

1) A 50-year-old male presents with back pain for a check-up. Radiographs of the pelvis show a lytic sclerotic lesion in the right iliac bone with cortical thickening and expansion. What is the most likely diagnosis?

   A. Fluorosis

   B. Metastasis

   C. Paget's disease

   D. Requires further evaluation with MRI

   E. Osteoid osteoma

2) A 21-year-old female presented with low back pain, which aggravated over the last 6 months. On evaluation, blood investigation showed an elevated alkaline phosphatase of 1500 IU/L, and a PTH of 1800 pg/mL. Which investigation would you perform next?

   A. MRI lumbosacral spine

   B. CECT neck

   C. Sestamibi scan

   D. USG neck

   E. MRI neck

3) A 70-year-old male with uncontrolled diabetes presented with low back pain, and thigh pain. Radiographs showed few fractures along the pubic rami and medial femoral neck. Few lytic lesions were also seen in the left iliac wing, and in the left proximal femur. What is the most likely diagnosis?

   A. Metastasis with pathological fractures

   B. Paget's disease (lytic phase)

   C. Secondary hyperparathyroidism from chronic renal failure

   D. Primary hyperparathyroidism

   E. Osteoporosis

4) A middle-aged male from India came for a routine evaluation. Radiographs show diffuse osteosclerosis with flowing osteophytes in the cervical spine, ossification of the posterior longitudinal ligament, and entheseal attachments in pelvic radiographs. Forearm radiographs also showed interosseous membrane ossification. What is the most likely diagnosis?

   A. DISH

   B. OPLL

   C. Ankylosing spondylitis

   D. Fluorosis

   E. Age-related degenerative changes

5) A 4-year-old child who was born prematurely and on long-term formula feeds presented with bowing of legs. Radiographs showed a widened growth plate, with flaring of metaphysis. What is the most likely diagnosis?

   A. Blount's disease

   B. Scurvy

   C. Rickets

   D. Hyperparathyroidism

   E. Infantile hypothyroidism (cretinism)

6) A 60-year-old woman presented with generalised body pain and fatigue. Radiographs of the spine and pelvis showed new-onset osteomalacia with multiple insufficiency fractures in the pelvis. On evaluation, she was found to have hypophosphatemia. Workup of vitamin D deficiency/resistance, renal tubular acidosis, and malabsorption were negative. What would you like to suggest next?

   A. Suggest calcium, vitamin D, and phosphate supplementation and follow-up

   B. Advise bone densitometry

   C. Nuclear scintigraphy

   D. Reassurance and follow-up

   E. Contrast-enhanced CT scan of the chest, abdomen, and pelvis

7) A 35-year-old male with many years of multiple joint pain presented with swellings of the distal leg near the heel bilaterally. USG showed a ruptured Achilles tendon bilaterally. Radiographs showed significant osteoporosis and arthritic changes. Spine radiographs also showed osteoporosis with intervertebral disc calcifications. What investigation would you like to do next?

   A. Serum uric acid

   B. DECT

   C. Serum/blood homogentisic acid

   D. MRI sacroiliac joints

   E. MRI whole spine and sacroiliac joints

8) In this patient, what is the most likely diagnosis?

   A. Gout or other deposition disease

   B. Ankylosing spondylitis

   C. Achilles tendinopathy

   D. Alkaptonuria

   E. Phenylketonuria

9) A 40-year-old diabetic woman who had undergone total thyroidectomy for a large goiter 5 months ago presented with seizures. CT scans showed few intracranial calcifications and vault thickening. Recent limb radiographs, which were taken for other indications, showed osteosclerosis and metaphyseal bands. What would you like to do next?

   A. Assess serum glucose levels

   B. USG kidneys to assess for chronic kidney disease

   C. Serum calcium, phosphorous, and PTH levels

   D. Sestamibi/4D CT scan

   E. DEXA scan

10) In the above patient, what is the most likely diagnosis?

    A. Hypoglycemic seizures with chronic anemia, and background Paget's disease

    B. Renal osteodystrophy

    C. Pseudohypoparathyroidism

    D. Hypoparathyroidism

    E. Hypothyroidism

Answers: (1) C, (2) D: To assess for parathyroid adenoma, (3) C, (4) D, (5) C, (6) C, (7) C, (8) D, (9) C, (10) C

Chapter 2.11
Crystal-Related Arthropathies

Sinan Al-Qassab

LEARNING OBJECTIVES

- Understand various crystalline deposition diseases affecting the musculoskeletal system

- Appreciate variety of imaging appearances of common crystalline arthropathies, their mimics and differentials

- Know typical sites affected by various crystal deposition disease

---

INTRODUCTION

Crystal deposition diseases are a spectrum of arthropathies secondary to an inflammatory response triggered by crystal deposition. They can mimic other arthropathies and occasionally may be challenging to diagnose. The most common of these crystal deposition diseases are gout, calcium pyrophosphate dihydrate deposition disease (CPPD or pseudogout), and calcium hydroxyapatite, and these will be discussed with some detail with practical pointers that will aid in achieving a sound and reasonable diagnosis.

GOUT

It is due to articular and periarticular deposition of monosodium urate crystals (MSU) as a result of hyperuricemia. These needle-like and negatively birefringent crystals on polarised light will elicit an inflammatory reaction responsible for the acute attacks.

Demographics

- Far more common in males.

- Peak in the 4th and 5th decades.

- Incidence in women increases following menopause.

- Premenopausal women are thought to be protected by oestrogen and its precursors, which promote urate excretion and protects against membrane lysis.

- May be familial, especially in females.

Aetiology

- Hyperuricemia: Underexcretion (more common) vs overproduction (less common) of uric acid.

- This may be primary due to inborn enzymatic deficiency, as is the case in Lesch–Nyhan syndrome or secondary to other diseases.

Underexcretion	Overproduction
• Chronic kidney disease	• Blood dyscrasia: myeloproliferative disorders, haemolytic anaemia
• Hyperparathyroidism	• Tumour lysis
• Drugs: Diuretics, salicylates	• Psoriasis
• Obesity	• Starvation
• Diabetes	
• Alcoholism	

Tip: Hyperuricemia does not mean gout, and normal uric acid does not exclude it.

Anatomical Sites Involved

- Asymmetric and monoarticular at presentation.

- Polyarticular, uncommon, particularly in women, in chronic disease.

- Lower limbs > upper limbs, smaller joints > larger joints.

DOI: 10.1201/9781003500247-20

- The 1st metatarsophalangeal joint is the commonest involved, approximately 50% at onset.

- Ankles, midfoot joints, and knees are involved early.

- Other joints can be involved including shoulders, hips, and sacroiliac joints.

- Axial involvement is rare.

- **Tendons and bursae usually at areas of dynamic stress such as the tibial insertion of the patellar ligament and Achilles tendon insertion.**

- Gout uncommonly presents to sarcoma MDTs as suspected soft tissue sarcomas. Previous history of hyperuricemia, knowledge of commonly involved sites such as patellar, quadriceps, and Achilles tendons, small joints, and tendon sheaths can clinch the diagnosis.

Clinical Stages of Gout

Asymptomatic hyperuricaemia	Please note that hyperuricaemia does not imply gout.
Acute gouty arthritis	Usually asymmetric monoarticular, classically involving the 1st MTP joint (podagra) with acute sever pain, swelling and redness that usually subsides in 3–10 days. During this phase, serum uric acid may be normal or low with normal or non-specific radiographic appearances of the joint.
Intercritical gout	Asymptomatic period between acute attacks that can last from months to years.
Chronic (tophaceous) gout	Characterised by tophi (Greek: chalk), which are white aggregates of urate in articular and periarticular tissues favouring areas of repetitive mechanical stresses and extensor surfaces. Tophi may demonstrate faint calcification; however, dense calcification is atypical and should raise concerns about co-existing conditions such as renal insufficiency and CPPD. Sometimes, gouty tophi can rupture or ulcerate, causing superimposed infection.

Imaging: Radiography
Normal or Non-Specific Appearances

Especially early in the disease. During the acute attack, there may be some soft tissue density, which is reflective of synovitis and effusion; however, this is non-specific and can be seen in other conditions such as trauma, septic arthritis, and other arthritidies.

Characteristic Findings in Chronic Gout

- Tophi: Small tophi are not visualised on plain radiographs. Large tophi may be seen as soft tissue densities. Faint calcification may occur. Dense calcification is atypical and should raise the suspicion of abnormalities in calcium metabolism as in renal insufficiency (Figures 2.11.1 and 2.11.2).

- Erosions: Usually eccentric juxtuarticular in location adjacent to tophi. Classically are rounded or oval, well circumscribed with overhanging margins, juxta-articular, and oriented along the long axis of the bone. They can also be intra-articular or intraosseous, having sclerotic margins and a "punched out" appearance (Figure 2.11.3).

- The joint space is usually well preserved until the advanced stages. Ankylosis is rare.

- Osteopenia is not typical of gout, although periarticular osteopenia may be seen during the acute attack, but this is transient.

- Focal sclerosis, which is thought to be due to calcification in intraosseous tophi. Bone infarcts and enchondromas have similar appearances on radiographs.

- New bone formation: Occasionally, gout may result in enlargement of the ends and shafts of the affected bone, fine periosteal new bone formation, and irregular bone spicules at muscle and tendon insertion sites.

- Bursitis can be seen as soft tissue densities with or without calcification, especially the olecranon and prepatellar bursae (Figure 2.11.4).

- Chondrocalcinosis is controversial and probably suggests co-existing CPPD.

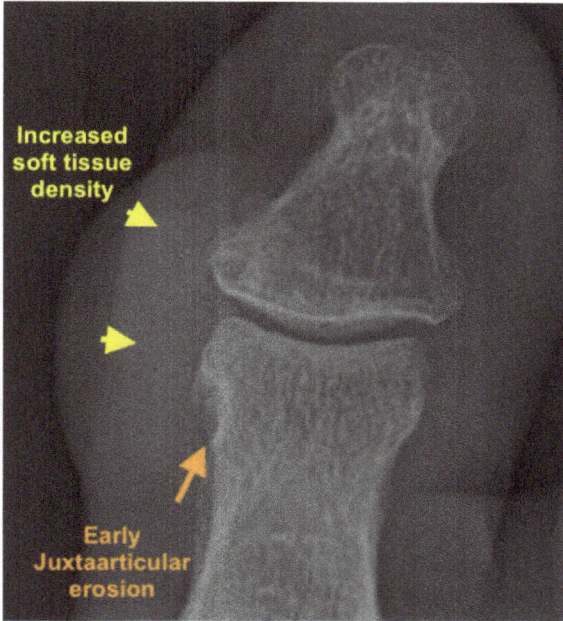

Figure 2.11.1 Early soft tissue gouty tophi on radiograph.

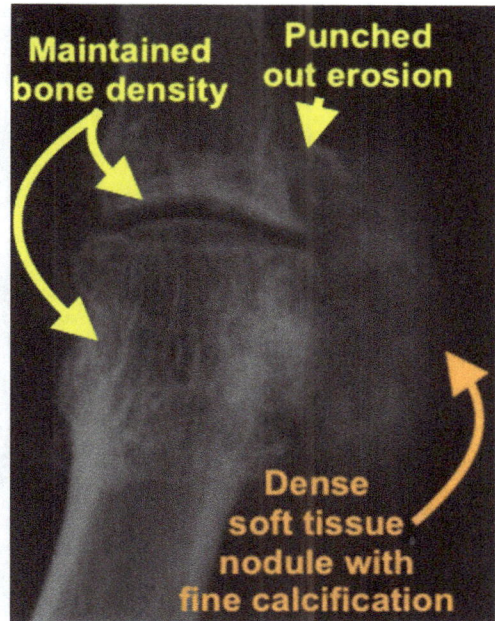

Figure 2.11.2 Dense gouty tophi with erosions and preserve bone density in adjacent bones.

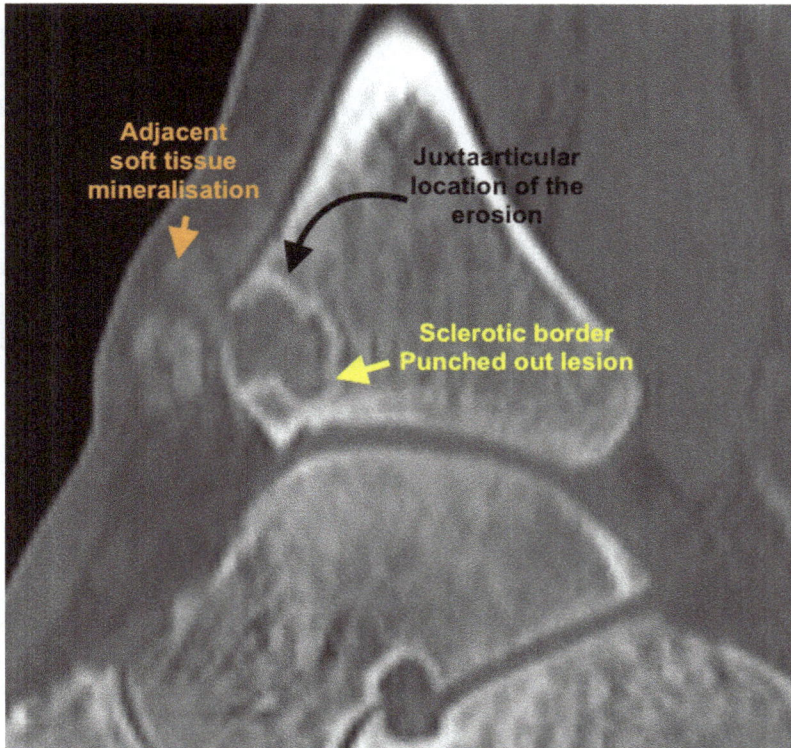

Figure 2.11.3 Erosive gout with adjacent soft tissue calcification on CT.

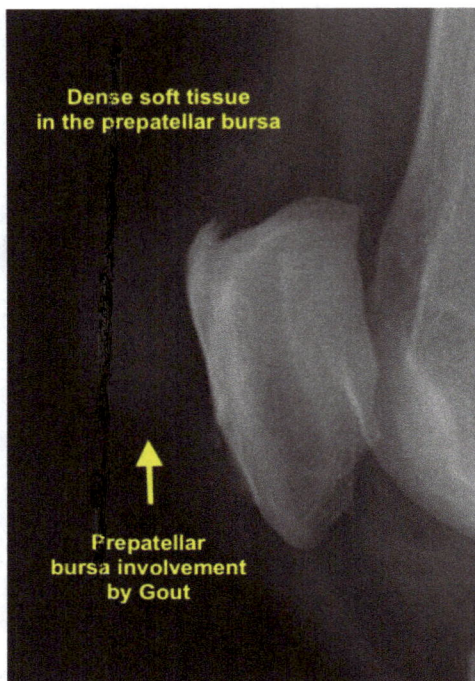

Figure 2.11.4   Gouty tophi in the prepatellar bursa.

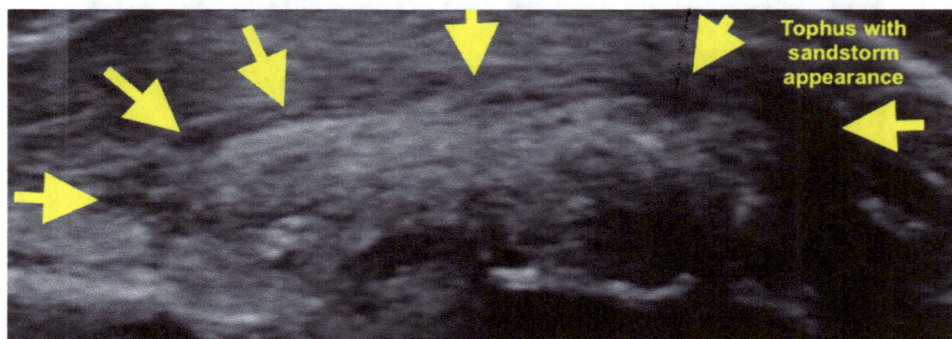

Figure 2.11.5   Sandstorm appearance of a prepatellar soft tissue tophus on ultrasound.

Ultrasound

- Joint effusions, synovitis, and hyperaemia.

- MSU aggregates are strongly reflective to US waves.

- Tophi can be seen as well-defined hyperechogenic lesions. They are less likely to cause "post-acoustic shadowing." They are surrounded by a thin hypoechogenic zone, representing foreign body reaction, which may demonstrate some vascularity on Doppler ultrasound (Figure 2.11.5).

- Microtophi can be seen as tiny hyperechoic foci in a joint effusion, giving the "snowstorm" appearance.

- Double contour sign: Hyperechoic inner line representing cortical bone and a second outer hyperechoic line representing MSU deposition separated by the anechoic articular cartilage.

- US may be used to guide joint aspiration and injection.

CT

- CT is superior in assessing bone architecture and configuration of erosions.

- The emergence of dual-energy CT (DECT) has revolutionised the diagnosis of gout where MSU deposits are depicted on the colour-coded images avoiding the necessity for invasive joint aspiration (Figure 2.11.6). It is the non-invasive imaging of choice.

- Limitations include technical issues when setting the parameters and artefact.

MRI

- MRI is not routinely used to investigate gout.

- When gout is encountered, MRI will show signs of inflammations, synovitis, joint effusion, and erosions.

- When tophi are large enough to visualise, they demonstrate low signal on T1W images and variable signal on T2W (Figure 2.11.7). They have variable contrast enhancement. They can mimic soft tissue sarcoma.

- MRI is also superior in assessment of the marrow.

CALCIUM PYROPHOSPHATE DIHYDRATE DEPOSITION

- CPPD is due to deposition of calcium pyrophosphate dihydrate crystals in cartilage, both hyaline and fibrocartilage, synovium, joint capsule, tendons, and ligaments.

- These crystals will induce an inflammatory reaction that will be responsible for the symptoms and arthritic changes.

- Different terms have been used: Pyrophosphate arthropathy when there are structural joint changes and pseudogout in symptomatic patients. However, this is all academic; they all identify the same pathology.

Epidemiology	Association	Location
• Middle-age and elderly population >50 years • Relatively equal prevalence • Rarely familial, autosomal dominant, early onset with severe disease	• Hyperparathyroidism • Haemochromatosis • Wilson's disease • Gout	• Knees • Wrists • Symphysis pubis • Elbows • Shoulders • Hips • Discovertebral joints

Clinical Presentation

- CPPD is a great mimicker.

- It is a triad: Pain, cartilage calcification, and degenerative joint disease. Pain can be abrupt and severe, mimicking gout, but it is typically milder (hence the term "pseudogout") and can last for weeks to months.

- Mimics septic arthritis, osteoarthritis, rheumatoid arthritis, or any other arthritis. Symptoms can be precipitated by trauma, surgery, or illness.

Cartilage calcification and degenerative changes will be discussed in more detail in the imaging section.

Imaging
Radiography

- Chondrocalcinosis is cartilage calcification which affects both hyaline and fibrocartilage. Hyaline cartilage calcification is seen as a thin line of calcification parallel to the articular cortex, while fibrocartilage calcification, as those seen in the menisci and triangular fibrocartilage in the wrist, appear coarse and irregular (Figures 2.11.8 and 2.11.9).

- Chondrocalcinosis may be absent when there is full-thickness cartilage loss and/or the menisci are severely degenerate or surgically excised, and the same applies to the TFCC.

- Tendon calcification commonly affects the Achilles, triceps, quadriceps, and supraspinatus tendons. It tends to be thin and linear and extends a considerable distance from the insertion, unlike calcium hydroxyapatite crystal deposition disease (CHA), which tends to extend for a shorter distance and tends to be denser and amorphous. Also, CHA does not usually deposit in cartilage except in extreme cases.

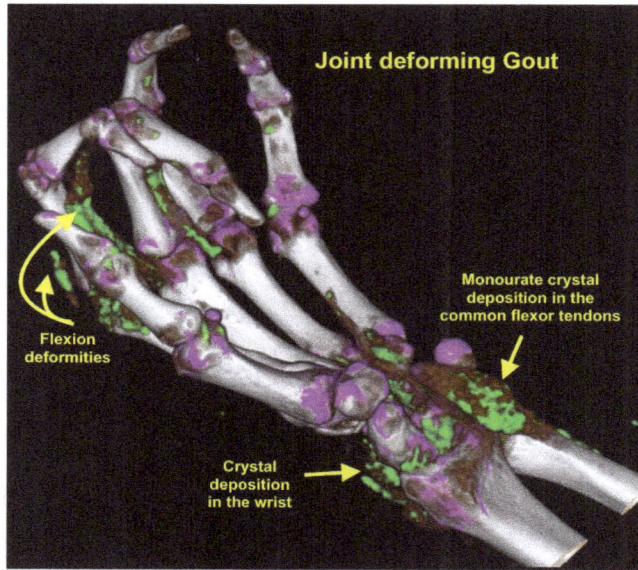

Figure 2.11.6   Joint deforming gout due to crystal deposition in common flexor tendons—utility of DECT.

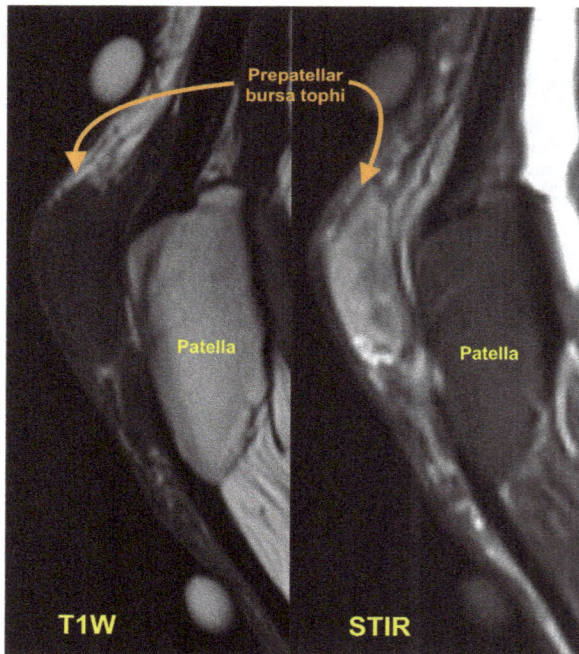

Figure 2.11.7   MRI appearances of the prepatellar soft tissue deposits on T1W and STIR.

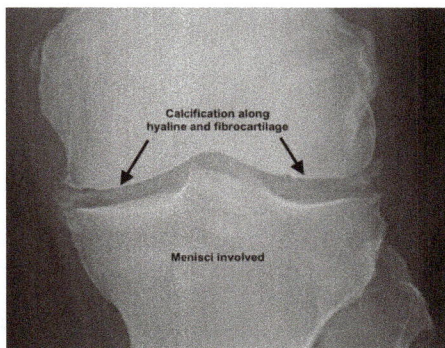

Figure 2.11.8 Chondrocalcinosis/CPPD in the menisci.

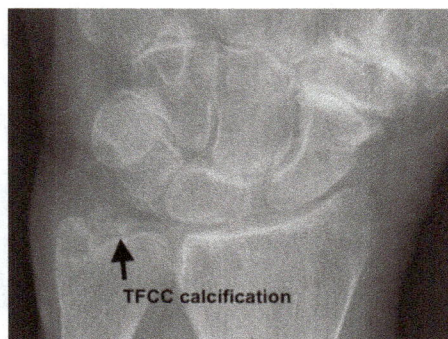

Figure 2.11.9 Chondrocalcinosis in the TFCC and severe degenerative changes in the STTJ and first CMCJ.

- Ligament calcification, particularly in the wrist, resulting in scapholunate advanced collapse (SLAC).

- Degenerative joint changes demonstrate the characteristic features of joint space narrowing, subchondral sclerosis, and cyst and osteophyte formation. However, there are a few indicators that will help distinguish CPPD from osteoarthritis:

  - Distribution: CPPD favours the upper limb and non-weight-bearing joints such as the metacarpophalangeal (particularly 2nd and 3rd), radiocarpal, elbow, and shoulder joints, as well as the patellofemoral joint in the absence of tibiofemoral compartments involvement.

  - Large subchondral cysts (geodes). Large geodes can also be seen in CPPD and psoriatic arthritis.

  - Severe, destructive joint disease which could be rapidly progressive and may mimic neuropathic joints; however, CPPD is usually painful.

  - Variable osteophyte formation despite severe joint space narrowing. Hook osteophytes in the MCP joints.

  - Linear calcification along joint spaces/fibrocartilage.

Ultrasound

- Ultrasound can present non-specific findings of joint effusion, synovitis, and guides with intervention.

- Tendon and ligament calcification can appear as focal hyperechoic areas with posterior acoustic shadowing.

CT

- CT is useful in depicting subtle calcification.

- It is particularly valuable in the spine where it is superior in demonstrating calcification in the retro-odantoid soft tissue, which results in retro-odantoid pseudotumour as well as calcification in the intervertebral disc and ligamentum flavum. Calcification around the odontoid process is termed "crowned dens" (Figure 2.11.10).

- It can also assess the degree of discovertebral degeneration.

MRI Is Least Useful for CPPD

- Chondrocalcinosis can be difficult to appreciate on MRI given that calcification and menisci, tendons, and ligaments demonstrate low signal on all sequences.

- MRI will show other features such as joint effusions, synovitis, erosions, and marrow oedema.

- MRI may show inflammatory changes in the spine, but the presence of disc or ligamentous calcification should draw the attention to the possibility of CPPD.

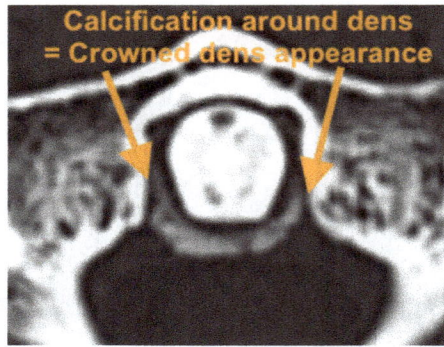

Figure 2.11.10 Crowned dens appearance on CT due to calcification of the transverse ligament of the atlas around the dens.

CALCIUM HYDROXYAPATITE DEPOSITION DISEASE

- Deposition of calcium hydroxyapatite crystals in periarticular and articular tissue. The most widely accepted theory is that it is secondary to focal degeneration, resulting in ischaemia that leads to tendinous tears and calcium deposition.

- HADD usually affects tendons and bursae around the joint.

- Different terms have been used including calcific tendinitis, calcific periarthritis, peritendinitis, and periarthritis calcarea.

Epidemiology	Association	Location
• Between 40 and 70 years • Relatively equal incidence between males and females • May be familial	• Trauma • Renal osteodystrophy • Collagen vascular disease • Multiple intra-articular steroid injections	• Shoulder: Most commonly affecting the supraspinatus tendon • Spine: Most commonly affecting the longus colli muscle. Less frequently intervertebral discs • Wrist: Extensor carpi ulnaris • Hips: Gluteal muscle insertion • Elbow: Triceps tendon and collateral ligaments

Clinical Presentation

- Patients may be asymptomatic.

- Some might present acutely with pain, swelling, and reduced range of movement. This is thought to be due to dissolvement of the calcium hydroxyapatite crystals (breakdown phase) rather than their deposition (formation phase).

- In cases of longus colli involvement, patients may have neck stiffness, pain on swallowing, and a sensation of globus hystericus.

- Symptoms might be chronic.

- It is important to note that the radiographic features do not correspond to the severity of clinical symptoms.

Imaging
Radiography

- Periarticular calcification is usually seen in tendons and bursae around the joints. The shoulder is the most affected joint, with the supraspinatus tendon being most commonly involved. The calcification usually extends for a short distance from the tendon insertion and is not continuous with the cortex. The calcification is amorphous or fluffy, well-circumscribed later in the course of the disease, and may be rounded, nodular, or curvilinear. It may be difficult to differentiate between supraspinatus tendon calcification and subacromial bursa calcification (Figure 2.11.11). The size and morphology of the calcification may change with time and may even completely resolve.

■ Adjacent bone: The adjacent bone is usually normal, but occasional erosions, sclerosis, and cysts have been described.

■ Intra-articular deposition of hydroxyapatite crystals may not be visible on radiographs. Articular involvement usually presents as osteoarthritis.

■ Milwaukee shoulder syndrome is a destructive arthropathy of the glenohumeral joint due to intra-articular HADD. It is more commonly seen in women over 50. It demonstrates severe loss of joint space, erosions, and subchondral sclerosis. Osteophytes are not prominent. It is usually associated with a large joint effusion and calcific debris within. There is superior subluxation of the humeral head due to rotator cuff tears, resulting in impaction and remodelling of the acromion (Figure 2.11.12). Despite the destructive radiological appearance, the clinical symptoms are mild.

■ Longus colli calcification can be seen as amorphous calcification on the lateral neck radiograph projecting anterior and inferior to the anterior tubercle of the atlas. There may also be widening of the retrophalangeal space.

Ultrasound

■ Ultrasound may demonstrate tendon and bursal calcifications as hyperechoic foci with posterior acoustic shadowing.

■ Ultrasound is also used to guide interventional procedures such as steroid injections and barbotage (described in detail in Chapter 2.15).

CT

■ CT is valuable in detecting small and faint calcification as well as in cases of challenging anatomy as in longus colli calcification.

■ It can also assess the degree of joint destruction and presence of calcific debris in Milwaukee shoulder.

MRI

■ On MRI, calcification is seen as foci of low signal on all sequences.

■ MRI may also show additional ancillary features such as rotator cuff tears, synovitis, joint effusions, and soft tissue oedema in case of longus colli calcification.

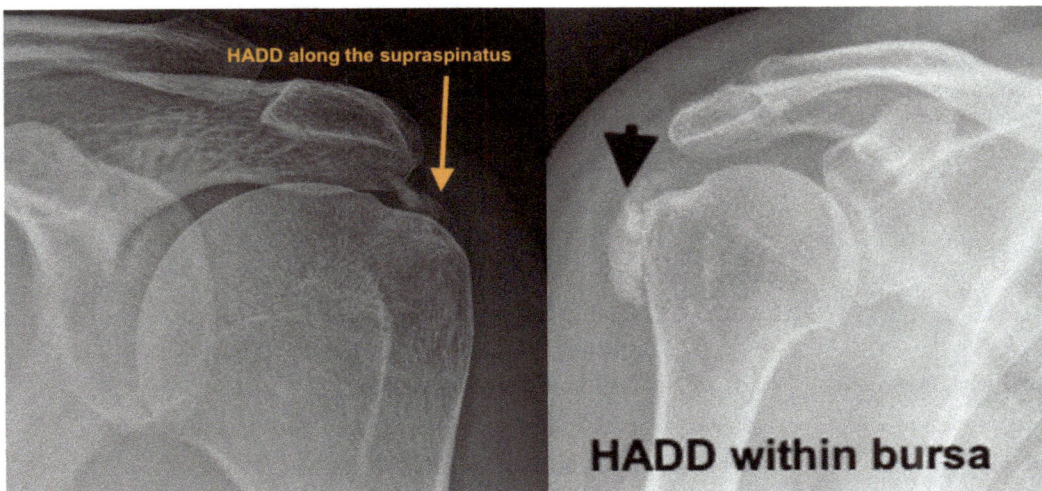

Figure 2.11.11 Hydroxyapatite crystal deposition along the supraspinatus tendon and in the subacromial bursa.

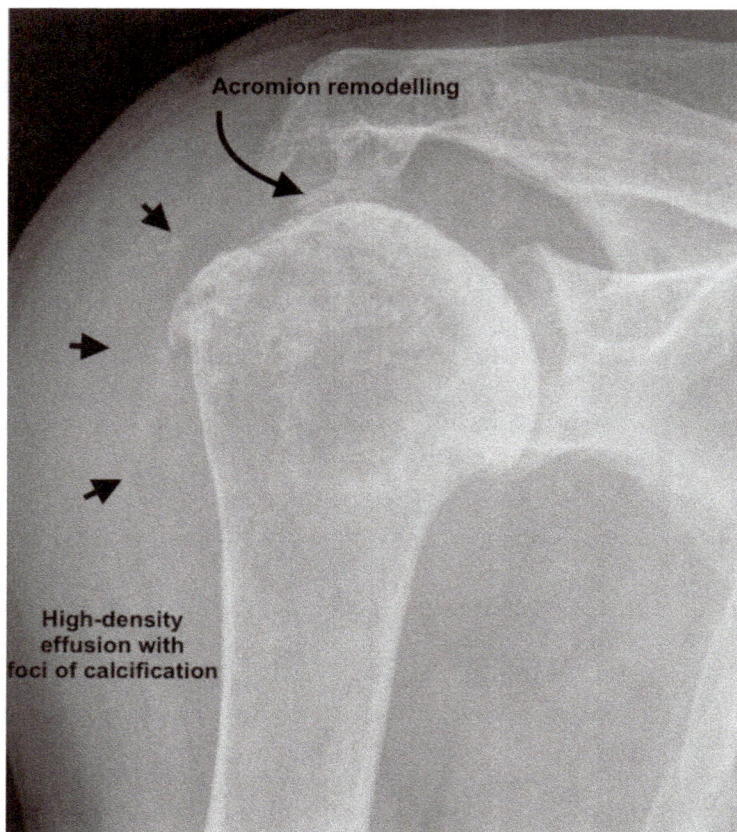

Figure 2.11.12 Intra-articular deposition of hydroxyapatite crystal (Milwaukee shoulder) causing severe loss of glenohumeral joint space, large joint effusion, and calcific debris within the joint. Note the lack of osteophyte formation and erosive changes in the acromion.

OCHRONOSIS

Ochronosis is a rare autosomal recessive metabolic disease due to deficiency of homogentisic acid oxidase resulting in urinary excretion of homogentisic acid and tissue deposition.

Epidemiology	Location
• Familial: Autosomal recessive • Seen in the 3rd and 4th decades • More common in males (2:1)	• Spine • Hips • Shoulders • Knees

Clinical Presentation

■ Usually asymptomatic till adult life but could be identified earlier.

■ Patients present with progressive pain and stiffness in the spine, shoulders, and hips.

■ Pain may resemble that of ankylosing spondylitis but usually less severe.

Imaging Appearance

- The spine is the most commonly affected location particularly in the lumbar and thoracic spine with intervertebral disc calcification, which is usually thin and parallel to the endplate, reduction in disc height, subchondral sclerosis, and cyst and small osteophyte formation.

- Eventually, this may result in ankylosis of the spine; however, unlike ankylosing spondylitis, there is reduction in disc height and there is no evidence of sacroiliitis.

- Calcification may also be seen in soft tissues including tendons, bursae, and menisci.

OTHER FAR LESS COMMON CRYSTAL DEPOSITION DISEASES INCLUDE

- Cholesterol deposition in rheumatoid arthritis and osteoarthritis

- Xanthine

- Cysteine

- Oxalosis

- Lysophospholipase (Charcot–Leyden)

CONCLUSION

Crystal deposition arthropathy is commonly encountered in routine medical practice. Occasionally, the imaging findings are incidental in asymptomatic patients, while some symptomatic patients may have normal imaging early in the course of the disease. Radiographs remain the main and initial imaging modality capable of providing confident diagnosis. However, occasionally the diagnosis is not clear, such as the case with some tophi where they might be mistaken for soft tissue tumours, intraosseous tophi mistaken for lytic bone lesions, or the arthropathy might mimic other joint diseases. Knowledge of the location, distribution, and imaging findings of individual crystal deposition disease is essential in achieving the diagnosis. Dual-energy CT has had a major impact in the diagnosis of gout and reduced the need for invasive procedures. Other imaging modalities may help as problem solvers or in cases of difficult anatomy. Occasionally, biopsy is required to rule out neoplastic lesions or infection.

SUGGESTED READING

- Radiological manifestations of the crystal related arthropathies. Daniel S Uri, William Martel. *Seminars in Roentgenology*, Volume 31, Issue 3, July 1996, 229–238

- Imaging in the crystal arthropathies. McQueen, Fiona M. et al. *Rheumatic Disease Clinics*, Volume 40, Issue 2, 2014, 231–249

- Imaging features of crystal-induced arthropathy. *Choi, Marc H. et al. Rheumatic Disease Clinics*, Volume 32, Issue 2, 2006, 427–446

SBA QUESTIONS

1) Which of the following statements is **true** regarding gout?

   A. Hyperuricaemia is essential to the diagnosis.

   B. Normal serum uric acid excludes gout.

   C. Erosions are seen early in the disease.

   D. Dense calcification is typical in tophi.

   E. The joint space is usually preserved until the advanced stages.

2) Which of the following is most suggestive of CPPD?

A. Tendon calcification

B. Chondrocalcinosis

C. Degenerative changes

D. Erosions

E. Tophi

3) Which of the following is **not true** regarding CHA?

A. Calcific tendinitis most commonly affects the supraspinatus tendon.

B. Calcification extends a long distance from the tendon insertion.

C. Calcific tendinitis affects gluteal muscle insertions.

D. Longus colli muscle involvement is common in the spine.

E. Milwaukee shoulder is a destructive form of the disease, most commonly seen in women.

Answers: (1) E, (2) B, (3) B

Chapter 2.12
Rheumatoid Arthritis and Multisystem Connective Tissue Diseases

Zoe Winston, Harun Gupta, and Michelle Ooi

LEARNING OBJECTIVES

- Understand radiological appearance of rheumatoid arthritis (RA) and other arthritidies
- Key differences in imaging findings between common inflammatory arthritidies

---

INTRODUCTION

Connective tissue diseases (CTDs) are a group of systemic autoimmune disorders characterised by chronic inflammation of the connective tissue containing collagen and elastin. This chapter will provide an overview of common CTDs with a focus on radiological musculoskeletal manifestations of rheumatoid arthritis (RA), seronegative CTDs (ankylosing spondylitis, psoriatic arthritis, reactive arthritis, and enteropathic arthritis), scleroderma, systemic lupus erythematosus, Sjögren syndrome, mixed CTD, and idiopathic inflammatory myopathies (dermatomyositis and inclusion body myositis).

RHEUMATOID ARTHRITIS

- Autoimmune symmetrical arthropathy (70% Rh factor +ve, 80% anti-CCP +ve).

- Synovium is the primary site of inflammation, with a predilection for the proximal joints of the hands (wrist, MCP, and PIP joints) and feet (MTP and PIP joints). The DIP joints tend to be spared. Small joints are involved in a variety of arthritidies (Figure 2.12.1) with diverse imaging appearances. The primary challenge for the radiologist is to differentiate inflammatory from non-inflammatory arthritis.

- Early signs include synovitis, tenosynovitis (extensor carpi ulnaris is usually first to be involved), periarticular osteopenia (usually predates erosion), and soft tissue swelling.

- Late signs (Figure 2.12.2) include marginal erosions (as a result of the synovitis), ulnar styloid erosion, uniform joint space narrowing, and symmetrical joint subluxation (boutonniere, swan neck ulnar subluxation at MCPJs, hitchhiker's thumb).

- Bone proliferation is **not** a feature.

- In the cervical spine, RA can result in atlantoaxial subluxation (Figure 2.12.3) as well as odontoid peg erosions with associated cervical myelopathy (Figure 2.12.4). Figure 2.12.5 shows an inflamed pannus.

- Peripheral nervous system involvement occurs in 30% of patients with RA, either secondary to nerve entrapment (carpal tunnel syndrome is the most common) or non-compressive neuropathies due to small vessel vasculitis (i.e. mononeuritis multiplex).

- Systemic manifestations of RA occur in 40% of patients.

- Pulmonary manifestations include rheumatoid nodules and pulmonary fibrosis (more commonly UIP pattern).

- Caplan syndrome (a.k.a. rheumatoid pneumoconiosis), characterised by the combination of pneumoconiosis (upper lobe predominant fibrosis) and RA.

- Felty's syndrome (characterised by RA, splenomegaly, and neutropenia) is rare and usually occurs in those with severe, long-standing RA with evidence of erosive disease.

DOI: 10.1201/9781003500247-21

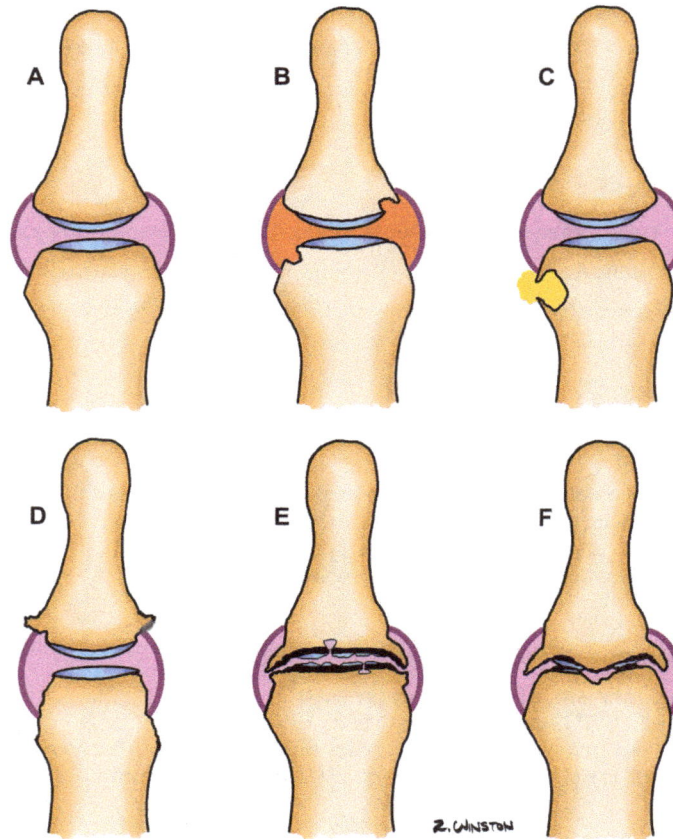

Figure 2.12.1 Illustration demonstrating erosions in various arthropathies in a distal interphalangeal joint (DIPJ) of the hand.

- **A**—Normal DIPJ with joint capsule (dark purple), synovial fluid (light purple), joint cartilage (blue).

- **B**—Rheumatoid arthritis with inflammatory pannus (orange), periarticular osteopenia, and marginal erosions in the bare areas adjacent to cartilage.

- **C**—Gout with an extra-articular erosion and soft tissue formation (yellow).

- **D**—Psoriatic arthritis with periarticular bone proliferation, enthesitis (grey), and erosions at tendonous insertions, resulting in a characteristic "pencil-in-cup" deformity.

- **E**—Osteoarthritis with articular cartilage damage, osteophytes, subchondral sclerosis, subchondral cyst formation, and joint space loss.

- **F**—Erosive osteoarthritis with central erosions, cartilage damage, joint space loss, and osteophyte formation resulting in a characteristic "gull-wing" deformity.

- Cardiovascular disease is the leading cause of death in patients with RA. Cardiovascular manifestations include an increased risk of cardiovascular disease, heart failure associated with pericarditis, myocarditis, and amyloidosis.

- In the weight-bearing hip joints, it can manifest as concentric joint space narrowing (Figure 2.12.6) in contrast to osteoarthritis where joint space narrowing occurs eccentrically (superior or medial joint space narrowing).

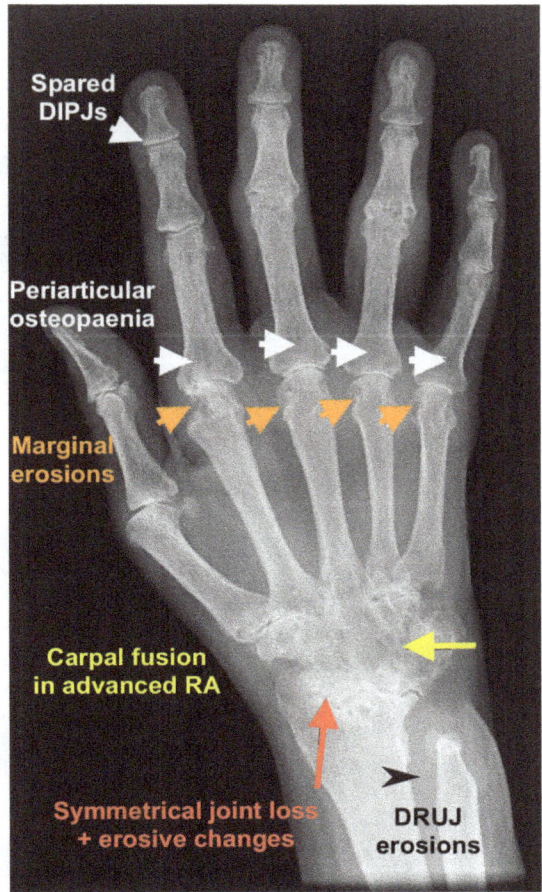

Figure 2.12.2 X-ray features of advanced rheumatoid arthritis affecting hand and wrist.

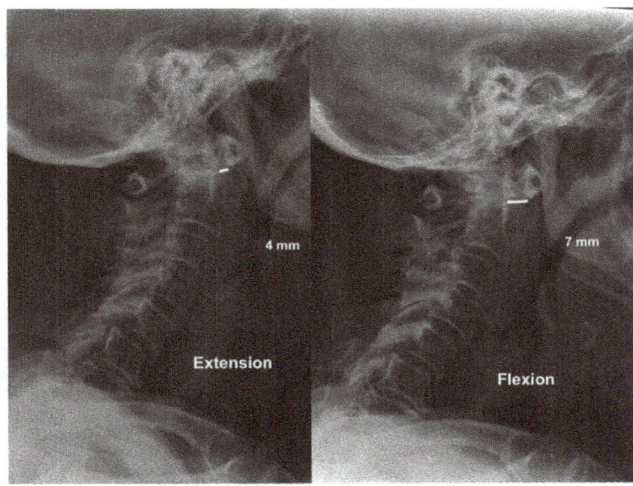

Figure 2.12.3 Atlantoaxial instability in rheumatoid arthritis on lateral X-rays of the cervical spine in extension and flexion showing increased predental space/anterior atlantoaxial interval.

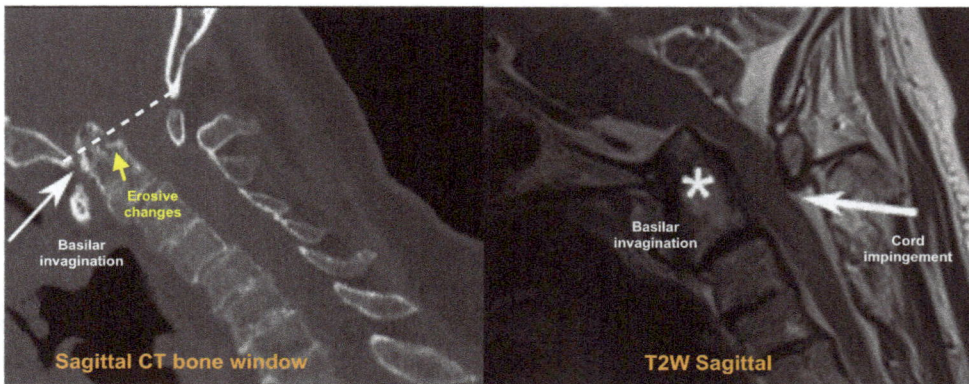

Figure 2.12.4   CT and MRI images showing basilar invagination causing narrowing of foramen magnum and cord impingement.

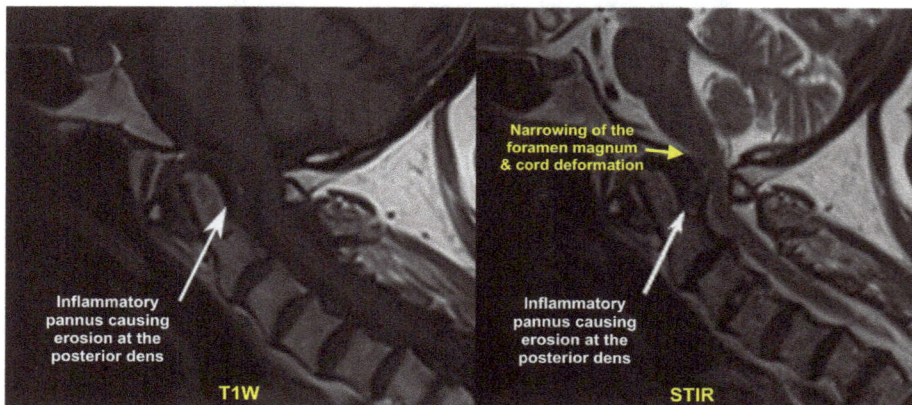

Figure 2.12.5   Inflammatory pannus resulting in severe canal stenosis and distortion of the cord contour.

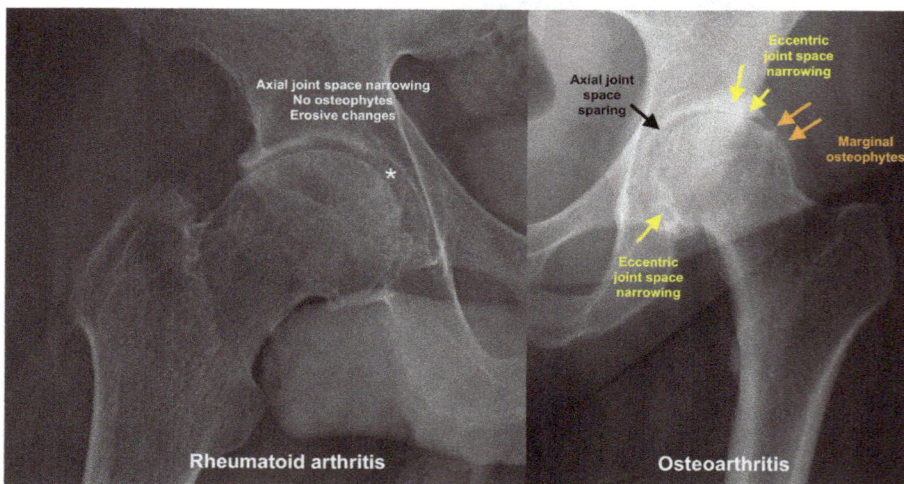

Figure 2.12.6   Radiographic features of rheumatoid arthritis versus osteoarthritis.

SERONEGATIVE CONNECTIVE TISSUE DISEASE

- Rheumatoid factor negative (seronegative)

- Broadly divided into four inflammatory arthropathies: Ankylosing spondylitis, psoriatic arthritis (PsA), reactive arthritis, and enteropathic arthritis

- May have similar appearances on imaging, all with a predisposition for the sacroiliac joint with iliac involvement usually predating the sacral involvement

- Associated with HLA-B27 gene

Detailed imaging features, criteria, and imaging assessment for axial and peripheral spondyloarthritis are discussed in Chapter 2.13. In this chapter, we will briefly describe features of seronegative spondyloarthritis, which will be complementary to the following chapter.

ANKYLOSING SPONDYLITIS

- Up to 90% of those with AS are positive for HLA-B27 gene

- 1%–2% of those with HLA B27 gene will develop AS

Vertebral body changes include Romanus lesions (vertebral body corner erosions), "shiny corners" (reactive sclerosis of the vertebral body corner erosions, appearing sclerotic on X-ray/CT and high T1/T2 signal on MR), "bamboo spine" (ankylosis with flowing syndesmophytes adjacent to vertebral bodies), syndesmophytes prone to fractures with minimal trauma ("carrot stick" fractures), "dagger sign" on frontal radiograph (calcification of the interspinous ligaments secondary to enthesitis), "trolley-track sign" (ossification of the apophyseal joint capsule appears as lateral vertical lines on frontal radiography) (Figure 2.12.7), and Andersson lesion (central vertebral body endplate erosions) are seen late in the disease process.

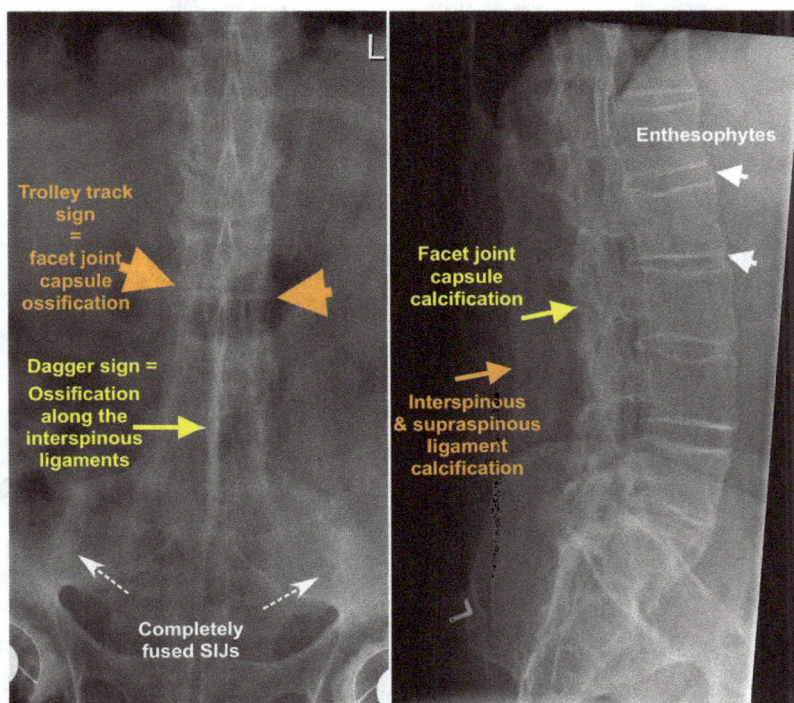

Figure 2.12.7   Radiographic features of chronic ankylosing spondylitis and important radiographic signs.

- CT is recommended for assessment in advanced ankylosing spondylitis and pain following even minor trauma due to risk of carrot stick fracture, which is unstable.

- Bilateral symmetrical sacroiliitis is a characteristic feature. MRI is the investigation of choice to detect and stage sacroiliitis. The most recent classification separates sacroiliac joint features into inflammatory (marrow oedema) and structural lesions (erosions, periarticular fatty metaplasia, bony bridging, and ankylosis) (Figure 2.12.8). MRI is also helpful in identifying the disease activity, which helps adjusting the medical therapy (Figure 2.12.9).

- Hips are the most common joint involved outside of the axial skeleton. Pelvic and spinal enthesitis are pathonomic features of seronegative spondyloarthritis (Figures 2.12.10 and 2.12.11).

- Extra-articular manifestation includes apical predominant interstitial lung disease, acute anterior uveitis, and cardiac abnormalities/aortic valve disease/heart block.

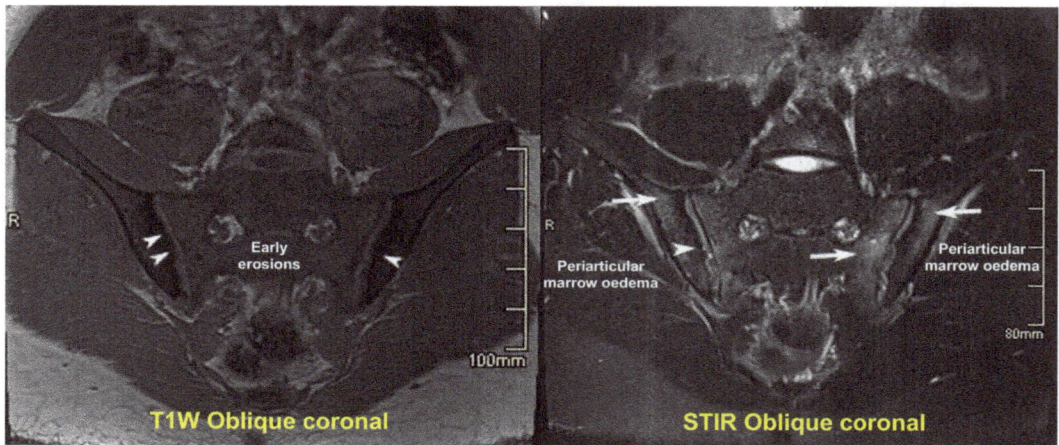

Figure 2.12.8 MRI features of bilateral acute sacroiliitis in a patient with ankylosing spondylitis.

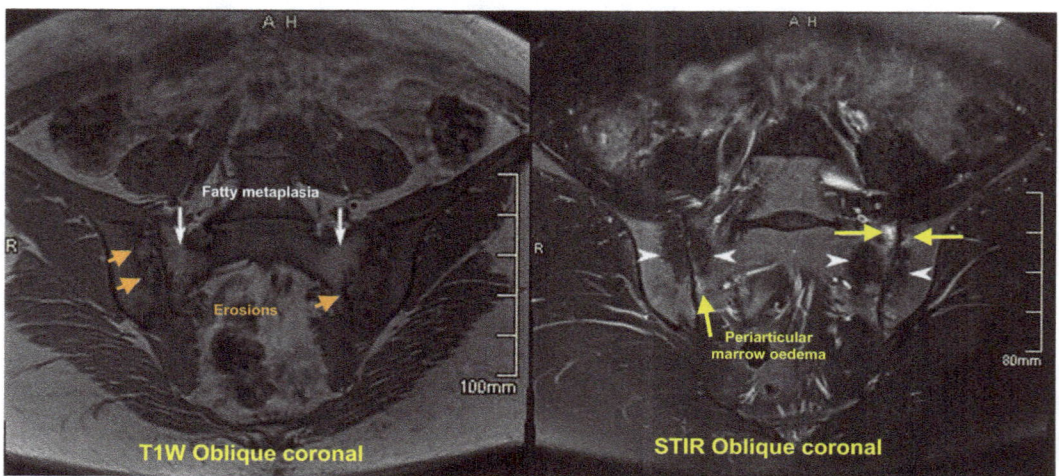

Figure 2.12.9 MRI showing features of acute-on-chronic sacroiliitis secondary to ankylosing spondylitis.

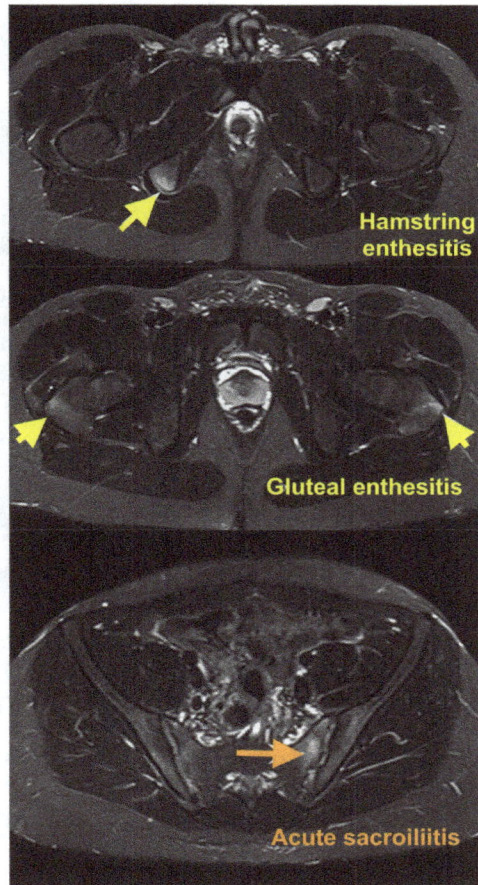

Figure 2.12.10 Pelvic MRI axial images showing right hamstring origin enthesitis, bilateral gluteal enthesitis, and left acute sacroiliitis.

PSORIATIC ARTHRITIS (PsA)

- Chronic inflammatory disease, affecting up to 40% of patients with psoriasis, most commonly involving the hands with skin/nail changes predating the arthropathy.

- Entheses (point of tendon/ligamentous insertion) are the primary site of inflammation, with secondary spread to the synovium, in contrast to rheumatoid arthritis where the inflammation begins in the synovium

- Multiple distributions: Oligoarticular <4 joints, asymmetric; polyarticular >5 joints and symmetrical (similar to RhA); distal (DIPJs only); axial (spine/SIJs).

- Imaging features include asymmetrical SIJ involvement, acro-osteolysis, periosteal bone proliferation, and in advanced cases, ankylosis.

- Unlike RhA, periarticular osteopenia is **not** a feature of PsA.

- Radiographic signs of PsA include pencil-in-cup deformity (central erosions), marginal erosions with new bone formation (mouse ears) (Figure 2.12.12), periosteal new bone proliferation ("fuzzy" or "whiskering" appearance) (Figure 2.12.13) and ivory phalanx (increased density of the entire phalanx), which has a high specificity for PsA.

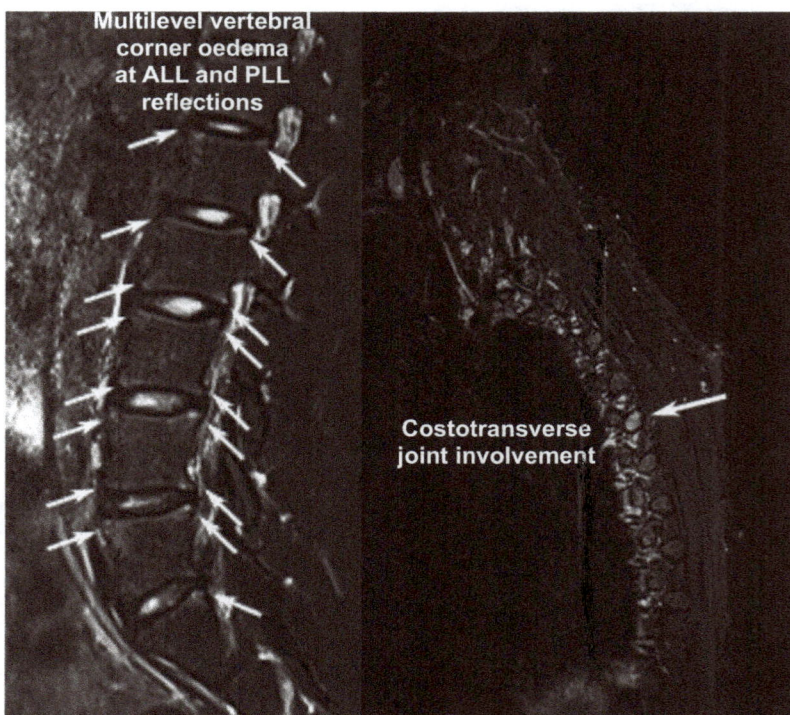

Figure 2.12.11 Vertebral corner oedema and costotransverse oedema on STIR image in a patient with ankylosing spondylitis.

REACTIVE ARTHRITIS

- Sterile inflammatory arthropathy, with a typical onset 1–4 weeks following urogenital or enteric infection, most commonly *Salmonella, Shigella, Campylobacter,* and *Chlamydia*

- Associated with urethritis and conjunctivitis.

- 60%–90% of patients with reactive arthritis are HLA-B27 positive.

- Affects males more than females, most commonly ages 25–30.

- Early changes include soft tissue swelling and periarticular osteopenia.

- Oligoarthritis more commonly affecting the lower extremities, classically the feet with calcaneal involvement. The upper extremities and hands are less often involved; however, when this occurs, the interphalangeal (IPJ) and metatarsophalangeal (MTPJ) joints can be affected.

- Imaging features are similar to that of psoriatic arthritis, including soft tissue swelling ("sausage digit"), asymmetrical sacroiliitis, enthesitis leading to marginal erosions, periostitis, and bone proliferation.

ENTEROPATHIC ARTHRITIS

- Spondyloarthropathy is the most frequent extra-intestinal manifestation of inflammatory bowel disease (IBD), occurring in approximately 20%–50% of those with IBD.

- In the axial skeleton, bilateral and symmetrical sacroiliitis is the most common finding and patients may be asymptomatic. Early features include joint space pseudo-widening with cortical erosions, sclerosis and ankylosis later in the disease process. Spondylitis presents with similar radiological findings to AS in advanced disease. HLA-B27 is associated with the progression to AS (Figure 2.12.14).

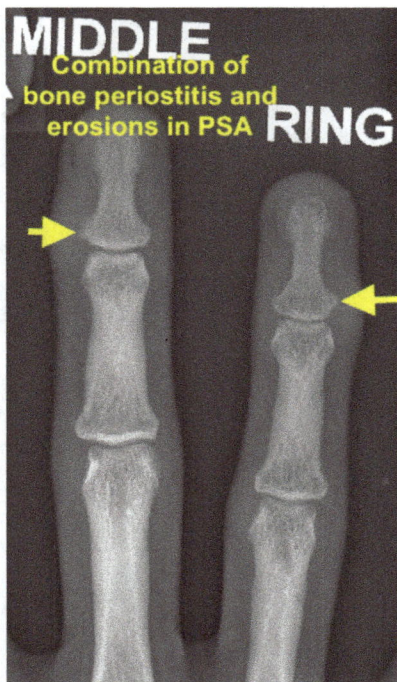

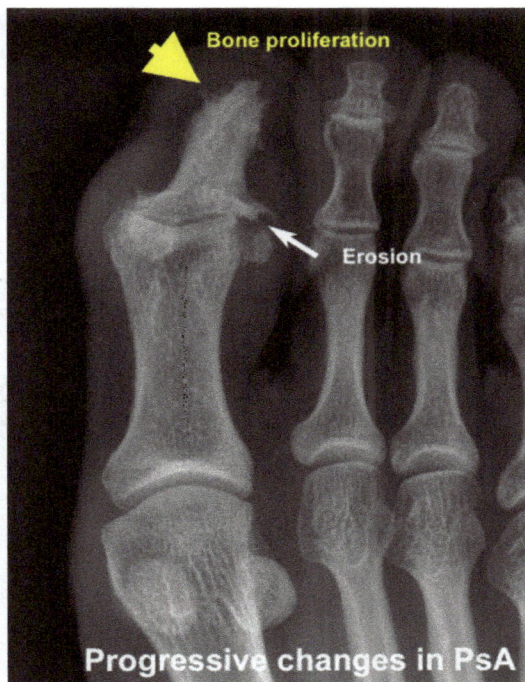

Figure 2.12.12 Radiographic features of psoriatic arthritis with bone proliferation (periostitis) and erosions affecting DIPJs.

Figure 2.12.13 Progressive radiographic features of psoriatic arthritis in the great toe distal phalanx.

- There are two main subtypes of peripheral joint involvement in enteropathic arthritis. Type 1 involves fewer than 5 joints, is acute and associated with IBD flares and other extra-intestinal manifestations of IBD. Type 2 is polyarticular (>5 joints), chronic, independent from IBD flares, and not associated with extra-intestinal manifestations of IBD.

- Enthesitis occurs in up to 50% of patients with IBD, most commonly at the Achilles insertion onto the calcaneum.

SCLERODERMA

- Scleroderma, otherwise known as systemic sclerosis, is a multisystem connective tissue disease with abnormal collagen deposition, small vessel vasculopathy, and organ fibrosis. There are two forms, limited and diffuse cutaneous scleroderma. The limited form is associated with CREST syndrome.

- Musculoskeletal involvement in between 10% and 60% of patients, characteristically involves the hands. Radiological findings in the hands include skin thinning, sclerodactyly, acro-osteolysis ("sharpened pencil" sign, thought to be secondary to vascular involvement/chronic inflammation), MCP/DIP joint erosions, digital ulceration, dystrophic soft tissue calcification (subcutaneous and periarticular), and flexion contractures. Other sites of bone resorption include the mandible, clavicle, ribs, radius, and ulna (Figure 2.12.15).

- Other systems commonly involved include thoracic (NSIP type interstitial lung disease, pulmonary hypertension being the most common cause of death), gastrointestinal (loss of oesophageal motility with a patulous oesophagus (Figure 2.12.16), "hidebound" small bowel appearance and antimesenteric pseudosacculation), small vessel pruning and telangiectasia.

217

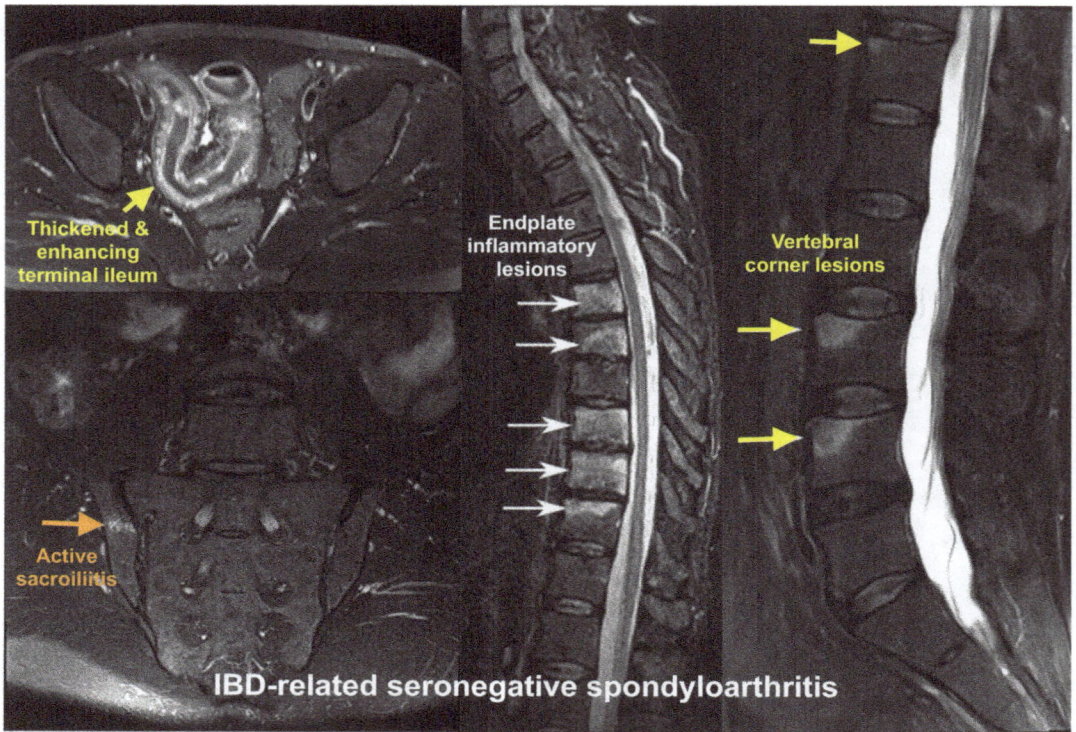

Figure 2.12.14 MRI features IBD-related seronegative spondyloarthritis—terminal ileitis, acute sacroiliitis, endplate-related (Andersson's lesions), and vertebral corner inflammatory lesions.

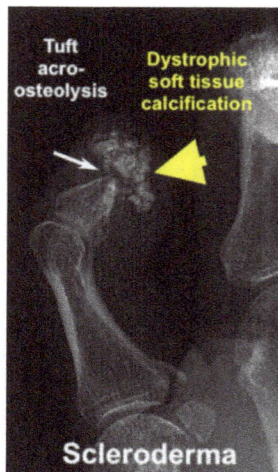

Figure 2.12.15 Radiographic features of scleroderma affecting the thumb in the form of dystrophic soft tissue calcification and tuft acro-osteolysis.

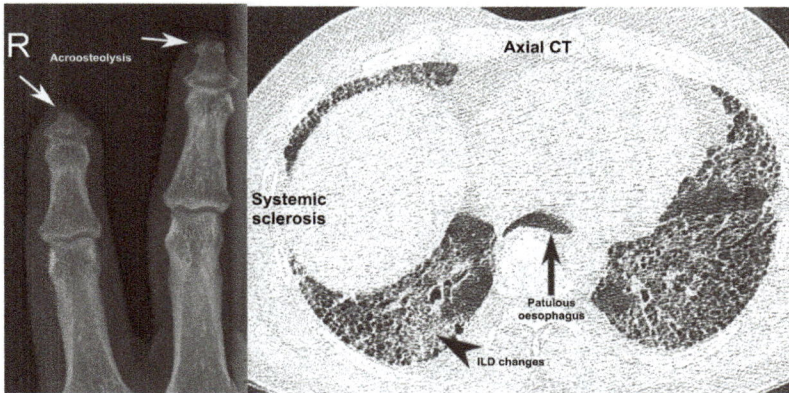

Figure 2.12.16 Systemic involvement in scleroderma presenting with acro-osteolysis (fingers), interstitial lung disease, and patulous oesophagus.

SYSTEMIC LUPUS ERYTHEMATOSUS (SLE)

- SLE is a chronic multisystem autoimmune disease, classically affecting women in their 2nd to 4th decades.

- Antinuclear antibody (ANA) positive in >95% patients (although less specific), double-stranded DNA and anti-Smith antibodies are more specific for SLE.

- Musculoskeletal involvement is seen in up to 90% of cases, most commonly affecting the small joints of hands and wrists as well as knees and shoulders. Osteonecrosis occurs in up to 15% of cases and can be multifocal, most commonly in the knees or hips.

- Three phenotypes:

  - Non-deforming and non-erosive (most common, usually a bilateral, symmetrical polyarthritis)

  - Deforming arthropathy (Jaccoud's arthropathy), characterised by ulnar deviation at the MTPJs with subluxation, which is reducible in early stages (Figures 2.12.17 and 2.12.18)

  - Erosive arthropathy ("Rhupus")

- Inflammatory tenosynovitis is present in up to 34% of patients, more common in the cohort with erosive arthropathy phenotype. Inflammatory myositis can also occur.

- Extra-musculoskeletal manifestations occur frequently, with respiratory involvement (21% of patients with SLE develop pleural effusions), renal involvement (50% of patients with SLE develop lupus nephritis), and cardiac involvement (75% of patients develop cardiac valvular disease).

- There is a strong association of SLE with antiphospholipid syndrome, co-existing in one-third of patients with SLE.

SJÖGREN SYNDROME

- Sjögren's syndrome is a chronic, multisystem, inflammatory, autoimmune condition characterised by lymphocytic infiltration of lacrimal and salivary exocrine glands, resulting in symptoms of keratoconjunctivitis (dry eyes) and xerostomia (dry mouth), symptoms known as "sicca."

- It can co-exist with other autoimmune conditions such as rheumatoid arthritis or thyroid disease, where it is known as secondary Sjögren's syndrome; the primary syndrome occurs alone.

- There are multiple musculoskeletal manifestations of Sjögren's syndrome, the most common being arthralgia in up to 96% of patients, and arthritis in approximately 16% of patients. The most affected joints are the MCPJs of the hand and wrist joints.

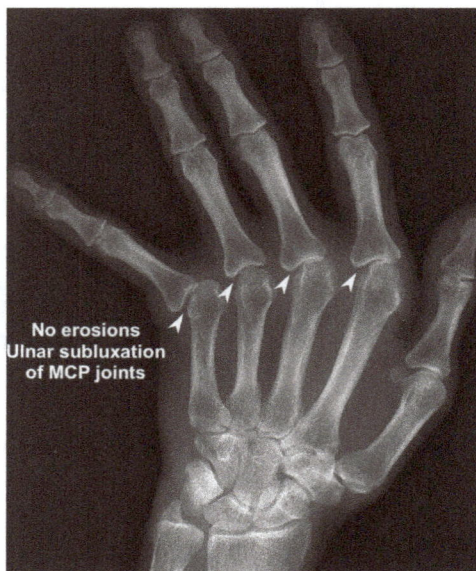

Figure 2.12.17 Radiographic features of Jaccoud arthropathy with non-erosive ulnar subluxation at the MCPJs.

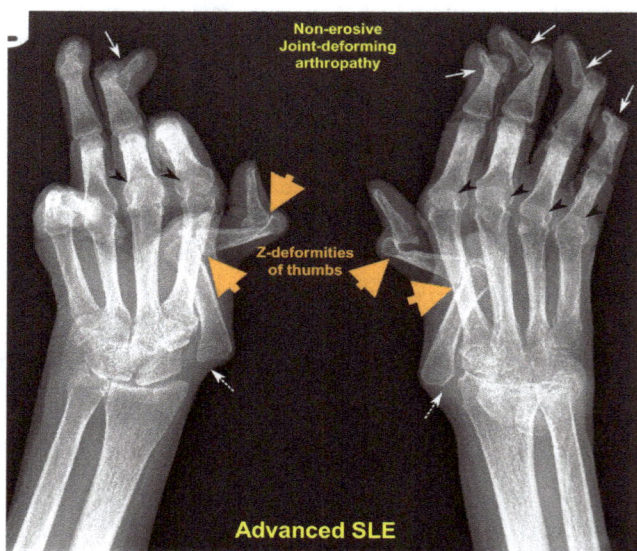

Figure 2.12.18 Radiographic features with advanced SLE demonstrating non-erosive deforming arthropathy involving the CMC joints, MCP joints, DIP joints, and Z-thumb deformity. Note the lack of erosion despite advanced disease.

■ The imaging features are of a symmetrical, fluctuating, non-erosive synovitis on ultrasound, usually with normal X-rays. In some patients, joint involvement can predate the development of sicca symptoms. Abnormal bone metabolism in Sjögren's syndrome can result in osteomalacia and osteopenia/osteoporosis.

- There is an association with inclusion body myositis and polymyositis, which may be asymptomatic.

- Other extra-glandular features include lymphadenopathy, NSIP pattern of interstitial lung disease, cutaneous vasculitis, and Raynaud's phenomenon association. There is also an increased risk of mucosa-associated lymphoid tissue (MALT) type non-Hodgkin's lymphoma.

MIXED CONNECTIVE TISSUE DISEASE (MCTD)

- Mixed CTD is a chronic, multisystem autoimmune condition predominantly affecting females (5:1) with an onset in their 4th decade, characterised by a high anti-U1-RNP antibodies with overlapping clinical features of rheumatoid arthritis, polymyositis, SLE, and systemic sclerosis. There is a strong association with Raynaud's phenomenon, with symptoms occurring in up to 93% of patients with MCTD.

- The musculoskeletal system is involved in up to 95% of patients with MCTD. Musculoskeletal system imaging features include synovitis, myositis, swollen fingers/hands, and arthritis, with erosion patterns similar to that of rheumatoid arthritis, and proximal myositis.

- Other systems involved include gastrointestinal (oesophageal dysmotility and dilation), respiratory (pleural effusions, NSIP pattern interstitial lung disease, pulmonary arterial hypertension), cardiac (pericarditis, myocarditis, and heart block), and renal (glomerulonephritis).

IDIOPATHIC INFLAMMATORY MYOPATHIES

- Two main subtypes: Dermatomyositis and Inclusion Body Myositis (see Table 2.12.1)

Dermatomyositis (DM)

- DM has two forms: the more severe juvenile form and the adult form.
- Classic imaging findings include various patterns of soft tissue calcification:

  - Skin/subcutaneous tissue (superficial nodule and lacy reticular patterns)

  - Intramuscular (deep tumourous pattern)

  - Fascial/peritendinous (deep linear/sheet-like pattern)

- Muscle weakness with evidence of myopathy on MRI can be seen in a bilateral, symmetrical pattern with a preference for proximal muscles of the lower and upper extremities.

- Skin, subcutaneous fat, and fascial involvement on MRI are key in differentiating DM from other inflammatory myopathies (Figure 2.12.19).

- Active muscle inflammation appears as high T2 signal with post-contrast T1 enhancement. In the chronic stage, fatty infiltration occurs, which is best seen on T1W MRI imaging.

- Clinically, dermatological manifestations of DM include skin rashes (heliotrope rash of the upper eyelids and sun exposed areas, Gottron's papules and "shawl sign").

Table 2.12.1 Key Differentiating Features between Dermatomyositis (DM) and Inclusion Body Myositis (IBM)

	Age	Rash	Muscle Distribution	Key Radiological Findings
DM	Children and adults	Yes	Bilateral + symmetrical proximal muscle involvement of upper and lower limbs	Skin, subcutaneous fat, and facial involvement Soft tissue calcification
IBM	Adults >50 years old	No	Bilateral + asymmetrical muscle involvement Anterior compartment of the thigh (vastus lateralis most involved with rectus femoris sparing) Posterior compartment of the calf (medial gastrocnemius most involved) Anterior compartment of the forearm (flexor digitorum profundus most involved with flexor carpi ulnaris, thenar, and hypothenar muscle sparing)	Severe atrophy and fatty infiltration Undulating fascia sign due to atrophy/fatty atrophy of the vastus laterals and intermedius

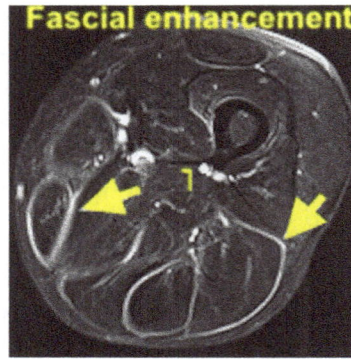

Figure 2.12.19 Fascial enhancement on T1W post-contrast axial image through mid-thigh in autoimmune fasciitis.

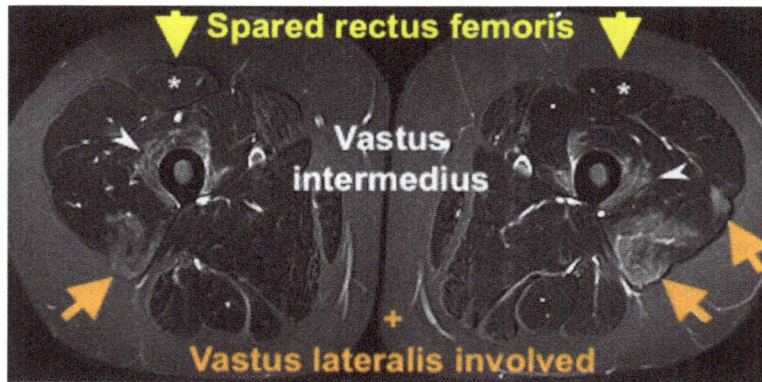

Figure 2.12.20 MRI in inclusion body myositis with sparing of bilateral rectus femoris and patchy involvement of bilateral vastus intermedius and lateralis.

Inclusion Body Myositis (IBM)

- IBM is a bilateral asymmetrical inflammatory myopathy, affecting males more than females, typically those over 50 years old.

- On MRI, muscle atrophy and fatty infiltration is more typical of IBM than muscle oedema. Unlike DM, there is no fascial or subcutaneous involvement.

- In contrast with DM, there is asymmetric involvement of more peripheral muscles. Muscle compartments most frequently affected include the anterior compartment of the thigh (vastus lateralis is most involved, with rectus femoris sparing) (Figure 2.12.20), the posterior compartment of the calf (medial gastrocnemius is most involved), and the anterior compartment of the forearm (flexor digitorum profundus is most involved with flexor carpi ulnaris sparing). Also sparing of the thenar and hypothenar muscles.

- The "undulating fascia" sign can be demonstrated on T1W MRI imaging, with severe atrophy and fatty infiltrating of vastus intermedius and lateralis, resulting in an undulating morphology of the fascia.

- IBM is diagnosed histologically by distinct inclusion bodies of amyloid-β protein in the nuclei and cytoplasms of affected muscle cells.

- Clinically, IBM is refractory to treatment.

At the end of the chapter, we provide an approach to diagnosing various arthropathies that affect hands. This will be helpful in tackling the new format of FRCR 2B short cases and table viva (Figure 2.12.21).

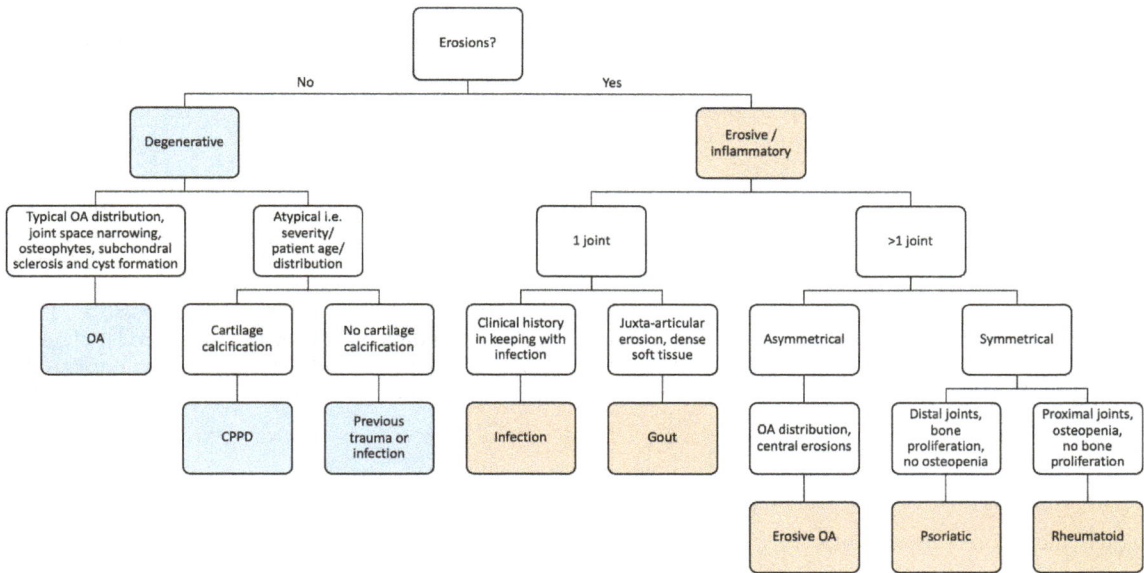

Figure 2.12.21 Diagnostic flowchart for the differential diagnosis of arthritis on hand radiographs. Osteoarthritis (OA) is diagnosed through the typical distribution, i.e. scapho-trapeziotrapezoid joint (STTJ), thumb carpometacarpal joint (CMCJ), distal interphalangeal joints (DIPJs), and proximal interphalangeal joints (PIPJs). Joint space narrowing, osteophyte formation, subchondral sclerosis, and cyst formation are key features of OA. Erosive/inflammatory arthropathy can be divided into monoarthritis or polyarthritis. Polyarthritis can then again be divided into asymmetrical and symmetrical distributions, with psoriatic and rheumatoid arthritis appearing more symmetrically, and erosive OA typically asymmetrical.

CONCLUSION

This chapter has outlined the key features of various connective tissue disorders including rheumatoid arthritis, seronegative arthritis (AS, PsA, reactive arthritis, and enteropathic arthritis), and other multisystem connective tissue disorders. Serological markers and imaging are used in conjunction with clinical examination to aid in the diagnosis of connective tissue disorders. Plain film provides a remarkable amount of information and remains the mainstay of modality in the initial workup for connective tissue disorder, followed by MRI.

SUGGESTED READING

- Resnick DL, Jacobson JA, Chung CB, Kransdorf MJ, Pathria MN. *Bone and Joint Imaging E-Book*. Elsevier Health Sciences; 2024 Feb 3.

- Walter WR, Samim M. Imaging Updates in Rheumatoid Arthritis. In *Seminars in Musculoskeletal Radiology* (Vol. 29, No. 02, pp. 156–166). Thieme Medical Publishers, Inc.; 2025 Apr.

SBA QUESTIONS

1) A 64-year-old patient presents with pain in their hands, ankles, and back. They have an X-ray of both hands, which shows preserved bone density and terminal tuft acro-osteolysis of the 2nd and 4th digits of the left hand. There are marginal erosions with new bone formation involving the DIPJs and extensive periosteal reaction adjacent to the right 3rd and 4th DIPJs. What is the most likely diagnosis?

   A. Osteoarthritis

   B. Rheumatoid arthritis

   C. Psoriatic arthritis

   D. Erosive osteoarthritis

   E. Calcium pyrophosphate dihydrate deposition disease

2) A 52-year-old patient with lower back pain is found on MRI imaging to have bilateral symmetrical sacroiliac joint space pseudo-widening with cortical erosions. They have also recently been complaining of abdominal pain and diarrhoea. What is the most likely diagnosis?

   A. Enteropathic spondyloarthropathy

   B. Reactive arthritis

   C. Ankylosing spondylitis

   D. Psoriatic arthritis

   E. Rheumatoid arthritis

3) A 55-year-old patient comes with muscle weakness, with difficulty standing from a sitting position. They have a facial rash. They undergo an MRI scan of the pelvis and bilateral lower limbs. There is bilateral, symmetrical, and patchy high STIR signal within the quadratus femoris and anterior compartment of the thighs. There is also high STIR signal involving the fascia and a reticular pattern in the subcutaneous fat. What is the most likely diagnosis?

   A. Polymyositis

   B. Immune-mediated necrotising myopathy

   C. Inclusion body myositis

   D. Dermatomyositis

   E. Cellulitis

Answers: (1) C, (2) A, (3) D

Chapter 2.13
Axial and Peripheral Spondyloarthritis and Mimics

Neel Raja, Mohsin AM Hussein, Siddharth Thaker, and Winston J Rennie

---

LEARNING OBJECTIVES

■ Delineate the key clinical features of axial spondyloarthritis (AxSpA), and peripheral spondyloarthritis, and their imaging appearances

■ Understanding the MRI scanning protocol, normal and abnormal appearances of relevant structures, and mimickers of pathology

---

Axial Spondyloarthritis

CLINICAL REASONING BEHIND IMAGING REQUESTS FROM RHEUMATOLOGIST

■ Confirm clinical suspicion, differentiate axSpA from mimics, and identify early disease

■ Assess disease activity and treatment response

■ Identify complications in long-standing disease

INTRODUCTION

Spondyloarthritis (SpA) is an umbrella term encompassing a group of seronegative inflammatory conditions which share common clinical, genetic, and radiological features, particularly an association with HLA B27 antigen. It is further divided into axial spondyloarthritis (ax-SpA), which affects the spine and sacroiliac joints, or peripheral spondyloarthritis, which affects peripheral musculoskeletal structures with variable degree of axial involvement. If left undiagnosed and therefore untreated, it may lead to significantly increased patient morbidity. SpA may be subclassified according to clinical manifestation of symptoms:

■ Ankylosing spondylitis (AS)

■ Psoriatic arthritis (PsA)

■ Inflammatory bowel disease (IBD)-associated arthritis

■ Reactive arthritis (ReA)

■ Undifferentiated spondyloarthritis (SpA)

Juvenile-onset SpA has more recently been included under this umbrella. The pathogenesis of axSpA varies depending on the underlying aetiology and discussion of the theorised immunology is beyond the scope of this book.

In addition to the prototypical ankylosing spondylitis, the other subclasses may also have varying degrees of axial (spine and SIJ) disease manifestation. For simplicity, the term "ax-SpA" in this chapter refers to the radiological patterns of axial involvement across all subtypes; it is appreciated that some authors may prefer the term "psoriatic arthritis with axial involvement," for example. The semantics are notoriously beloved to an MSK radiologist, but knowledge beyond this is unlikely to be required for the 2B exam! This chapter will briefly discuss some of the clinico-radiological classification systems, before delving into the various imaging appearances of axSpA.

CLASSIFICATION CRITERIA

There have been numerous classification criteria for SpA over the years, of which we will focus on two in particular. The Modified New York criteria for AS (mNYC) published in 1984, is the original but old criteria and has two positive outcomes: probable or definite. These conclusions are reached based on two sets of criteria: clinical and imaging (radiography, **NOT** MRI).

DOI: 10.1201/9781003500247-22

Clinical Criteria

■ Low back pain persisting for ≥3 months, reduced by exercise and not relieved by rest

■ Limited motion in the lumbar spine in coronal and sagittal planes

■ Limited chest expansion compared with normal values for age and sex

Radiological Criteria

■ Bilateral sacroiliitis ≥ grade 2 or unilateral sacroiliitis ≥ grade 3 on radiograph (Figure 2.13.1)

- **Either all 3 clinical criteria *or* the radiologic criteria alone = Probable AS**

- **The radiologic criteria and ≥ 1 of the clinical criteria = Definite AS**

Ferguson's view is a specific radiographic view in which the patient is prone with a PA view and the X-ray tube is angled cephalad (towards head) by 30–35° centred on the sacrum. A central pelvic image is obtained, with a divergent beam demonstration the entire SIJ articular surface (Figure 2.13.2).

The main drawback of the mNYC is that radiographic change occurs late in the disease process (lag between the onset of clinical symptoms and diagnosis is 7 to 9 years). Since the publication of the Assessment in SpondyloArthritis International Society criteria for classification of axSpA, which uses MRI instead of radiographs. There has been an increased use of MRI due to its ability to detect inflammatory and post-inflammatory changes much earlier in the disease than radiographs.

Similarly, this criterion relies on a combination of clinico-radiological features and two distinct diagnostic arms, provided patients are under the age of 45 have a history of ≥ 3 months of back pain:

■ Sacroiliitis on MRI + ≥1 SpA feature (Imaging arm)

■ HLA-B27 positive + ≥2 SpA features (Clinical arm)

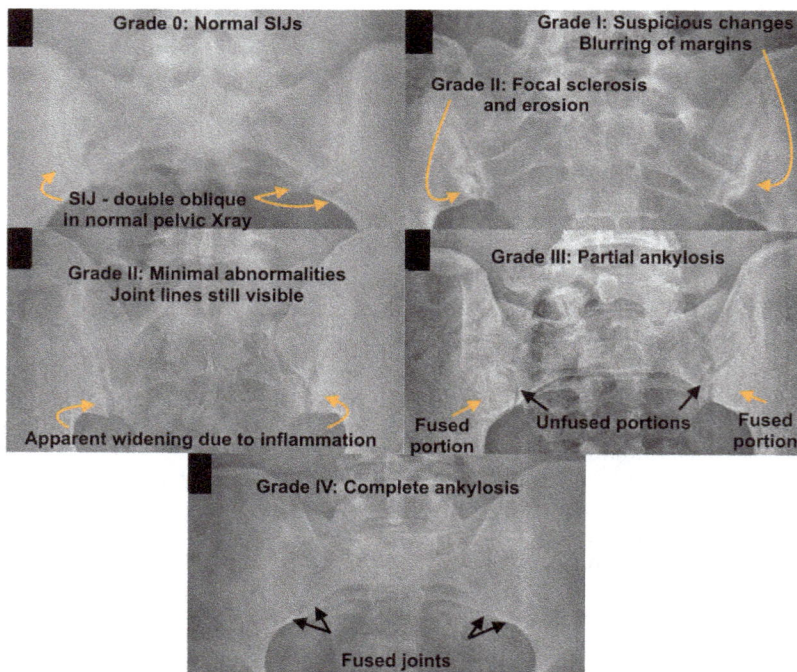

Figure 2.13.1 Various grades of sacroiliitis on X-rays according the mNYC criteria.

The SpA features included are inflammatory back pain, arthritis, enthesitis, uveitis, dactylitis, psoriasis, Crohn's/colitis, good response to NSAIDs, family history for SpA, HLA-B27 antigen positivity, and elevated CRP.

SACROILIAC JOINT (SIJ) MRI SEQUENCES IN axSPA

■ The specific imaging sequences used to image the SIJs in the context of axSpA vary between institutions, due to coils available and scanner specifications; however, below is a suggested imaging protocol recommended by the European Society of Skeletal Radiology (ESSR) Arthritis Subcommittee

• Coronal oblique (which we refer to as coronal for the rest of the chapter), angled tangent to the posterior cortex of the S2 sacral segment (Figure 2.13.3)

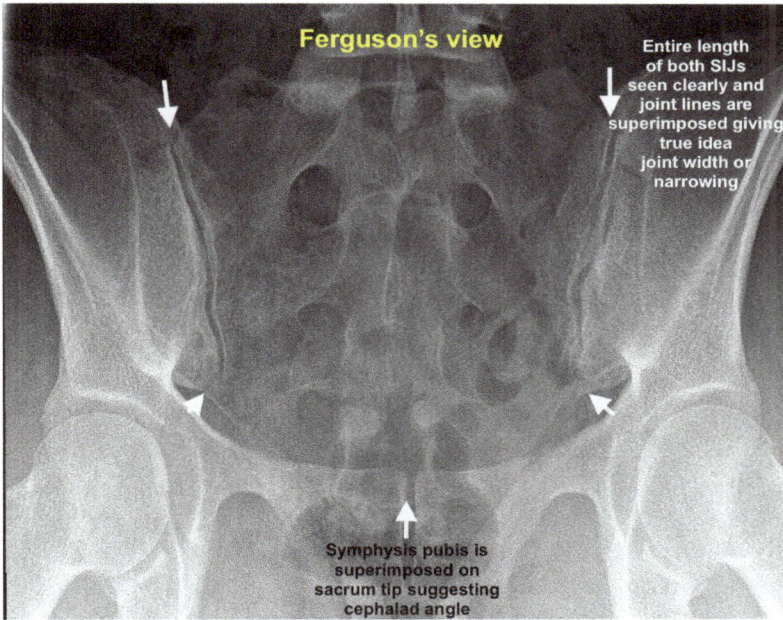

Ferguson's view

Entire length of both SIJs seen clearly and joint lines are superimposed giving true idea joint width or narrowing

Symphysis pubis is superimposed on sacrum tip suggesting cephalad angle

Figure 2.13.2 Ferguson's view of the SIJs.

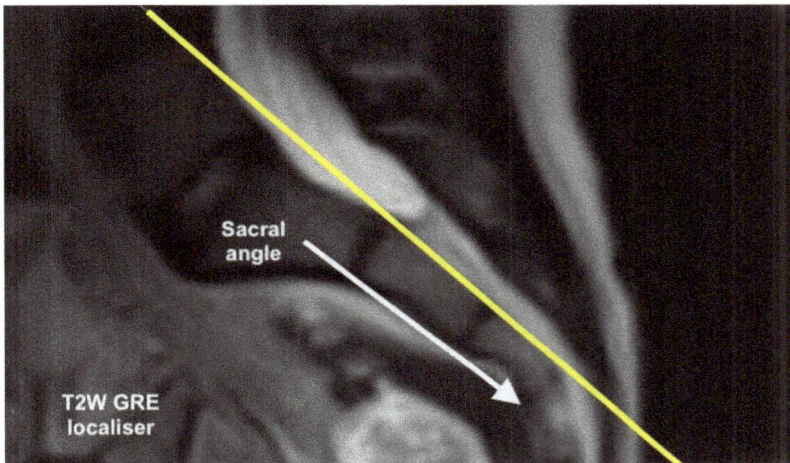

Sacral angle

T2W GRE localiser

Figure 2.13.3 Orientation of the localiser to obtain true coronal oblique plane on T2W GRE.

Table 2.13.1 Normal and Abnormal Appearances of SIJs on Different MRI Sequences

Sequence	Normal Appearances	Abnormal Appearances
T1W coronal and axial	• Homogeneous marrow signal on both sides of the SIJs • Smooth cortical contours on both sides of the SIJs, with intervening articular cartilage • Preserved joint space	• Juxta-articular bone marrow oedema • Juxta-articular geographic fat metaplasia • Subchondral sclerosis • Erosions +/− associated bone marrow oedema
STIR coronal and axial	• Homogeneous marrow fat suppression on both sides of the SIJs • Low signal ligaments	• Ankylosis • Enthesitis • Capsulitis • Tissue back fill

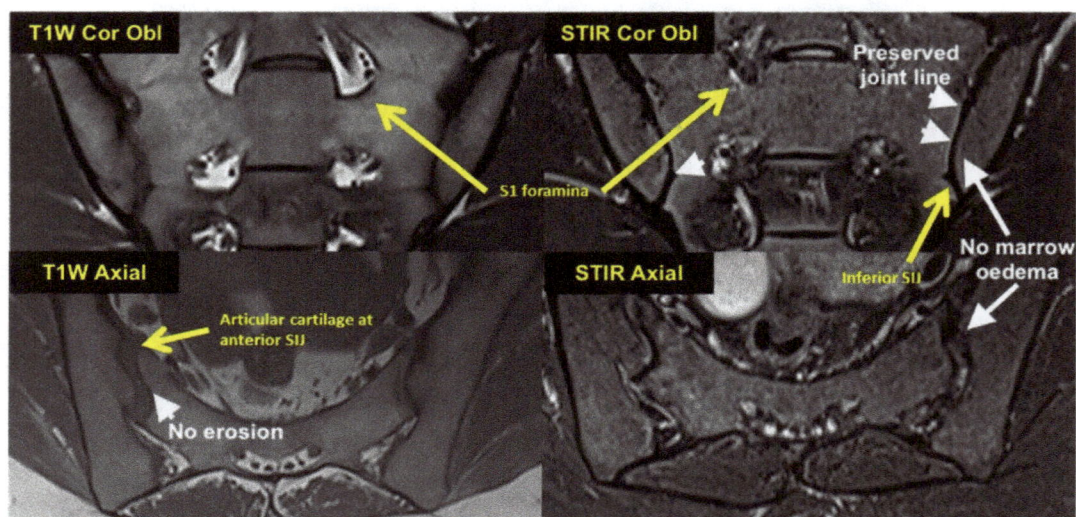

Figure 2.13.4 Normal SIJ appearances.

- T1W spin echo sequence through the SIJs

- Coronal STIR sequence through the SIJs

- Axial T1W and STIR sequences through the SIJs

- Visualisation in two perpendicular planes (Figure 2.13.4)

- An additional cartilage sequence is sometimes utilised

axSPA Sacrolitis on MRI

- The SIJ is formed by a fibrous part at its superior aspect and a synovial part at its inferior aspect.

- The synovial part is a boomerang-shaped joint, with anterosuperior and posteroinferior portions (Figure 2.13.5).

- It is bounded by hyaline type cartilage (weaker) along its sacral side and fibrocartilage (stronger) along its iliac side. Understanding this histology makes interpretation of imaging findings easier.

- Enthesitis, resultant osteitis, and new bone formation are key elements of the pathogenesis in axSpA, which can aid MRI interpretation.

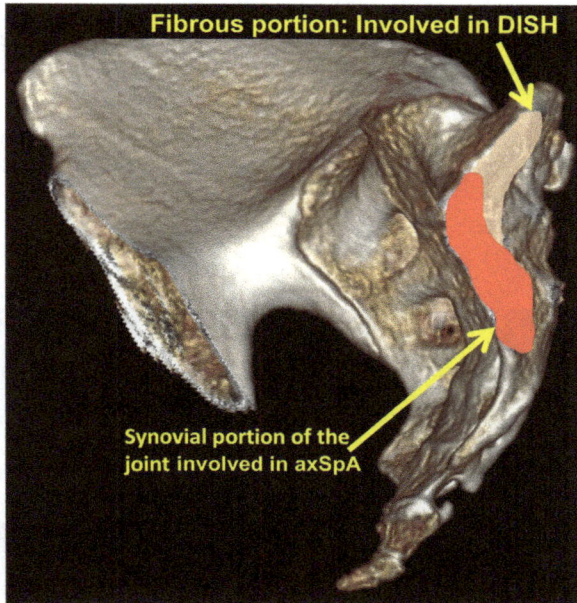

Figure 2.13.5 Sagittal oblique 3D reconstruction demonstrating the left SIJ (cut) with the fibrous and synovial regions shaded.

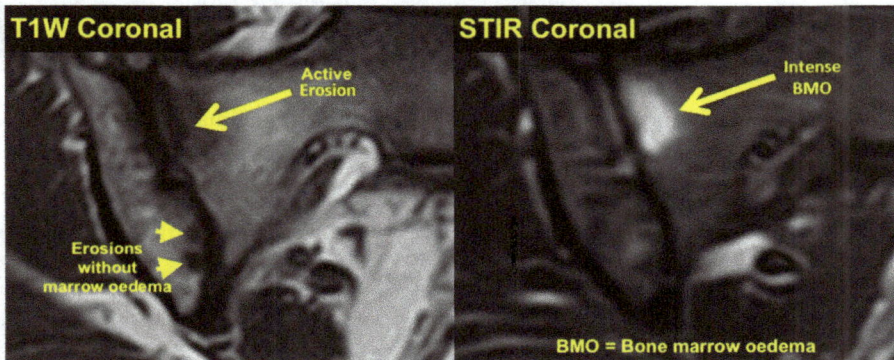

Figure 2.13.6 Coronal T1W and STIR images showing active erosions with bone marrow oedema and quiescent erosions with surrounding marrow oedema.

- Entheses: Sites of tendinous/ligamentous attachment to bone—are primarily involved.

- During inflammatory phase, there is enthesitis and resultant inflammatory osteitis at the bone interface, which are seen as increased signal on fluid-sensitive sequences (Figure 2.13.6).

- Inflammation at the SIJ can result in cartilage degeneration and subchondral bone resorption in the first instance (erosion). Varying degrees of subchondral bone marrow oedema will be present during this phase.

- If inflammation is allowed to continue unchecked, then subacute/chronic or "structural" changes begin to occur.

229

- In the SIJs, these consist of **juxta-articular fat metaplasia** (geographic high signal on T1W imaging) (Figure 2.13.7), **subchondral sclerosis** (low signal on all sequences), **tissue backfill** (Figure 2.13.8), **aberrant endochondral ossification** (bone budding), and **bone bridge formation**, ultimately leading to **ankylosis** (Figure 2.13.9).

- Tissue backfill is a term used to describe the intermediary post-inflammatory fibrofatty tissue (high signal on both T1W and fluid-sensitive sequences) present at the site of excavated erosion, adjacent to a remodelled articular surface.

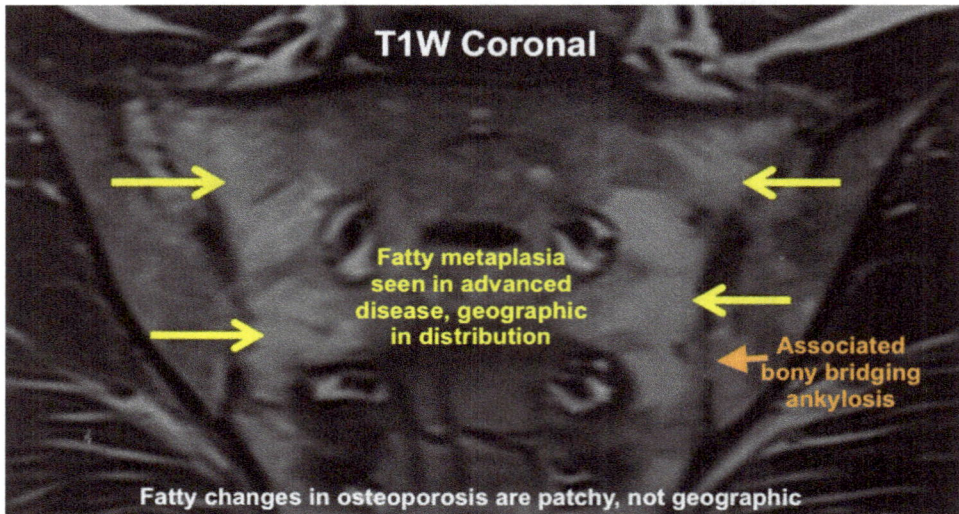

Figure 2.13.7   Fat metaplasia and early bony ankylosis on T1W coronal image.

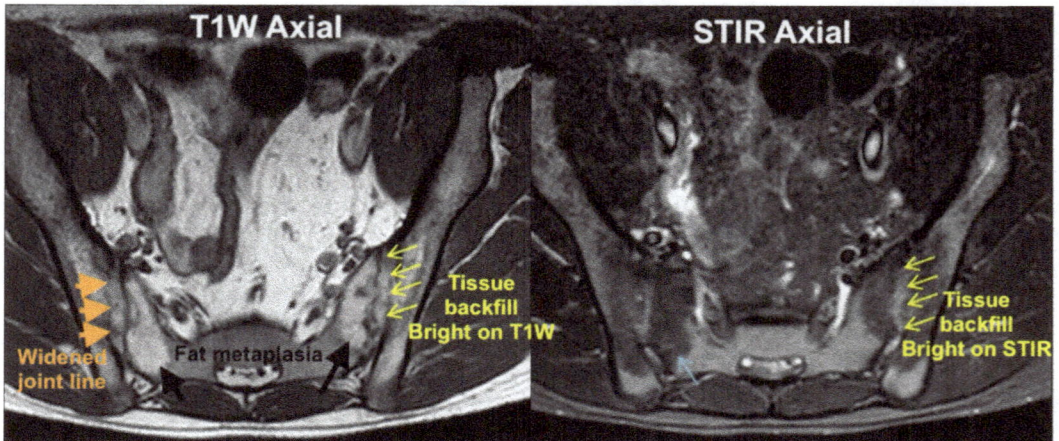

Figure 2.13.8   Tissue backfill (yellow arrows), formation of a pseudojoint line (amber arrows) away from the original joint line, and juxta-articular fat metaplasia (black arrows) on MRI.

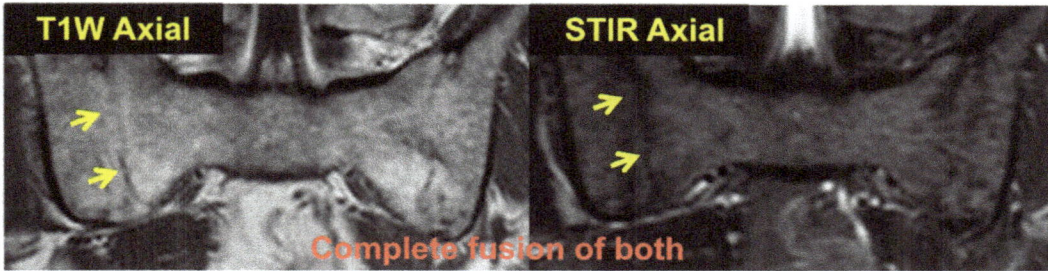

Figure 2.13.9 Complete bony ankylosis.

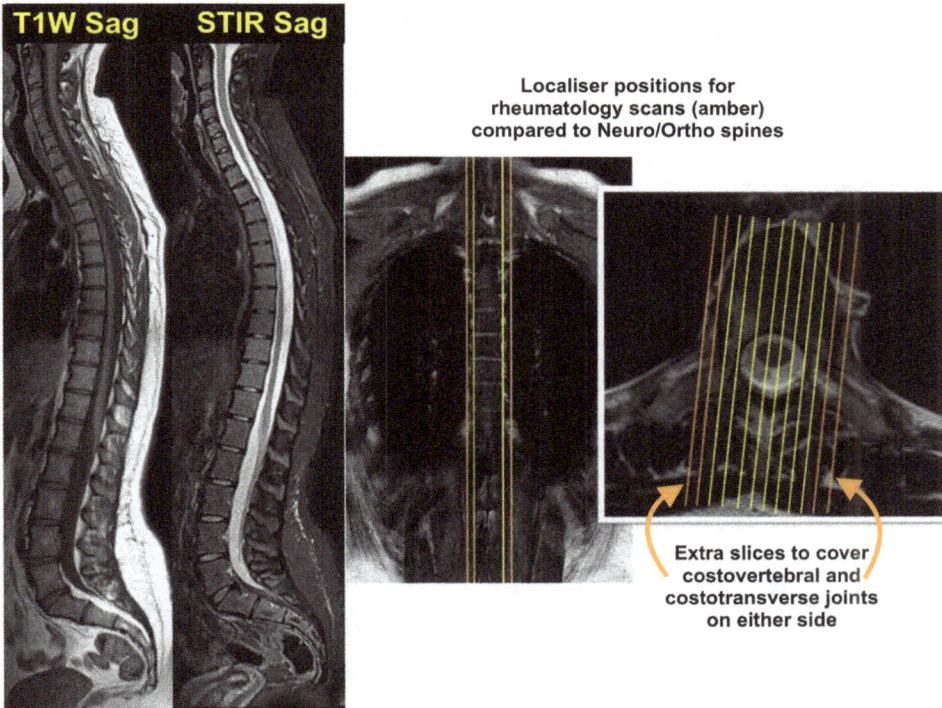

Figure 2.13.10 Whole-spine sagittal scans for rheumatological indications. Note scout images demonstrating the extended field of view required for axSpA scanning protocol.

Spine MRI Sequences in axSPA

Standard spine MRI imaging protocol in suspected axSpA is variable. We recommend following NICE guidance to use appropriate protocol. A suggested protocol to visualise commonly implicated anatomy is axSpA is provided as follows (Figure 2.13.10):

- Sagittal T1W images of the whole spine acquired in 2 blocks (cervicothoracic + thoracolumbosacral), the key differentiation with standard MRI of the spine is that it has extended lateral slices to image the costovertebral (CVJ) and costotransverse (CTJ) joints. Standard MRI spine planning is performed from pedicle to pedicle focusing on the spinal cord and disc elements.

- Sagittal STIR images with the same coverage.

Spinal Manifestations of axSPA

The pathogenesis underpinning the spinal changes in axSpA is similar to that in the SIJs, so it should come as no surprise that the imaging features are similar and progress with similar chronology.

Corner Inflammatory/Fat Lesion

■ Inflammation of the enthesis between the annulus fibrosus of the intervertebral disc and the adjacent vertebral body ring apophysis/endplate results in the characteristic corner inflammatory lesion (Figure 2.13.11, STIR image).

■ Over time, the bone marrow oedema is replaced by fat metaplasia (Figure 2.13.11, T1W) and eventually sclerosis, giving rise to the radiographic "shiny corner sign" or Romanus lesion (Figure 2.13.11, CT image).

Central Inflammatory Lesion

■ Sometimes referred to as an Andersson lesion, erosion of the vertebral body endplates in axSpA occurs due to discovertebral inflammation (sterile spondylodiscitis).

■ Typically occurring centrally and resulting in the irregularity and bone marrow oedema of the endplates, the intradiscal signal is preserved.

Table 2.13.2 Normal and Abnormal Appearances of the Spine on Different MRI Sequences

Sequence	Normal Appearance	Abnormal Appearance
T1W Sag	• Homogeneous marrow signal • Smooth cortical contours, particularly at the vertebral body corners and endplates • Preserved CVJs and CTJs	• Corner inflammatory lesions (CILs) • Central inflammatory lesions (Andersson lesion) • Corner fat lesions (CFLs) • Erosions +/– associated bone marrow oedema
STIR Sag	• Homogeneous marrow fat suppression • Low signal ligaments	• Oedema, juxta-articular fat metaplasia or ankylosis at CVJs or CTJs • Enthesitis • Syndesmophytes

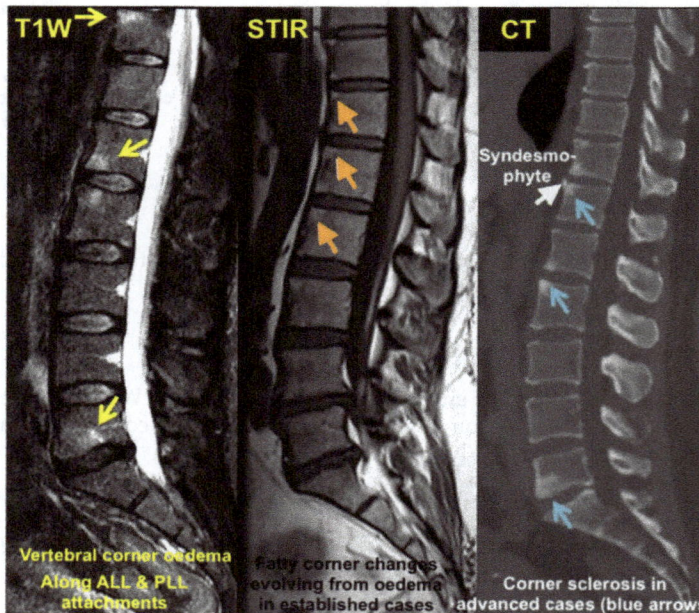

Figure 2.13.11 Evolving corner changes from vertebral corner oedema to fatty change to sclerosis.

- Early lesions exhibit hemispherical bone marrow oedema surrounding a *central* endplate erosion before progressing to fat metaplasia in the same morphology (Figure 2.13.12), then eventually sclerosing and ankylosing.

- These can be differentiated from Schmorl's nodes due to their central location at the endplate and both Modic change and infective spondylodiscitis, by the preserved intradiscal signal.

Costovertebral and Costotransverse Joint Involvement

- The CVJ and CTJ, along with their associated entheses, can also be affected similarly.

- CVJ inflammatory change is characterised by bone marrow oedema in both the head of the rib and the portions of the vertebral body/bodies to which it articulates (Figure 2.13.13, STIR).

- This affected marrow eventually undergoes fat metaplasia (Figure 2.13.13, T1W) then sclerosis (Figure 2.13.13, CT).

- The CTJs, between the thoracic vertebral transverse process and costal tuberosity, are ligament rich and enthesis rich joints which are commonly overlooked due to being on the far lateral sections of our scanning protocol.

Syndesmophytes

- The term syndesmophyte is used to describe heterotopic ossification within the deep portion of a spinal ligament (most commonly the anterior longitudinal ligament) and the annulus fibrosus.

- These classically appear as fine ossifications arising directly from the vertebral body corner with a vertical orientation, i.e. perpendicular to the endplate (Figures 2.13.11 and 2.13.13).

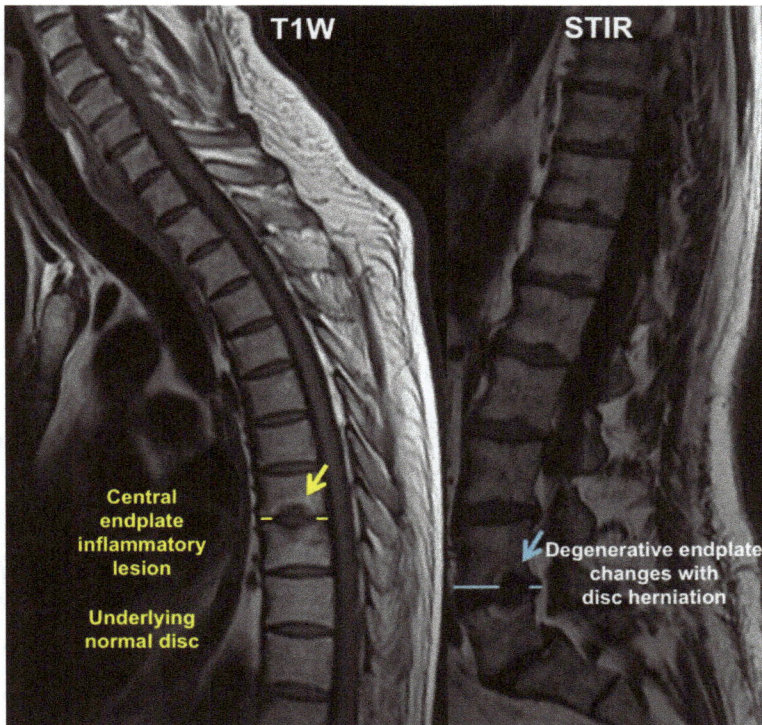

Figure 2.13.12 Central endplate erosion with adjacent fat metaplasia versus Schmorl's node, which is eccentrically located on the endplate.

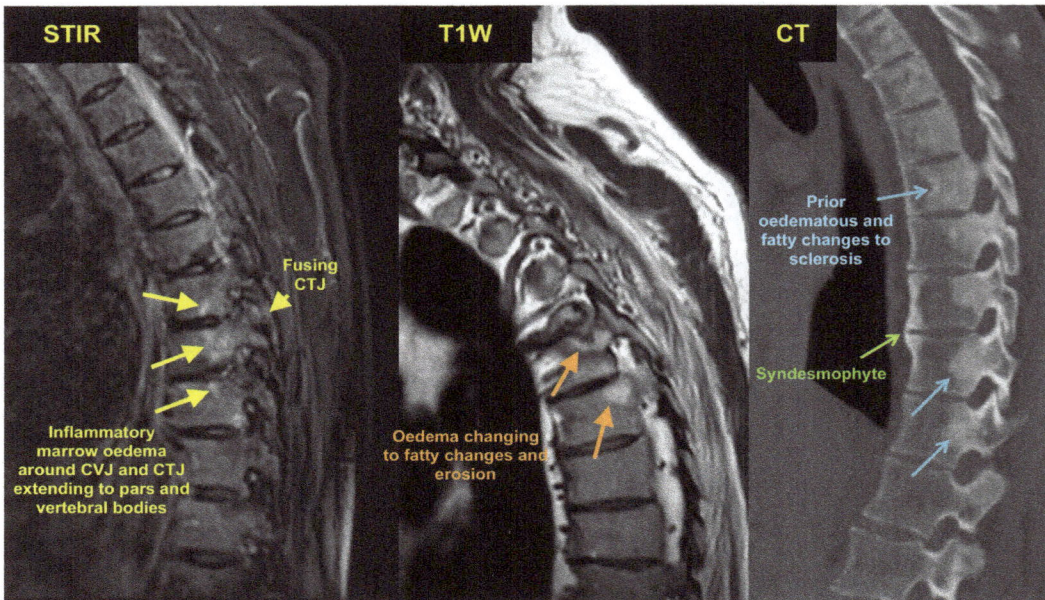

Figure 2.13.13 Inflammatory changes in various stages around the costovertebral joints (CVJ) and costotransverse joints (CTJ)—not shown, progressing from inflammatory (oedema on STIR), to fatty (T1W), and ultimately to sclerotic phase (CT). Also appreciate the syndesmophyte along the anterior longitudinal ligament (green arrow).

■ These are in contrast to osteophytes formed in osteoarthritis or DISH-like processes, which are "chunky" and arise slightly away from the level of the endplate, with a horizontal orientation. Examples are shown in the diffuse idiopathic skeletal hyperostosis section shortly.

■ Of the four subtypes, ankylosing spondylitis and IBD related spondyloarthritis are classically bilateral and symmetrical; psoriatic and Reiter's spondyloarthritis are typically bilateral and asymmetric on radiographs.

Mimics of axSPA

Tip: One of the most common interpretative errors made during MRI assessment is the attribution of *any* type of bone marrow oedema, marrow heterogeneity, or sclerosis to axSpA.

STIR MRI sequences are extremely sensitive albeit non-specific for bone marrow oedema unless correlated with its anatomical location and clinical features.

■ Bone marrow oedema at the inferior aspect of the SIJ must be viewed with an increased suspicion of axSpA, given the synovial nature of this joint portion.

■ In contrast, isolated bone marrow oedema at the anterosuperior aspects of the joint is typical of that related to mechanical stress or degenerative inflammatory change.

■ Sacroiliac joint osteoarthritis is the most common pathology affecting the sacroiliac joints and is often an incidental finding radiologically, especially when reading CT scans.

• Aetiologies include high body mass index (BMI), pregnancy, adjacent hip or spine degenerative change, chronic gait abnormalities, lumbosacral transitional vertebra, and high levels of physical activity.

• Like other joints, it is depicted by joint space narrowing, osteophytes, and subchondral sclerosis.

• A useful discriminator is vacuum phenomenon depicting gas (predominantly nitrogen, due to its low solubility) within the joint occurring secondary to negative pressure from joint mobility and degenerative change. This is less likely to be observed in inflammatory conditions which "fill" the joint with inflammation.

- It is important to note that osteoarthritis is the ultimate end point for all progressive arthropathies; hence it may be seen in conjunction with inflammatory changes depending on the time point of scanning.

■ Mechanical-type bone marrow oedema related to degenerative change and altered biomechanics in the spine or SIJ can similarly appear as bone marrow oedema or fat metaplasia in the vertebral body corners. (Look for hypermobility or athletic activities in the clinical history.) These are characteristically anterior in location and oriented along the end-plate as opposed to axSpA where the orientation is along the anterior vertebral cortex flowing the ALL.

Imaging Features

■ Osteophytosis, degeneration of the intervertebral disc associated with irregular endplate (Figure 2.13.14), and variable degree of marrow oedema around them

■ Involvement of the anterosuperior portion of the SIJ (Figure 2.13.14)

■ Vacuum phenomenon in the SIJ

■ Preserved joint space till late

Diffuse Idiopathic Skeletal Hyperostosis

■ Flowing ossification between at least four contiguous thoracic vertebral bodies, with preservation of the intervertebral disc heights and lack of ankylosis of the facet joints and posterior elements. It is non-erosive and usually an incidental finding unrelated to pain (Figure 2.13.15, thoracic CT image).

■ Patients are older than those with axSpA (middle-aged, male predilection).

■ Concurrent metabolic disorders (e.g. diabetes mellitus, dyslipidaemia, obesity).

■ Note: These co-morbidities are also related to psoriasis and the overlap with psoriatic axSpA is a key differential diagnosis.

■ Key imaging appearance: New bone formation, coarse and flowing, located to the right of the midline in the thoracic spine (Aortic pulsation on the left side is thought to prevent new bone formation on the left side).

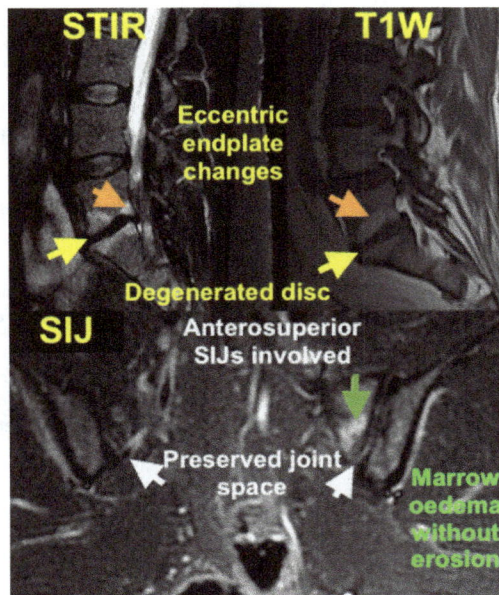

Figure 2.13.14 Degenerative/mechanical changes in the L5/S1 disc and endplates and left SIJ.

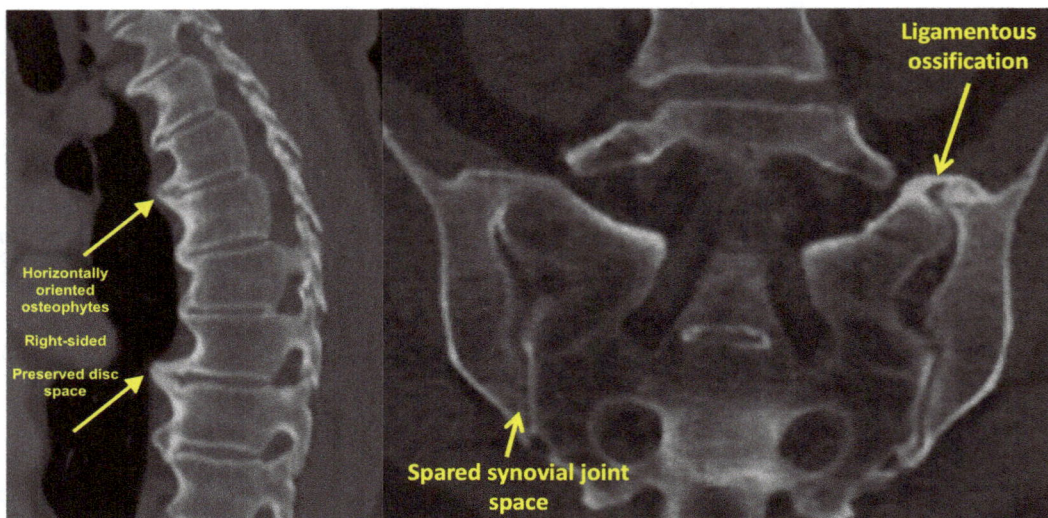

Figure 2.13.15 DISH changes in the thoracic spine and sacroiliac joints.

- Associated with ossified posterior longitudinal ligament (OPLL) in the cervical spine and resultant degenerative lumbar disc and facet disease.

- Ligamentous ossification can also occur at the SIJs, more often at their superior aspects (Figure 2.13.15).

- **Tip:** The axSpA-related syndesmophytes are delicate and parallel the anterior cortices of the vertebral bodies. Facet joint, CVJ, and CTJ ankylosis also favours axSpA over DISH. Despite exuberant ligamentous ossification, SIJ articular surfaces are characteristically uninvolved in DISH.

- The two diseases can co-exist, which gives rise to a diagnostic conundrum.

Osteitis Condensans Ilii

- Triangular areas of dense sclerosis on the iliac sides (predominantly) of the anteroinferior SIJs on radiographs (Figure 2.13.16).

- Scleortic signal intensity can be seen on both sides of the SIJ on MRI. The term OCI may be a misnomer given the MRI findings and was classically coined in the days of plain radiography.

- OCI may be discovered during active investigation for low back pain or incidentally during investigations for other processes, classically affecting women in pregnancy or puerperal period.

Septic Arthritis

Infection of the sacroiliac joint is not uncommon and may share overlapping radiological features with acute sacroiliitis in the early stages, osteitis, joint effusion, and capsulitis. It is a key differential diagnosis for unilateral sacroiliitis and is a "do not miss" condition (Figure 2.13.17).

- Infection has a more exuberant inflammatory response with osteitis being much more pronounced.

- Articular erosion and destruction is more apparent. A key feature is involvement of both sides of the joint.

- Soft tissue oedema is more pronounced in the periarticular soft tissues. A key feature is involvement of tissues far external from the SIJ.

- Pyogenic collections may extend into the surrounding muscles (pyriformis and iliacus) and later extend in to the epidural space.

- In isolated unilateral septic arthritis, top differentials of tuberculosis infection and history of intravenous drug use need to be assessed.

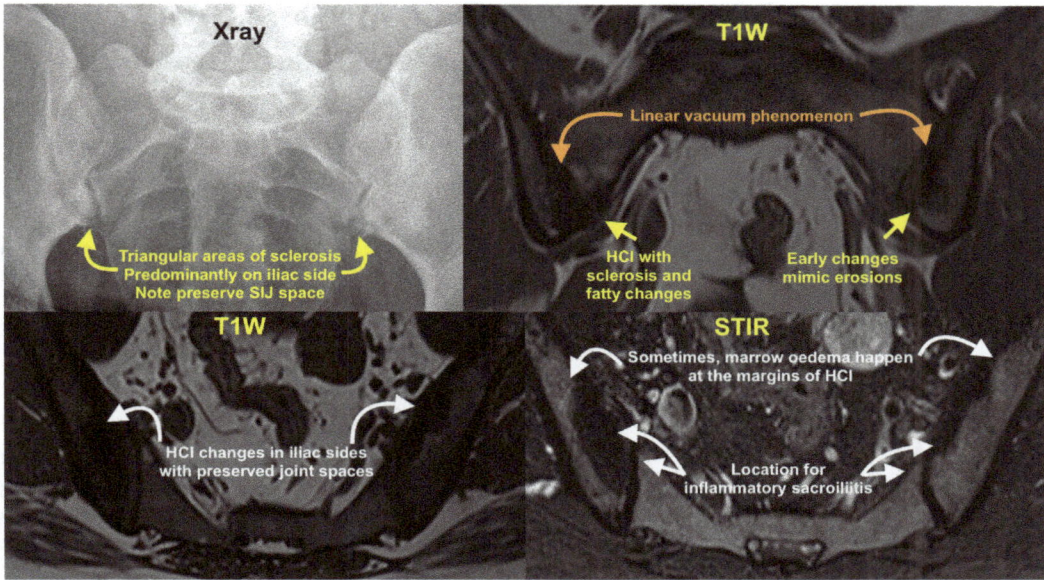

Figure 2.13.16 Hyperostosis condensans ilii on X-ray and MRI.

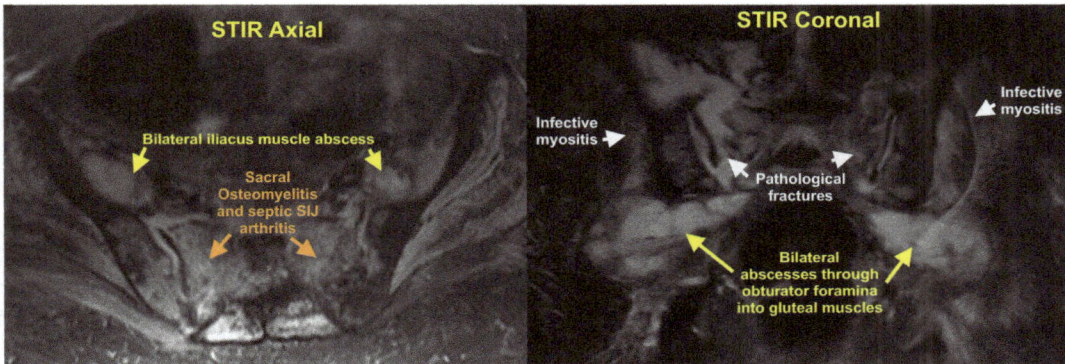

Figure 2.13.17 STIR axial and coronal images showing sacral osteomyelitis with bilateral SIJ septic arthritis, pathological fractures through sacral alar, bilateral iliacus, and obturator abscesses.

Peripheral Spondyloarthritis

- Peripheral spondyloarthritis (pSpA), its family of disorders, and their imaging appearances

CLINICAL REASONING BEHIND IMAGING REQUESTS FROM RHEUMATOLOGIST

- Confirm clinical suspicion of inflammatory arthritis in patients with joint pain and appropriate clinical histories
- Differentiate primary degenerative, erosive osteoarthritis, crystalline arthropathy from inflammatory arthropathies
- Assess disease status and identify complications in chronic cases

Introduction

Peripheral spondyloarthritis (pSpA) describes the peripheral involvement in joints of patients within the aforementioned seronegative spondyloarthropathy subtypes; ankylosing spondylitis (AS), psoriatic arthritis (PsA), reactive arthritis (ReA), and inflammatory bowel disease (IBD) related arthritis. The latter three conditions are those which are often implicated in patients with appendicular skeletal manifestations, and the imaging findings of these conditions will be discussed in this section and summarised in Table 2.13.3.

PSORIATIC ARTHRITIS

PsA refers to the inflammatory arthropathy which can be associated with the inflammatory dermatological condition psoriasis, variants of which include plaque and guttate. Globally, there is significant variation in both the incidence and prevalence of PsA likely depending on the diagnostic/classification criteria used by the rheumatologist, as well as genuine geographic variation in the distribution of the disease. Patients tend to be affected in their 5th decade, and there is no significant gender predominance. Clinically, the presence of psoriasis, an inflammatory arthritis and negative rheumatoid factor serology are classic for this disease. HLA-B27 is positive in approximately 30% of patients.

PsA most commonly affects the hands, specifically the interphalangeal joints, followed by the feet. As with the other seronegative spondyloarthritidies, enthesitis is a hallmark feature, which manifests peripherally with marginal erosions at the bare areas along with periosteal new bone formation, eventually leading to a pencil-in-cup deformity, referring to the proximal phalanx head as the pencil and middle phalanx base as the cup. Dactylitis, another feature of PsA, can be appreciated on radiographs as increased soft tissue density at the digits, which can further improve one's confidence in correctly raising PsA as a possibility (Figure 2.13.18).

Due to bone proliferation associated with this disease, the cortices close to the affected joints can become thick and/or irregular or even ankylose. PsA is one of many differentials for causes of acro-osteolysis of the terminal tuft and if the disease is left unchecked, can progress to arthritis mutilans. It is also in the differential diagnosis of "ivory phalanx," which is dense isolated phalangeal sclerosis from exuberant peri- and endosteal new bone formation. Typically the nail is also involved in the same digit, typically the hallux.

REACTIVE ARTHRITIS

ReA, as its name suggests, typically occurs following a systemic infection, usually genitourinary or gastro-intestinal in origin. It is usually a transient disease with mono- and occasionally oligoarthritis and has a predilection for large joints. Imaging findings are suggestive of but not pathognomonic of ReA, consisting of enthesitis once more, with the associated osseous changes being similar to that of PsA. A differentiating feature is that ReA favours the lower limb, whereas PsA favours the upper limb. A purely radiologic diagnosis is difficult to make, and the stock phrase of "clinical correlation recommended" is once again able to rear its head. The history of conjunctivitis and urethritis associated with arthritis can help: "Can't see, can't pee, and can't climb a tree."

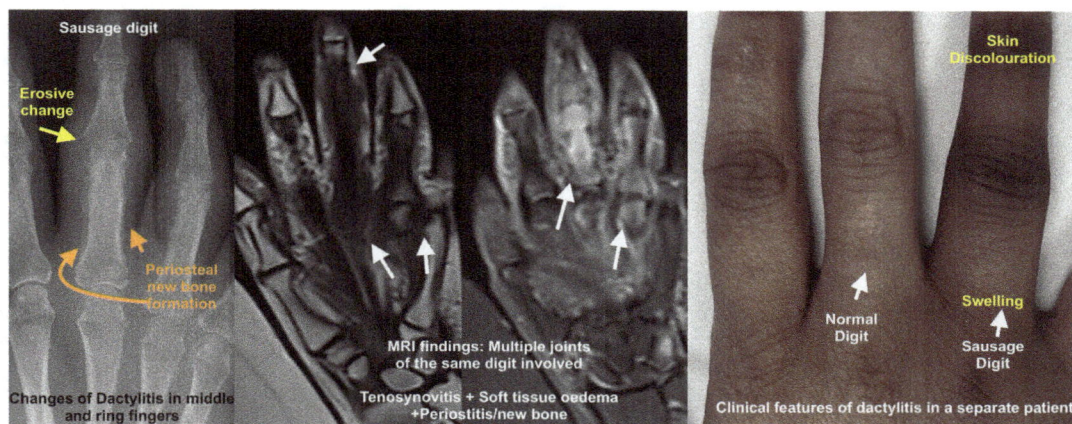

Figure 2.13.18 X-rays show features of dactylitis, erosions and periosteal new bone formation, corresponding MRI features, and clinical picture of a sausage digit. (Image courtesy of Dr James Francis, Consultant Rheumatologist, Leicester, UK.)

Table 2.13.3 **Features of Various Peripheral Spondyloarthritidies**

Psoriatic Arthritis	Reactive Arthritis	IBD-Related Arthritis
Skin psoriasis, RF -ve, HLA-B27 +ve (60%), 50s	Post-infection (genitourinary or gastrointestinal), classically with conjunctivitis/urethritis, HLA-B27 (80%), "can't see, pee, climb tree"	Ulcerative colitis, Crohn's disease, F > M
Symmetric polyarthropathy or asymmetric oligoarthropathy, small joints	Mono- or oligoarthritis, large joint(s)	Asymmetric, 2 patterns: oligoarthritis (knee), polyarthritis (small joints)
Hands > feet, SIJs/spine	Lower limb > upper limb, knee most commonly	Knee, ankle
Ill-defined bare area erosions, uniform joint space narrowing, pencil in cup, periostitis, dactylitis, acro-osteolysis	Ill-defined erosions, uniform joint space narrowing, periostitis	Dactylitis, enthesitis, periarticular osteopenia, joint effusions, erosions (rare)

INFLAMMATORY BOWEL DISEASE-RELATED ARTHRITIS

IBD-related arthritis or enteropathic arthritis (EA) is the seronegative arthritis which a minority (10%–20%) of patients with IBD, ulcerative colitis/Crohn's disease, also suffer. There are two postulated types: type 1 which is a self-limiting oligoarthritis affecting large joints and parallelling IBD activity, and type 2 which is a polyarthritis, which can last for months to years, preferentially affecting the small joints, classically metatarsophalangeal joints, with less correlation to the IBD activity. Common imaging findings include dactylitis, enthesitis, periarticular osteopenia, joint effusions, and, rarely, erosions, which are not specific for IBD related arthritis and can be demonstrated across the board in pSpA (Table 2.13.3).

CONCLUSION

Spondyloarthritis is a diagnosis heavily reliant on robust imaging strategies, in terms of both the MRI sequences acquired and ensuring that the reporting radiologist or registrar knows which anatomical sites are key to assess. Once these are achieved, we hope that this chapter will provide the reader with the confidence to differentiate true axSpA changes from mimics caused by other diseases and provide the referring clinicians with clear reports, thereby providing patients with a timely diagnosis and potentially allowing earlier treatment initiation, reducing morbidity.

SUGGESTED READING

- Rennie WJ, Cotten A, Jurik AG, Lecouvet F, Jans L, Omoumi P, Del Grande F, Dalili D, Bazzocchi A, Becce F, Bielecki DK, Boesen M, Diekhoff T, Grainger A, Guglielmi G, Hemke R, Hermann KGA, Herregods N, Isaac A, Ivanac G, Kainberger F, Klauser A, Marsico S, Mascarenhas V, O'Connor P, Oei E, Pansini V, Papakonstantinou O, Zejden A, Reijnierse M, Rosskopf AB, Shah A, Sudol-Szopinska I, Laloo F, Giraudo C. Standardized reporting of spine and sacroiliac joints in axial spondyloarthritis MRI: From the ESSR-Arthritis Subcommittee. *Eur Radiol*. 2025 Jan;35(1):360–369. https://doi.org/10.1007/s00330-024-10926-x. Epub 2024 Jul 19. PMID: 39030373.

SBA QUESTIONS

1) A 45-year-old man has a CT abdomen and pelvis for acute appendicitis. The scan is negative for appendicitis but reports an abnormality of the sacroiliac joints. Which feature would favour an infective sacroiliitis over axial spondyloarthritis?

   A. Subchondral erosions

   B. Subchondral sclerosis

   C. Asymmetric iliacus muscles

   D. Vacuum phenomenon

   E. Joint ankylosis

2) A 32-year-old highly active sportsman presents to his GP with inflammatory back pain. An MRI of his whole spine and sacroiliac joints is suspicious for bilateral symmetric sacroiliitis. Which other feature is most likely to support a diagnosis of axial spondyloarthritis?

   A. Ossifications of the iliac crest

   B. Flowing osteophytes of 6 contiguous thoracic vertebrae

   C. Oedema at the costotransverse joint

   D. Vertebral corner oedema within the lumbar spine

   E. Subarticular sclerosis of the sacroiliac joints

3) A 49-year-old woman with pain and stiffness in the small joints of both hands had radiographs performed. Which feature would most favour a diagnosis of psoriatic arthritis over rheumatoid arthritis?

   A. Periarticular bone proliferation

   B. Marginal erosions

   C. Periarticular osteopenia

   D. Symmetrical joint involvement

   E. Sparing of the distal interphalangeal joints

Answers: (1) C, (2) C, (3) A

Chapter 2.14
Osteoarthritis

Tsz Shing Joshua Wong, Siddharth Thaker, and Harun Gupta

LEARNING OBJECTIVES

- Understand the appropriate use of radiographs, MRI, ultrasound, and CT for evaluating osteoarthritis

- Review the radiological differentiation of degenerative and inflammatory arthropathy in joint space narrowing

- Identify typical radiological features and distribution pattern in axial and peripheral joint osteoarthritis

- Differentiate osteoarthritis from mimics such as inflammatory arthropathy, septic arthritis, and subchondral insufficiency fracture

- Understand the radiologist's role in the management of osteoarthritis

---

ABBREVIATIONS

ACJ: acromioclavicular joint
CMCJ: carpometacarpal joints
DIPJ: distal interphalangeal joints
MCPJ: metacarpophalangeal joints

MTPJ: metatarsophalangeal joint
PIPJ: proximal interphalangeal joints
SIJ: sacroiliac joint
TMJ: temporomandibular joint.

INTRODUCTION

Osteoarthritis (OA) is the most common form of arthritis and one of the most prevalent age-related pathologies, making early detection crucial (see Figure 2.14.1).

- General radiologists frequently encounter OA in daily practice. A strong grasp of its radiological features is vital for accurate diagnosis and exclusion of other possible differentials.

- Arthropathies are a frequent focus in examinations, and proficiency in diagnosing OA while distinguishing degenerative from mimics is key to exam success.

APPROACH TO ARTHRITIS

- When assessing joint space narrowing on initial radiographs, the primary role of the radiologist is to differentiate degenerative joint disease from inflammatory arthropathy.

- OA typically presents with asymmetric joint space narrowing, osteophyte formation, and subchondral sclerosis.

- Atypical clinical scenarios, such as involvement of uncommon joints or unusual age of onset, should prompt consideration of alternative diagnoses, such as prior trauma, crystal arthropathy, or haemophilic arthropathy.

- *Early identification of inflammatory arthropathy is crucial for effective disease management and minimising functional impairment.*

The key radiological features of inflammatory arthropathy include bone erosions and osteopaenia, which may progress to osteoporosis over time. Although this chapter does not delve into specific inflammatory arthropathy subtypes (see Chapters 2.12 and 2.13 for details), a practical approach to distinguishing these conditions is as follows:

- Proximal small joint involvement suggests rheumatoid arthritis.

- Distal joint involvement with bony proliferation: Think seronegative spondyloarthropathy, which can be further classified into axial spondyloarthropathy (spine and sacroiliac joints) and peripheral spondyloarthropathy.

DOI: 10.1201/9781003500247-23

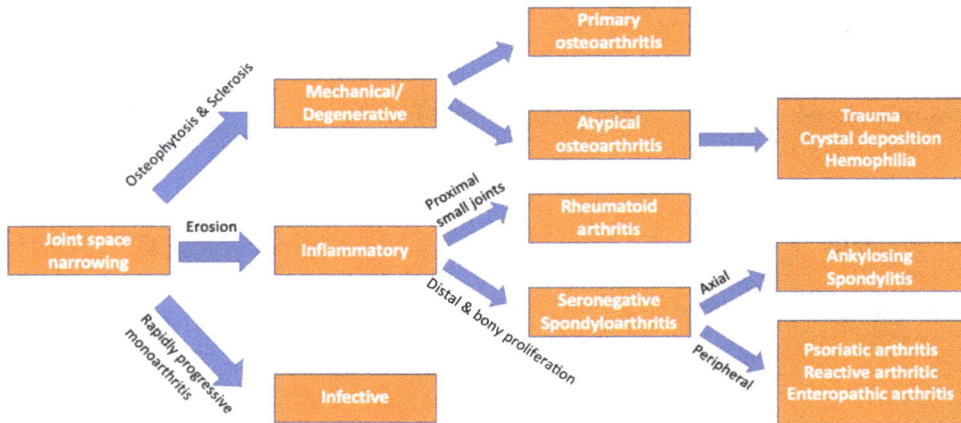

Figure 2.14.1 Flowchart illustrating the radiological evaluation of arthritis. (Modified from Jacobson JA, Girish G, Jiang Y, Resnick D. *Radiographic Evaluation of Arthritis: Inflammatory Conditions. Radiology*, 2008.)

Table 2.14.1 **Primary and Secondary Causes of Osteoarthritis**

Type	Description
Primary (Idiopathic)	• Has a strong genetic basis • Commonly affects middle-aged women and older population • Typically has asymmetrical joint predilection
Secondary	Resulting from a variety of causes: • *Mechanical Stress*: Repeated occupational strain or obesity • *Joint Injuries*: Post-traumatic OA is a leading cause in younger individuals • *Previous Surgeries*: History of joint-related procedures • *Crystal Arthropathy*: Gout or CPPD • *Inflammatory Arthritis*: For example, rheumatoid arthritis or seronegative spondylarthritis • *Metabolic Disorders*: Haemochromatosis, etc.

- If there is a rapidly progressive inflammation and destruction confined to a single joint, infectious arthritis should be strongly suspected.

- In patients under 40 with joint space narrowing, localised disease suggests post-traumatic or post-surgical causes, while generalised disease raises suspicion for inflammatory, crystal, or haemophilic arthropathy.

CAUSES OF OSTEOARTHRITIS

Although the exact pathophysiology of OA remains unclear, it primarily involves articular cartilage degeneration driven by alterations in local mechanical factors. OA affects all components of the joint, including the bone, ligaments, menisci, joint capsule, synovium, and muscles. This leads to various changes including bony remodelling, ligament laxity, meniscal degeneration, muscle weakness, and synovitis.

Pathophysiology of OA versus Inflammatory Arthropathy

OA arises from wear-and-tear processes, whereas inflammatory arthritis, such as rheumatoid arthritis, is caused by immune-driven mechanisms that result in systemic inflammation and synovial overgrowth (see Table 2.14.2).

THE ROLE OF IMAGING IN OSTEOARTHRITIS

In most clinical settings, X-rays are the preferred initial imaging technique for diagnosing and managing known or suspected OA.

Table 2.14.2 Degenerative versus Inflammatory Arthritis

Feature	Degenerative Arthropathy	Inflammatory Arthropathy
Synovium	Normal or mildly thickened due to mechanical reaction	Inflamed synovium
Cartilage damage	Localised damage due to mechanical wear and tear at load-bearing zones	Destruction to all cartilage driven by immune-mediated mechanisms
Joint	Asymmetric due to focal cartilage wear	Uniform due to generalised cartilage destruction
Bony remodelling	Subchondral sclerosis due to mechanical stress	Periarticular osteopenia due to inflammation
Osteophytosis	Prominent as a response to cartilage loss	Rare or absent
Erosions	Absent; intact bony surfaces	Marginal erosions due to pannus and cytokine activity

- Widely available and low cost: Make it the preferred choice for monitoring disease progression in patients undergoing conservative treatment.

- Limitations: Inability to detect early degenerative changes, low specificity for soft tissue abnormalities, and potential projectional discrepancies that may affect interpretation.

Ultrasound is not commonly used for evaluating OA due to the limited penetration of sound waves, which hinders assessment of dense bone and deep articular structures.

- It can identify secondary signs of degeneration, such as osteophytes, synovitis, and joint effusion.

- Ultrasound is valuable for guiding injections (e.g. steroid and local anaesthetic injections, and hyaluronic acid injections) in the management of joint degeneration.

Cross-sectional imaging is typically used when there is diagnostic uncertainty or to investigate alternative diagnoses.

CT provides high sensitivity for detecting bony degenerative changes and is particularly valuable for assessing spondylolisthesis, facet joint degeneration, and soft tissue calcifications. However, its use is limited by higher ionising radiation exposure and suboptimal soft tissue evaluation, making it unsuitable for routine OA assessment.

MRI is occasionally employed when alternative diagnoses are suspected, or a more detailed evaluation of bone and soft tissue structures is required. It provides comprehensive imaging of articular cartilage, menisci, ligaments, muscles, synovium, bone marrow, cysts, and fluid collections. MRI also can detect early morphological changes in OA before radiographic findings appear; the clinical significance of these pre-radiographic features remains uncertain.

General Radiological Features of Osteoarthritis

OA most commonly affects weight-bearing joints involving the knees and hips, as well as the hands. In younger patients or cases involving less common sites, such as the shoulder, elbow, or ankle, prior trauma or another form of arthritis is often the underlying cause.

Key Diagnostic Points

- A confident diagnosis of OA can be made when joint space narrowing, subchondral sclerosis, osteophytes, and subchondral cystic changes are present, while erosions and periarticular osteopenia are absent.

- If joint space narrowing, subchondral sclerosis, and osteophytes are not all observed, alternative diagnoses should be considered (see Table 2.14.3 and Figures 2.14.2 to 2.14.4).

- Suspect crystal arthropathy in patients with osteoarthritis changes in atypical locations.

- MRI can provide additional insights into disease progression and symptoms, with findings such as bone marrow lesions and synovitis offering valuable information (see Table 2.14.4 and Figure 2.14.5).

Table 2.14.3 Typical Radiographic Features of Osteoarthritis

Type	Description
Joint space narrowing	• Usually asymmetric • Least specific, as this is seen in many other conditions
Subchondral sclerosis	• Sclerotic changes at joint margins due to reactive subchondral remodelling • Less apparent in patients with diffuse bony demineralisation
Osteophytosis	• Due to bony remodelling • Common in degenerative joint disease but less in patients with osteoporosis
Subchondral cysts	• Due to passage of joint fluid into bone occurs through a defect in the cartilage • Non-specific findings, as it can also be seen in other conditions (e.g. RA, CPPD, avascular necrosis)
Bony remodelling	• Certain joints, such as the TMJ, ACJ, SIJ, and symphysis pubis, are more susceptible to degenerative bony remodelling, which can mimic erosions

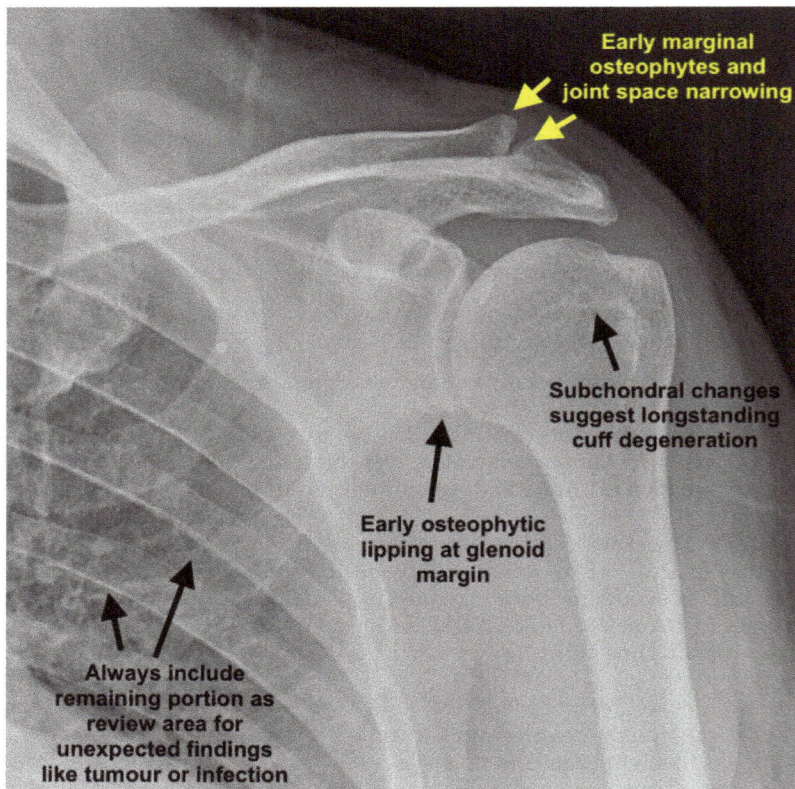

Figure 2.14.2 Mild glenohumeral or acromioclavicular osteoarthritis.

Specific Radiological Distribution of Osteoarthritis

Certain joints are more affected than the others, having a review area when reporting your outpatient plain films will help with your reporting accuracy and diagnostic confidence. Joint space width in the knees and ankles should be measured on weight-bearing radiographs. Table 2.14.5 shows typical radiological features and distribution pattern in axial and peripheral joints.

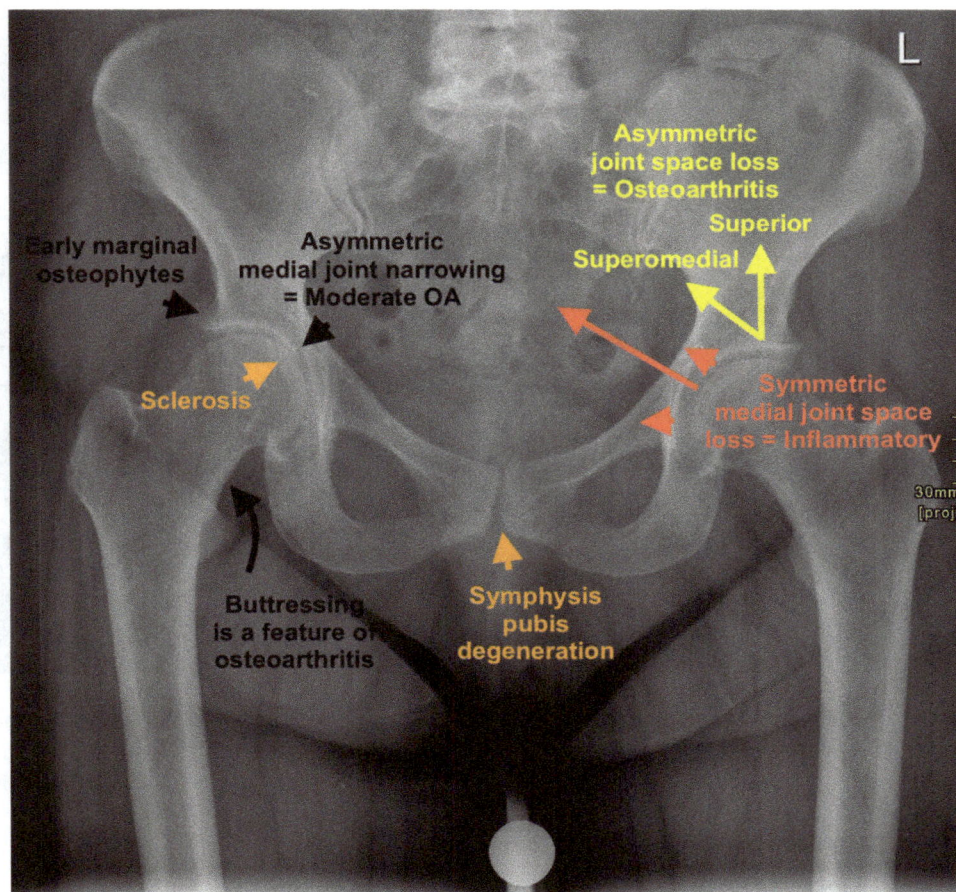

Figure 2.14.3 Moderate right and mild left hip osteoarthritis. Also appreciate buttressing along the medial wall of femoral neck as an early feature of osteoarthritis. Patterns of hip joint space narrowing in osteoarthritis (asymmetric superior or superomedial) and inflammatory arthropathy (symmetric medial where femoral head approaches and goes beyond acetabular teardrop and medial wall).

Radiological Classification of Osteoarthritis Severity

OA severity can be classified using the Kellgren and Lawrence system on radiographs (Table 2.14.6). A radiological diagnosis is confirmed at grade 2, even when the condition shows minimal severity. Figure 2.14.6 shows a visual progressions of OA.

IMPORTANT MIMICKERS OF OSTEOARTHRITIS AND WAYS TO DIFFERENTIATE THEM

Distinguishing osteoarthritis from its mimickers is a critical skill for radiologists, as many conditions—ranging from inflammatory and erosive arthritis to septic arthritis and subchondral insufficiency fractures—share overlapping clinical and imaging features. Accurate differentiation is essential for appropriate diagnosis and management, avoiding potential pitfalls in interpretation.

Inflammatory Arthritis

When erosions occur with joint space loss and osteophytes, it is important to differentiate degenerative from inflammatory conditions (Figure 2.14.7). Inflammatory joint disease is characterised by symmetrical joint space loss and erosions. There is a wide range of differentials when it comes to erosive arthritis, which is covered in Chapters 2.12 and 2.13.

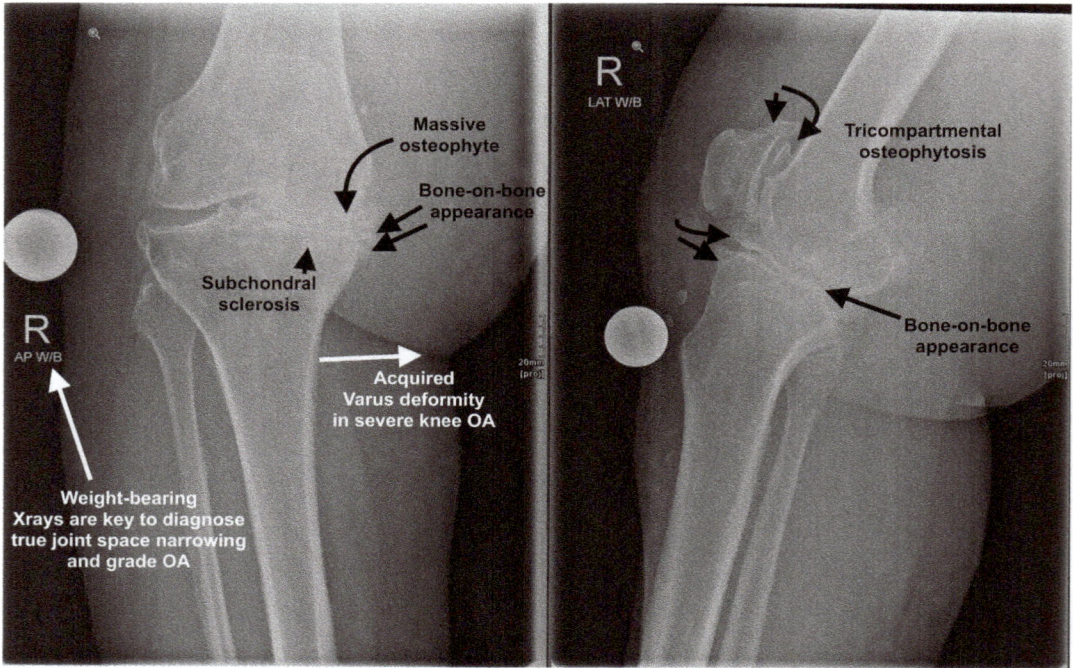

Figure 2.14.4 Severe medial and moderate knee osteoarthritis with complete loss of joint space, bone-on-bone appearances and extensive bony remodelling.

Table 2.14.4 MRI Features of Osteoarthritis

Type	Description
Bone marrow lesions	• Appear as oedema-like lesions at the subchondral surface, due to inflammatory and reactive changes
Synovitis	• Thickened and irregular synovium • Non-specific and can be present in up to half of OA cases • May correlate with pain, severity, and disease progression
Secondary features	• Cartilage loss and subchondral bone irregularity • Joint effusion • Cysts (e.g. parameniscal cysts) and bursitis (e.g. trochanteric bursitis) • Intra-articular loose bodies • Tendonitis (e.g. insertional tendonitis of the greater trochanter)

Erosive OA

Erosive OA, a subset of OA, exhibits both clinical and radiological features resembling rheumatoid arthritis. It predominantly affects elderly, postmenopausal women and is characterised by sudden inflammatory episodes that present with joint pain, swelling, and erythema.

■ The condition most commonly involves the DIPJ symmetrically, followed by the PIPJ and 1st CMCJ while typically sparing the MCPJ and larger joints.

■ A distinguishing feature of erosive OA is the presence of erosions, which set it apart from conventional OA (Figure 2.14.8).

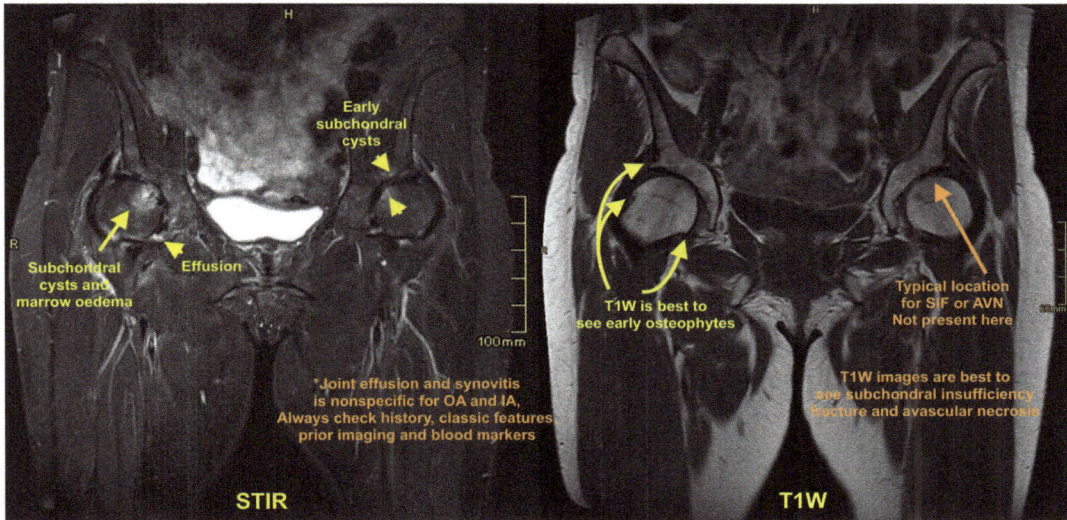

Figure 2.14.5 Typical MRI features of hip osteoarthritis. Also note importance of T1W images in the diagnosis of suspected subchondral insufficiency fracture or avascular necrosis (not shown).

Table 2.14.5 **Typical OA Locations and Appearances**

Region	Description
Hand	Most commonly affects the following sites, in descending order: • DIPJ • 1st CMC • PIPJ • MCPJ Hand OA tends to display symmetric joint space narrowing, unlike the typical asymmetry seen in other joints. • Osteophytes in hand OA • Heberden's nodes: DIPJ • Bouchard's nodes: PIPJ • Imaging: X-rays sufficient for diagnosis
Shoulder	• Associated with chronic rotator cuff tears, prior trauma, or inflammatory arthropathy. • Primary shoulder OA typically affects the ACJ first then glenohumeral joint. • Imaging: X-rays for bone evaluation; US and MRI may be required for labral and rotator cuff assessment.
Elbow	• Associated with trauma or repetitive stress. • Radiographic features include joint space narrowing, osteophytes most commonly in the olecranon and coronoid process, joint effusion, and intra-articular loose bodies. • Imaging: X-rays and CT for bone evaluation; MRI may be required for soft tissue assessment.
Spine	• Spine OA affects synovial joints, involving facet, SI, uncovertebral (C3–C7), atlantoaxial, and occasionally costovertebral joints. • Radiographic features include osteophytic lipping (endplate osteophytosis), intervertebral disc narrowing, subchondral sclerosis, and vacuum phenomenon (gas in intervertebral disc), which is pathognomonic for degenerative disc changes. • Complications: Spinal canal narrowing, neural foraminal stenoses, and degenerative spondylolisthesis. • Imaging: X-rays and CT for bony details; MRI for paravertebral soft tissue and nerve involvement.
Hip	• Associated with acetabular dysplasia, femoroacetabular impingement, prior trauma, or inflammatory arthropathy. • Frequently bilateral joint involvement with predominantly superior lateral and medial joint space narrowing. • Axial space loss with osteophytes suggests OA; without osteophytes suggests RA.

(Continued)

Table 2.14.5 (Continued) Typical OA Locations and Appearances

Region	Description
Knee	• Most common form of OA. • Commonly affects medial tibiofemoral compartment and/or patellofemoral joint asymmetrically; can involve all three compartments in severe cases. • May result in genu varum (bow-legged) or genu valgum (knock-knee) deformities. • Imaging: weight-bearing X-rays preferred; MRI for soft tissue e.g. meniscus injury or bursitis.
Ankle	• Associated with trauma, repetitive stress, or inflammatory conditions. • Most commonly affecting the tibiotalar and subtalar joints. • May result in chronic ankle instability. • Imaging: weight-bearing X-rays preferred; US/MRI for soft tissue, e.g. ligamentous, tendon or bursae related pathologies.
Foot	• Associated with repetitive stress, trauma, obesity. • Most commonly affects 1st MTPJ (hallux rigidus) and talonavicular joints. • Imaging: X-rays sufficient for diagnosis.

Table 2.14.6 The Kellgren and Lawrence System for Osteoarthritis Classification

Type	Description
Grade 0	No radiographic evidence of osteoarthritis
Grade 1	Doubtful changes: Minimal osteophytes; no clear joint space narrowing
Grade 2	Definite osteophytes; possible joint space narrowing
Grade 3	Moderate osteophytes; joint space narrowing; some sclerosis and possible deformity of bone ends
Grade 4	Large osteophytes; marked joint space narrowing; severe sclerosis and definite bone deformity

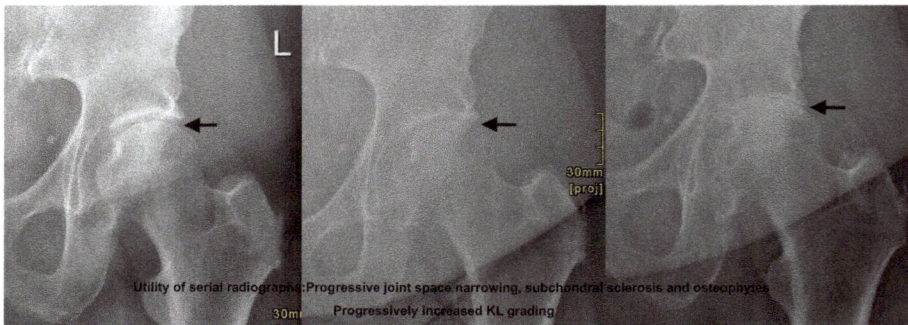

Figure 2.14.6 Serial imaging of the same patient demonstrates progressive degenerative changes in the left hip from mild to severe OA.

■ A hallmark radiological finding is the "gull-wing" or "seagull" deformity, caused by central erosions combined with marginal osteophytes.

■ In some cases, this appearance can mimic a pencil-in-cup deformity. As the disease progresses, late-stage presentations may include interphalangeal joint ankylosis.

Septic Arthritis

When a single joint is affected, it is important to consider septic arthritis (Figure 2.14.9), particularly in the presence of underlying risk factors.

■ It often manifests as rapidly progressive monoarthritis with various potential causes, such as haematogenous spread, trauma, or recent joint instrumentation and can lead to rapid, irreversible joint destruction if untreated.

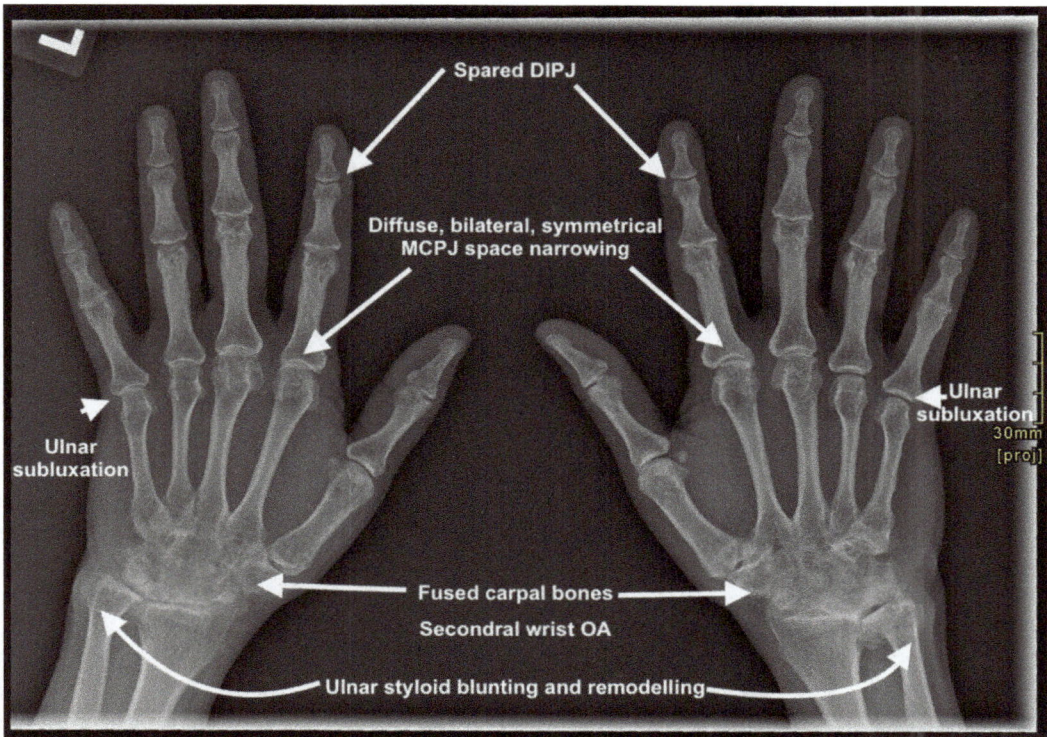

Figure 2.14.7 Severe rheumatoid arthritis in both wrists, characterised by classical features (see images), ankylosis, and de-ossification of carpal bones.

- Early radiological findings may appear normal on X-ray, with joint effusion being the only detectable sign, while advanced stages may show joint space narrowing, cartilage destruction, and eventually ankylosis.

- **A normal plain film does not exclude septic arthritis, and clinical assessment, blood markers, and if appropriate joint aspiration are crucial for confirmation.**

- Although MRI is a reasonable tool for further evaluation, **management should NOT be delayed while awaiting imaging**.

- MRI can provide additional details including synovitis, bone marrow oedema, and articular or bone erosion. In adults, the knees are the most commonly affected joints, while in children, it is typically the knees or hips.

SUBCHONDRAL INSUFFICIENCY FRACTURE/STRESS FRACTURE

Subchondral insufficiency fracture (SIF) is a type of stress fracture due to excessive mechanical stress applied to weight-bearing subchondral bone, most commonly occurs in the knee and femoral head.

- Many patients describe a sudden onset of severe pain in the absence of major trauma.

- Like most stress fractures, SIF can be normal in initial radiographs before demonstrating signs of fracture such as subchondral radiolucency, callus formation, and subchondral sclerosis followed by collapse.

- MRI shows low T1 signal intensity through the subchondral surface, indicating subchondral bone plate fracture and local ischaemia, with associated ill-defined florid bone marrow oedema.

- SIF may be complicated by secondary osteonecrosis, resulting in osteochondral collapse and concomitant secondary degeneration.

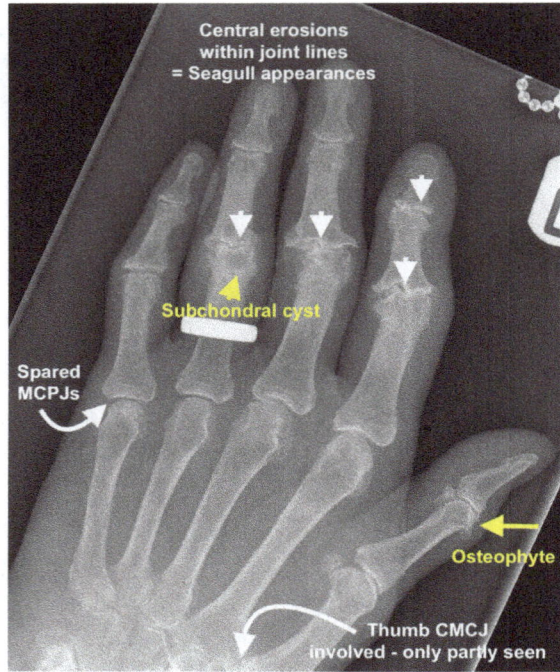

Figure 2.14.8 Erosive osteoarthritis with PIPJ and DIPJ involvement, spared MCPJs, central erosions giving rise to "gull-wing" deformity.

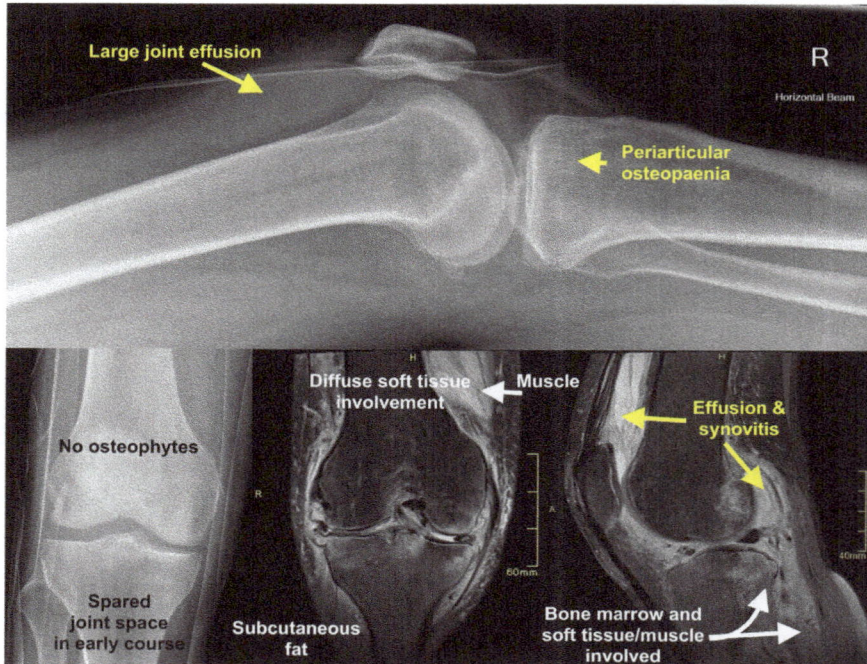

Figure 2.14.9 X-ray and MRI features of septic arthritis.

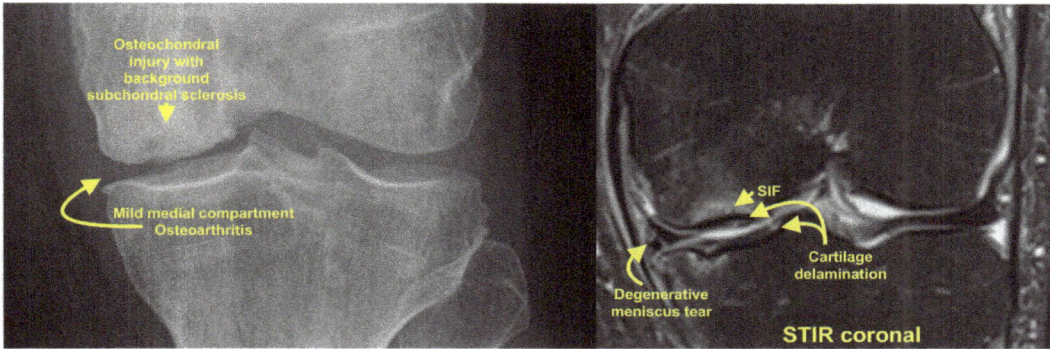

Figure 2.14.10   Subchondral insufficiency fracture complicating the medial compartment knee osteoarthritis.

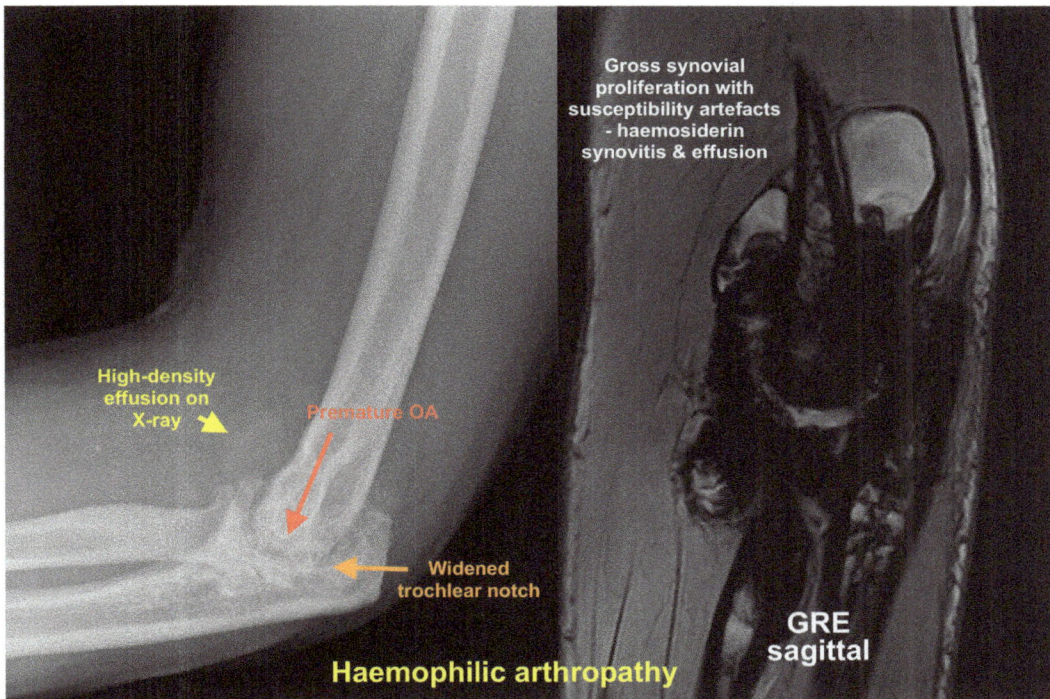

Figure 2.14.11   X-ray and MRI appearances of the haemophilic arthropathy affecting the elbow.

■ Subchondral insufficiency fracture of the knee is typically unilateral and generally affects the medial femoral condyle but can sometimes extend to the tibial plateau (Figure 2.14.10).

HAEMOPHILIA

■ X-linked recessive disease mainly affecting males, spontaneous or minor trauma related repeated-haemarthrosis since childhood causes intra-articular free iron and haemosiderin deposition, reactive synovial proliferation, cartilage degradation, and premature OA.

■ Knee, ankle, and hip in the lower limb and elbow and shoulder in the upper limb are commonly involved.

■ X-rays: High-density joint effusion, periarticular osteopaenia, multiple erosions, enlarged epiphysis, widened intracondylar notch in knees and trochlear notch in elbows (Figure 2.14.11), and features of OA.

- MRI: For early disease, joint effusion, synovitis, erosions, and cartilage damage; haemosiderin-related synovitis causing blooming artefacts; or susceptibility-related signal drop on GRE (Figure 2.14.11). Differential diagnoses are GCT and synovial osteochondromatosis.

THE ROLE OF THE RADIOLOGIST IN THE MANAGEMENT OF OA

Radiologists playing a pivotal role in diagnosing, prognosticating, monitoring, and guiding treatment for OA. Additional imaging is warranted in cases of atypical presentations or unusual radiographic findings. Radiologists must have a solid understanding of the utility of various imaging modalities in diagnosing additional or alternative joint abnormalities. Image-guided interventions, such as intra-articular injections using ultrasound or fluoroscopic guidance, can be performed by radiologists in managing symptomatic peripheral and axial joint degeneration.

CONCLUSION

With an ageing society, the complexity of radiological manifestations of OA will continue to increase. Having a solid understanding of the diverse presentations, mimickers, and appropriate imaging recommendations are vital to guide patient treatment. The ability to distinguish degenerative changes from other important mimics is crucial for early diagnosis and timely treatment. Familiarity with advanced imaging modalities enhances diagnostic accuracy, streamlines patient pathways, and contributes to improved outcomes.

SUGGESTED READING

- Roemer, F. W., Demehri, S., Omoumi, P., Link, T. M., Kijowski, R., Saarakkala, S., Crema, M. D., & Guermazi, A. (2020). State of the art: Imaging of osteoarthritis-revisited 2020. *Radiology*, 296(1), 5–21. https://doi.org/10.1148/radiol.2020192498

- Sakellariou, G., Conaghan, P. G., Zhang, W., Bijlsma, J. W. J., Boyesen, P., D'Agostino, M. A., Doherty, M., Fodor, D., Kloppenburg, M., Miese, F., Naredo, E., Porcheret, M., & Iagnocco, A. (2017). EULAR recommendations for the use of imaging in the clinical management of peripheral joint osteoarthritis. *Annals of the Rheumatic Diseases*, 76(9), 1484–1494. https://doi.org/10.1136/annrheumdis-2016–210815

- Uson, J., Rodriguez-García, S. C., Castellanos-Moreira, R., O'Neill, T. W., Doherty, M., Boesen, M., Pandit, H., Möller Parera, I., Vardanyan, V., Terslev, L., Kampen, W. U., D'Agostino, M. A., Berenbaum, F., Nikiphorou, E., Pitsillidou, I. A., de la Torre-Aboki, J., Carmona, L., & Naredo, E. (2021). EULAR recommendations for intra-articular therapies. *Annals of the Rheumatic Diseases*, 80(10), 1299–1305. https://doi.org/10.1136/annrheumdis-2021–220266

SBA QUESTIONS

1a) A 60-year-old female presented to the rheumatology clinic with bilateral hand pain and stiffness. Radiographs of both hands demonstrate joint space narrowing and irregularity with central erosions and large osteophytes at the proximal and distal interphalangeal joints. There is associated soft tissue swelling but no periosteal reaction. Normal appearances of the metacarpophalangeal joints. What is the most likely diagnosis?

    A. Gout

    B. Psoriatic arthritis

    C. Erosive osteoarthritis

    D. Rheumatoid arthritis

    E. Osteoarthritis

1b) Which joint is least likely to be involved in erosive osteoarthritis?

    A. DIP

    B. PIP

    C. MCP

    D. 1st MCP

    E. 1st IP joint of the thumb

2) A 70-year-old male has presented with worsening bilateral knee and hip pain. Which radiographic feature is more suggestive of a diagnosis of rheumatoid arthritis rather than osteoarthritis?

A. Protrusio acetabuli

B. Joint effusion

C. Tendon enthesopathy

D. Periarticular osteopaenia

E. Intra-articular loose body

3a) A 31-year-old semi-professional rugby player presented with insidious onset of left knee pain. He is systematically well and denies any prior trauma. Knee radiograph demonstrates small joint effusion and mild degenerative changes in the medial tibiofemoral and patellofemoral joints. What is the next best course of action?

A. Refer for US

B. Refer to physiotherapy

C. Refer to rheumatology clinic

D. Trial intra-articular joint injection

E. Refer for MRI

3b) What is the most likely finding on MRI?

Condition	Description
Horizontal tear of the posterior horn medial meniscus	• Peripheral meniscal vertical tears are common in young athletes. Horizontal tears are often associated with osteoarthritis.
Full-thickness cartilage loss with subchondral cyst formation	• **Full-thickness cartilage loss** and **subchondral cysts** are features of **advanced OA**. While this patient does have mild degenerative changes on radiographs, full-thickness cartilage loss is unlikely in a 31 year old with no prior trauma or long-standing joint degeneration.
Bone marrow oedema in the medial tibial plateau	• Bone marrow oedema is a common finding in early degenerative changes or mechanical overload, especially in athletes. Early osteoarthritis is often accompanied by bone marrow oedema on MRI.
Synovitis with pannus formation	• This patient has no systemic symptoms or radiological features to suggest inflammatory arthritis.
Anterior cruciate ligament tear	• The patient denies any prior trauma and presents with **insidious onset of pain** that is inconsistent with the clinical picture of an ACL tear.

A. Horizontal tear of the posterior horn medial meniscus

B. Full-thickness cartilage loss with subchondral cyst formation

C. Bone marrow oedema in the medial tibial plateau

D. Synovitis with pannus formation

E. ACL tear

Answers: (1a) C, (1b) C, (2) D, (3a) E, (3b) C

Chapter 2.15
Principles of Interventional Musculoskeletal Radiology

Patrick Baker and Kenneth Lupton

LEARNING OBJECTIVES

- Appreciate various types of musculoskeletal interventions available for various indications and appropriate choice of a relevant imaging technique to obtain the objective of the intervention

- Understand relevant need of asepsis, anticoagulation, consenting, and pre-procedural checks

- Understand the choice of approach and needle placement, and post-procedural care

---

INTRODUCTION

Interventions in musculoskeletal (MSK) radiology have several diagnostic and therapeutic applications. Depending on pathology, procedures can be undertaken using ultrasound, fluoroscopy, or computed tomography (CT), and indications are generally divided into three broad categories.

- Diagnostic sampling: Soft tissue or bone biopsies (when suspected sarcoma, please refer the patient to a dedicated sarcoma service), aspirations of fluid collections or joint effusions, and uncommonly fine needle aspiration/biopsy

- Therapeutic indications: Imaging-guided steroid and local anaesthetic injections to joints, tendons, bursae, and other soft tissue/bony abnormalities (majority of the requests), calcific tendinopathy barbotage, and uncommonly, platelet-rich-plasma (PRP) and hyaluronic acid injections

- Complex palliative or definitive treatments: Tumour ablations, cementoplasty, and vertebroplasty

Whilst a detailed description of all MSK guided intervention is beyond the scope of this text, the following chapter aims to give an overview of important considerations and general principles of commonly performed MSK procedures rather than providing FRCR-specific information. Occasionally, fluoroscopy images may be used to initiate the discussion about pathologies on MR arthrograms.

General Principles

- Always consider risks versus benefit for all interventional procedures.

- Have clear rationale for an intervention including its intended benefits and potential complications.

- Check the patient capacity, allergies, optimise medications, and assess patient ability to tolerate the procedure in ALL patients. It requires close collaboration between the requesting clinician and the radiologist performing the procedure.

Consent

- The patient must have the capacity to consent to a procedure.

- If not, follow the Trust-specified guidance on consenting the patient without mental capacity. It must be in the patient's best interests, and appropriate legal documentation MUST be completed.

- Consent can be verbal or written. Adequate information regarding the procedure, alternative options and risks must be provided. A record MUST made in the radiology report.

- It is good practice for the patient to have access to procedural information including benefits and risks in advance of their appointment to ensure sufficient time for consideration.

Anticoagulation

- Most MSK procedures, especially superficial procedures, have low risk of significant bleeding. Generally, no specific pre-procedural instructions regarding coagulation checks or cessation of antiplatelet/anticoagulant medications are required in such cases.

DOI: 10.1201/9781003500247-24

- Complex procedures including spinal interventions, bone interventions including biopsies, cementoplasties, and ablations have increased risk of bleeding or significant complication (e.g. epidural haematoma). It is recommended to ensure that coagulation status is optimised.

- Departmental guidelines will vary for the specific acceptable clotting parameters for each procedure. It is prudent to review and have a working understanding of these in your department. Appropriate bridging plan must be in place by the clinical team to prevent potential complications, e.g. stroke in the case of anticoagulation for AF.

HOW TO CHOOSE THE IMAGING MODALITY FOR A PROCEDURE

Ultrasound allows the real-time visualisation of needle placement to target soft tissue lesions or to facilitate injection/aspiration to joints, ganglia, bursae, or other regions. There is no ionising radiation risk.

- Superficial soft tissue lesions can usually be targeted using a high frequency linear or small footprint (hockey-stick) probe.

- The probe approach can be in plane or out of plane. In plane is generally preferred as it allows visualisation of the needle along its length. For smaller or superficial joints such as the thumb carpometacarpal and acromioclavicular joints, out of plane is used for ease of positioning where the needle appears as a bright dot in the image as it passes beneath the ultrasound probe.

- Disadvantage: Inability to image beneath bony structures poses challenge for deep structures.

CT offers the ability to guide needle placement for bony or deep joint intervention. It can be used to perform procedures such as sacroiliac injections, facet joint injections, and spinal nerve root blocks as well as bone biopsies.

- Disadvantage: Stringent patient positioning, intermittent needle tip visualisation during CT fluoroscopy, and the use of ionising radiation.

Fluoroscopy can track needle in real time and is particularly useful in joint-based injections such as in the glenohumeral and hip joint arthrograms and injections. It requires injection of radiopaque contrast to confirm intra-articular location of the needle tip. It also uses ionising radiation.

Positioning

- It varies depending on the site and nature of the procedure as well as factors such as patient mobility.

- Complex procedures may take longer and require prolonged patient lie, e.g. CT-guided spinal biopsy.

- Specific pathologies such as malignant lesions with pathological fracture or suspected spondylodiscitis are inherently painful and adds to the complexity of interventions requiring sedation.

Procedure-Specific Considerations for Consent before the Procedure
Musculoskeletal Biopsy

- Contraindications include: (1) an inaccessible lesion, (2) overlying skin/soft tissue infection, (3) uncontrolled bleeding diathesis, and (4) an uncooperative patient.

- Procedural risks include: (1) pain, (2) bleeding/bruising, (3) neurovascular injury, (4) adjacent soft tissue injury, and (5) non-diagnostic biopsy are possibilities. Additionally, the patient should be consented for neurological compromise for lesions of the spine and large peripheral nerves (including neural nerve sheath tumours).

- Biopsies for suspected sarcomas require special consideration for potential biopsy track-seeding. The track often requires surgical excision during definitive operative intervention to reduce the risk of local recurrence. Therefore, it is essential to plan the procedure via a dedicated bone/soft tissue sarcoma multidisciplinary team (MDT) meeting.

Steroid and Local Anaesthetic Injection

- Injectable corticosteroids come in the form of particulate and non-particulate formulations, the former having a longer tissue dwell time, potentially prolonging the beneficial treatment effect. Non-particulate formulations are preferred for high-risk injections, e.g. cervical nerve root blocks.

- Local complications include "steroid flare" whereby symptoms are exacerbated for a period of several days prior to any improvement, infection, tendon rupture, and skin dimpling/discolouration due to subcutaneous fatty atrophy.

- Systemic effects can include facial flushing, changes in menstrual cycle, hypertension, and hyperglycaemia in diabetic patients.

- Local anaesthetic risk of chondrotoxicity with frequent intra-articular injection should be considered. Lidocaine, bupivacaine, and ropivacaine are frequently used local anaesthetic agents. Ropivacaine is the least chondrotoxic.

- If the patient is undergoing surgery in near future, discussion with the referring surgeon is advised, as steroids can increase the risk of infection.

TECHNICAL ASPECTS OF COMMON MUSCULOSKELETAL INTERVENTIONS
Ultrasound
Ultrasound-Guided Biopsy

- Ultrasound is the commonly used imaging modality for needle guidance in soft tissue sampling.

- Once an appropriate entry site has been chosen, a mark on the skin is made at the planned entry site, and under strict aseptic technique, local anaesthetic is infiltrated to the skin and soft tissues overlying the lesion and along the planned biopsy path. A small skin incision is then made to facilitate passage of the biopsy needle into the lesion, thus enabling samples to be obtained and sent to histopathology.

- Several biopsy needles are available with varying total needle length, obtainable sample length, and needle gauge. The exact choice will depend on the depth and size of the lesion (Figure 2.15.1).

- Finally, the biopsy can be performed either coaxially or non-coaxially. The coaxial technique causes less damage to the overlying soft tissues. Generally, non-coaxial systems are used, likely because they are cheaper.

Therapeutic Injections

Steroid and local anaesthetic are commonly injected into bursae, tendon sheaths, and joints to reduce inflammation. Two of the most frequently targeted bursae are subacromial and trochanteric bursae.

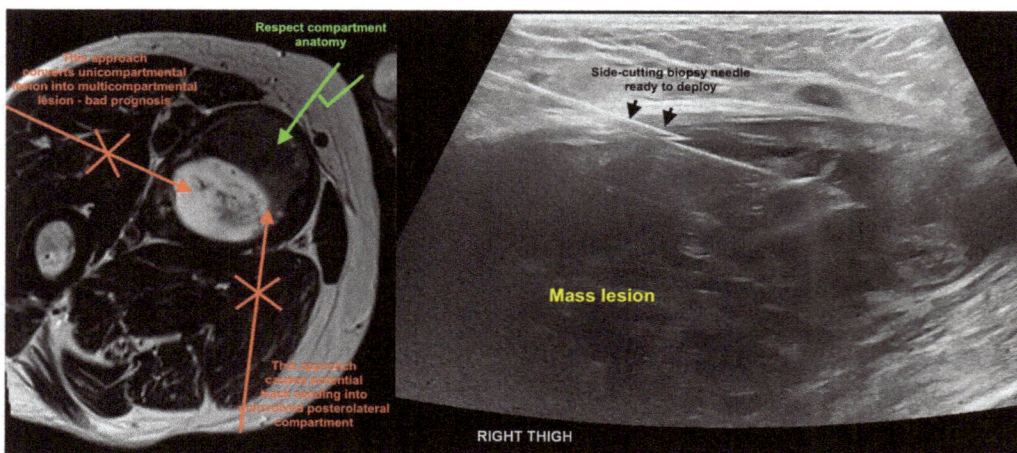

Figure 2.15.1 MRI image showing appropriateness of the biopsy track choice and ultrasound-guided biopsy procedure.

Subacromial Subdeltoid Bursa

- In-plane approach (Figure 2.15.2).

- Position the patient semi-supine with the arm in the neutral position and elbow slightly flexed over the waist.

- The needle is placed in the bursa, which immediately overlies the supraspinatus tendon. During injection, the bursa should distend slightly, and turbulent flow of the injectate should be seen flowing away from the needle tip.

Trochanteric Bursa

- In-plane approach (Figure 2.15.3).

- Position the patient in the lateral decubitus position (side to be injected facing up).

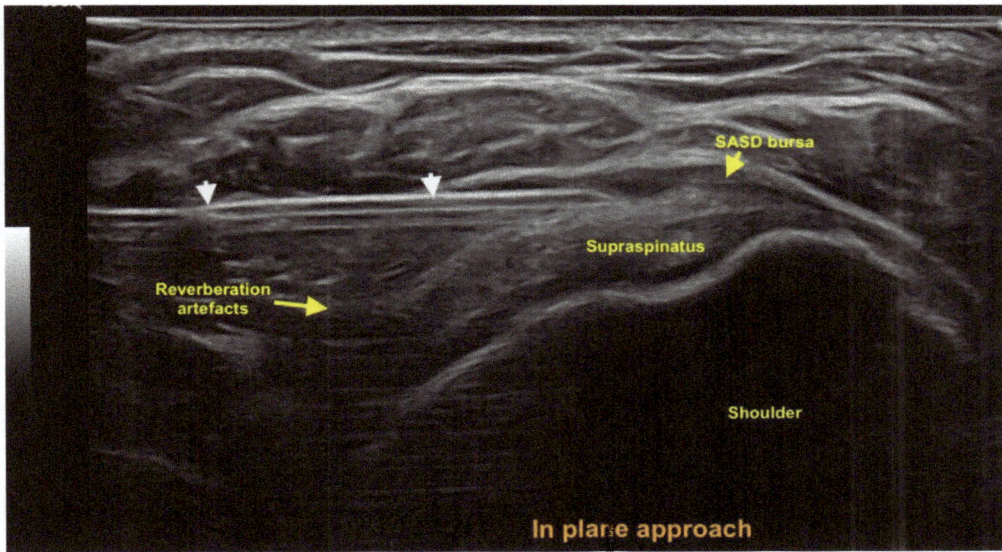

Figure 2.15.2 Ultrasound-guided subacromial subdeltoid bursal injection (in-plane approach).

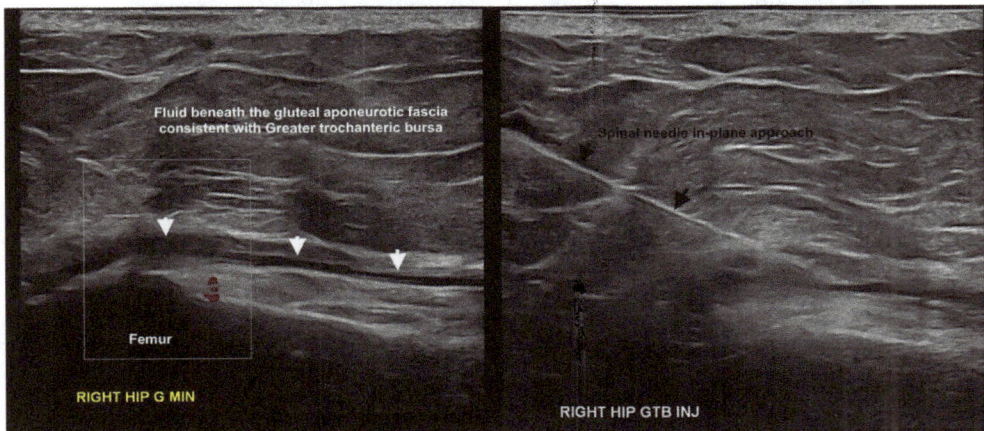

Figure 2.15.3 Ultrasound-guided trochanteric bursa injection (in-plane approach).

- The greater trochanter should be readily identifiable as a pyramidal shaped bony protuberance (in the transverse plane) with the gluteus medius tendon posteriorly, the gluteus minimus tendon anteriorly, and the trochanteric bursa overlying them.

- Often, a spinal needle is required due to deep location of the bursa.

Small Joints

- Small joints in the hands and feet can pose specific challenges due to limited space.

- An out-of-plane approach is preferred for "cliff-like" joints with limited space (Figure 2.15.4). The needle and its tip are visualised in cross-section giving a bright dot appearance.

- Occasionally, it is easier to perform injections under fluoroscopy for accurate intra-articular positioning and confirmation with contrast agent. Figure 2.15.5 gives examples of both ultrasound- and fluoroscopy-guided steroid injection to the STT complex.

Large Joints

- Commonly performed injections include glenohumeral joint, hip joint, iliopsoas tendon, and ankle joint injections (Figure 2.15.6).

- Lower-frequency probes are useful due to deep location.

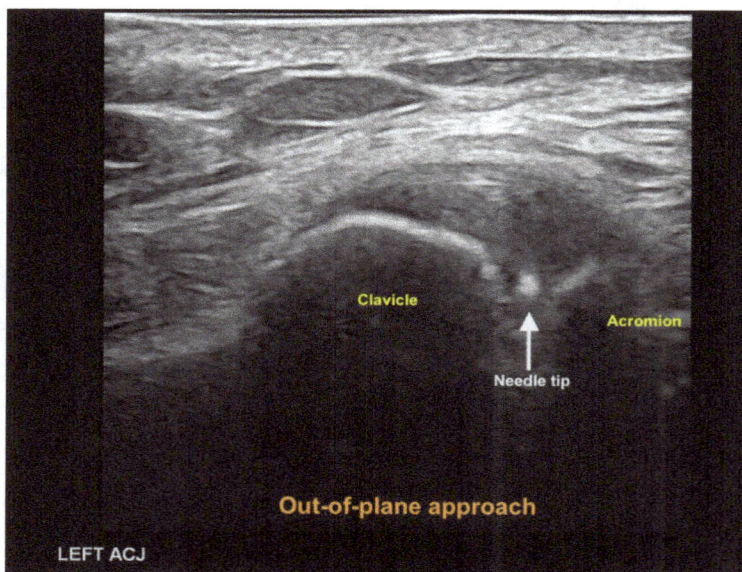

Figure 2.15.4   Ultrasound-guided acromioclavicular joint injection using out-of-plane approach.

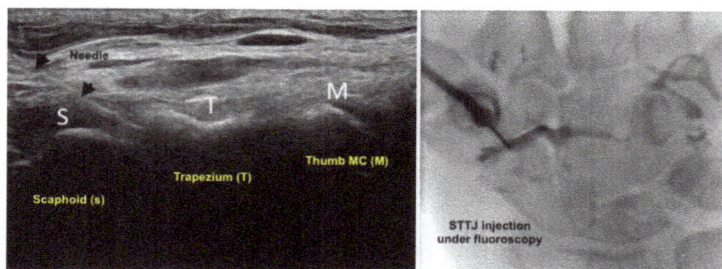

Figure 2.15.5   Ultrasound- and fluoroscopy-guided injection of the scapho-trapezio-trapezoid joint.

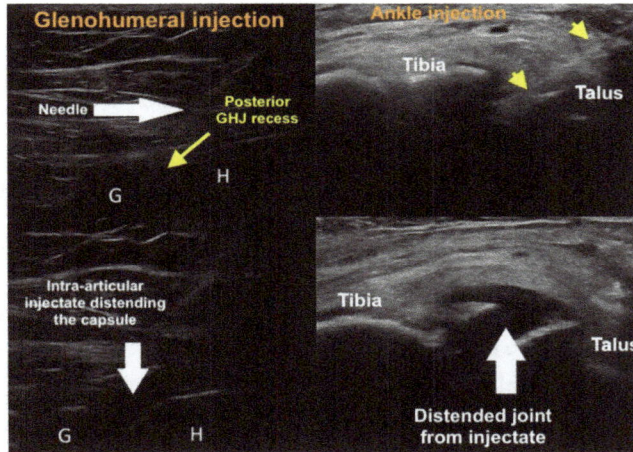

Figure 2.15.6 Ultrasound-guided injection of the glenohumeral joint and the ankle joint in two separate patients.

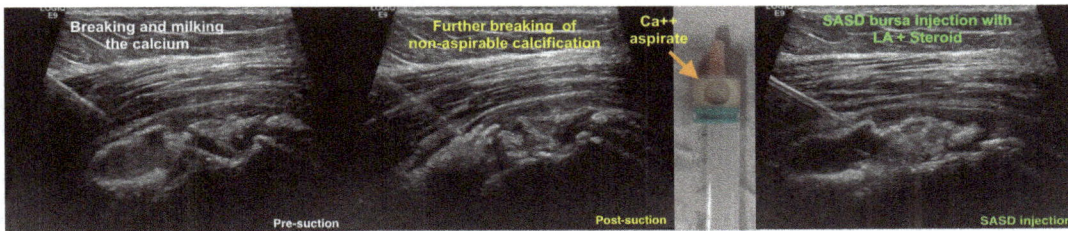

Figure 2.15.7 Ultrasound-guided barbotage of the calcific supraspinatus tendinopathy with 19-gauge needle.

- Longer needles are generally used (21-G or spinal needle).
- It is good practice to aspirate before injecting the medication to prevent inadvertent vascular injection when the needle tip is difficult to visualise.

Barbotage

- It is commonly performed for symptomatic relief of rotator cuff calcific tendinopathy.
- Under ultrasound guidance, a needle (usually 19-G) attached to a syringe of sterile saline/lignocaine is inserted directly into the calcific deposit (Figure 2.15.7).
- The calcific deposit is broken down and lavaged with the solution.
- In such cases with mature deposit, dry needling can be performed to break up the calcium and stimulate natural resorption.
- Following the procedure, steroid and local anaesthetic is injected to the subacromial subdeltoid bursa providing post-procedural pain relief.
- Barbotage can be uncomfortable for the patient, and it is often easiest to perform in the semi-supine position with the arm in the neutral position where access allows.

CT

CT-Guided Bone Biopsy

- For bony lesions, ultrasound can be used to guide needle placement if there is cortical breach and an accessible soft tissue component (often improving diagnostic yield).

- CT is the most common imaging method to visualise the lesion and surrounding structures.

- Under sterile technique, local anaesthetic is infiltrated to the superficial soft tissues and along the biopsy track down to the periosteum overlying the region of interest.

- Judicious subperiosteal local anaesthetic administration is recommended, as if this is achieved, the procedure is generally well tolerated.

- Intraprocedural analgesia and sedation with rapid acting opiates (e.g. fentanyl) and benzodiazepines (e.g. midazolam) can be administered as supplementary agents.

- A small skin incision is made to allow biopsy needle passage.

- It is recommended to use a coaxial technique with the coaxial needle placed at the edge of a lesion, through which the sampling needle can be passed.

- The needle gauge for bone biopsy is generally larger than that used for soft tissue biopsy, and a variety of needles are available including hand- and battery-powered drill biopsy sets.

- Battery-powered drills can be especially helpful in dense sclerotic lesions, which may be harder to access (Figure 2.15.8).

- **If primary bone sarcoma is in question, the patient should be referred to a dedicated bone tumour centre.**

- Spinal biopsies also require special consideration given the proximity of neurovascular structures.

- These are usually performed in the context of vertebral metastatic disease or spinal infection (Figure 2.15.9). However, the diagnostic yield of the latter is often relatively low, particularly if the patient has been on antibiotics prior to sampling.

- It is therefore prudent to ensure that in suspected spondylodiscitis, blood cultures have been taken to attempt to isolate a causative organism, as this may negate the need for the more intrusive biopsy and the associated risks. Various approaches include transpedicular, intercostovertebral, and intercostal routes.

CT-Guided Injections

- CT can be used to confirm accurate needle placement for injection.

- Sacroiliac joint, pubic symphysis, and facet joint injections are examples of where CT is of particular use, as shown in Figure 2.15.10.

- CT-guided nerve root injections are also widely performed (Figure 2.15.11). Contrast is usually injected after perineural needle placement to assess perineural and epidural spread.

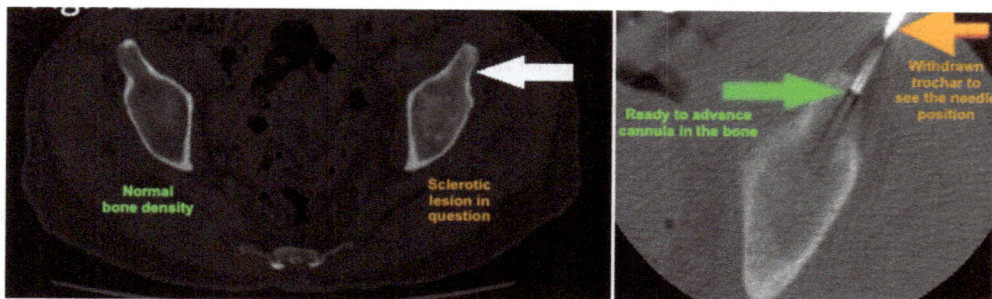

Figure 2.15.8 CT-guided bone biopsy. Note: the coaxial needle has been partially withdrawn to reduce beam hardening artefact at the edge of cortex and provide a more accurate image of the biopsy needle tip.

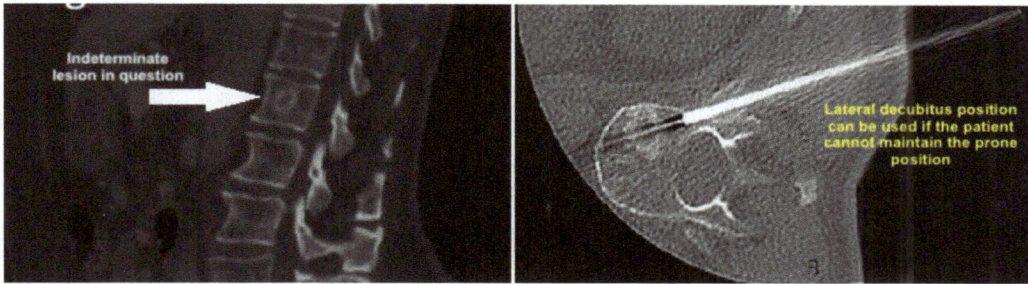

Figure 2.15.9 CT-guided T12 vertebral biopsy using intercosto-vertebral approach in lateral decubitus position. Histology: Metastatic pancreatic adenocarcinoma.

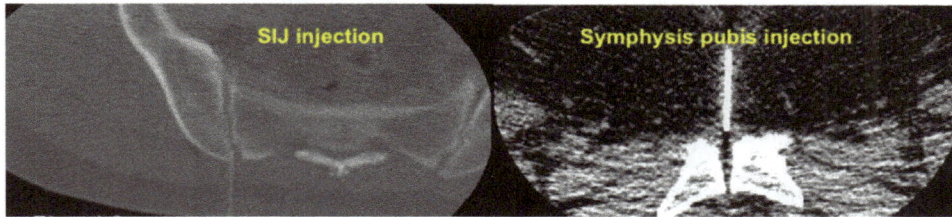

Figure 2.15.10 CT-guided sacroiliac joint injection and symphysis pubis injection in two different patients.

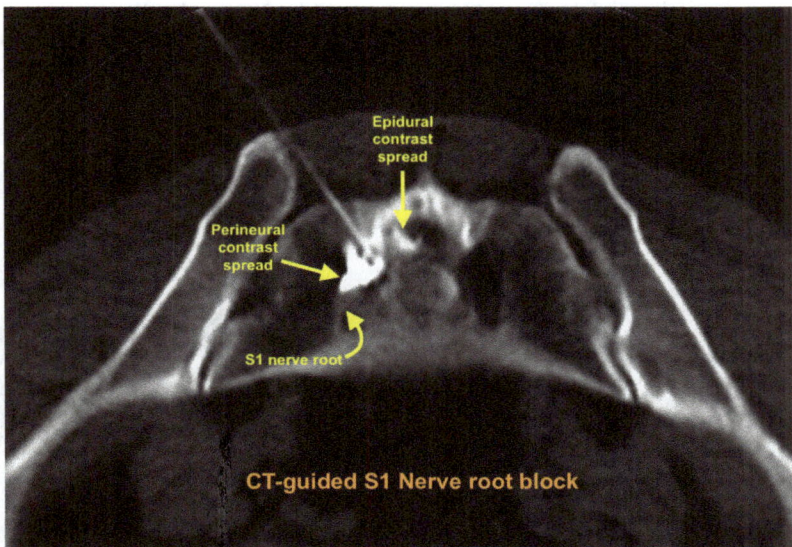

Figure 2.15.11 CT-guided left S1 neural block.

CT-Guided Radiofrequency Ablation

- RFA has become the mainstay of treatment in osteoid osteoma.
- Under CT guidance, an electrode with an active tip is inserted to the nidus of the lesion.

- A radiofrequency current is then passed through the electrode resulting in resistive heating in the tissue adjacent to the active tip inducing cell apoptosis and thus treating the lesion (Figure 2.15.12).

Fluoroscopy

- Fluoroscopy is quick and easy to perform, enabling real-/near-real-time monitoring of needle position.

- It is used to facilitate injection of gadolinium for MRI arthrography, joint steroid injections, shoulder hydrodistension for adhesive capsulitis/frozen shoulder.

- The injection of a small amount of radiopaque contrast prior to gadolinium and its dispersal/spillage away from the needle tip in characteristic patterns confirms satisfactory intra-articular location (Figure 2.15.13).

- Arthrography has the advantage over conventional MRI of improving visualisation of cartilage and labral structures.

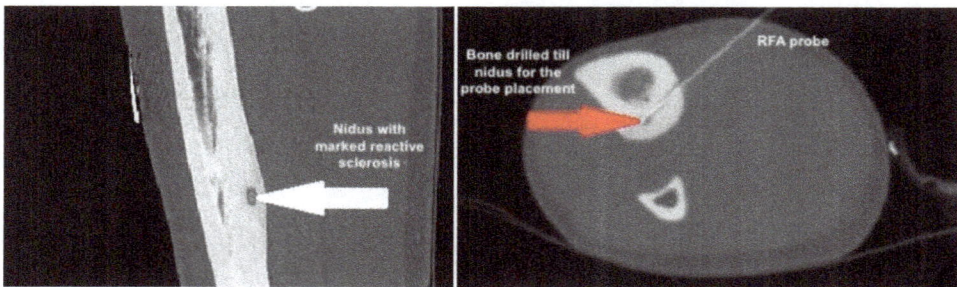

Figure 2.15.12 CT-guided radiofrequency ablation of the tibial osteoid osteoma. The lesion is accessed using a co-axial drill biopsy, and thereafter the radiofrequency electrode is inserted with the active tip (red arrow) in the centre of the lesion. The radiofrequency ablation is performed at 90 °C for 5 minutes.

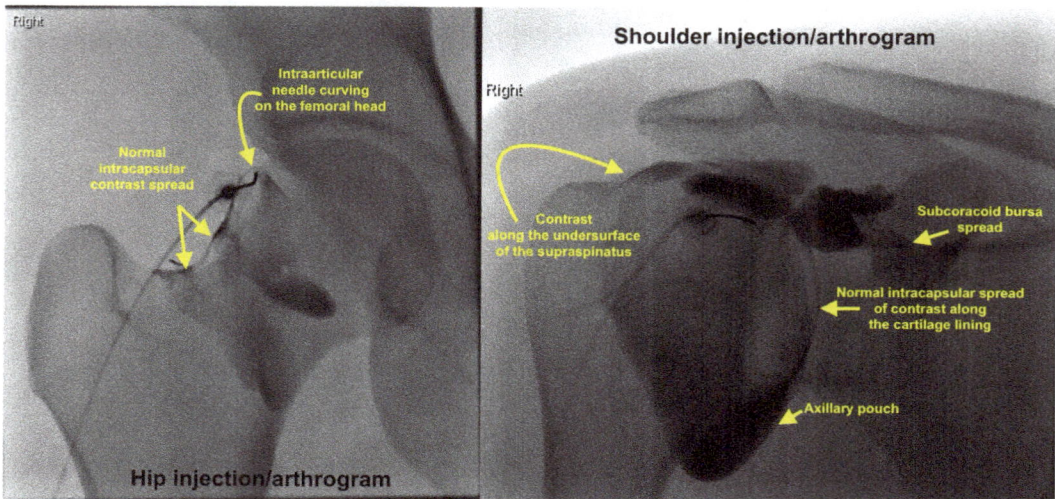

Figure 2.15.13 Needle position and contrast spread on fluoroscopy-guided hip and shoulder injections/arthrograms.

- The fluoroscopic contrast injection can also provide diagnostic information in certain circumstances. If the contrast extends into the midcarpal joint during radiocarpal joint injection, it suggests a scapholunate ligament tear. If the contrast extends from the wrist joint to the distal radioulnar joint, it suggests central perforation or a tear in the TFCC. If the contrast extends from the glenohumeral joint into the subacromial space, it suggests a rotator cuff tear (Figure 2.15.14). MRI appearances of such pathologies are given in Chapter 2.16.

- Fluoroscopy-guided nerve root injections are commonly performed via transforaminal approach and confirming location with a characteristic extension of contrast along the nerve root and epidural space (Figure 2.15.15).

- Procedures such as glenohumeral joint hydrodistension can also be performed for adhesive capsulitis. This involves the injection of approximately 30–40 mL of sterile saline into the joint (along with a smaller volume of steroid and local anaesthetic), stretching the joint capsule and aiming to improve stiffness and pain as well as to facilitate further physiotherapy (Figure 2.15.16).

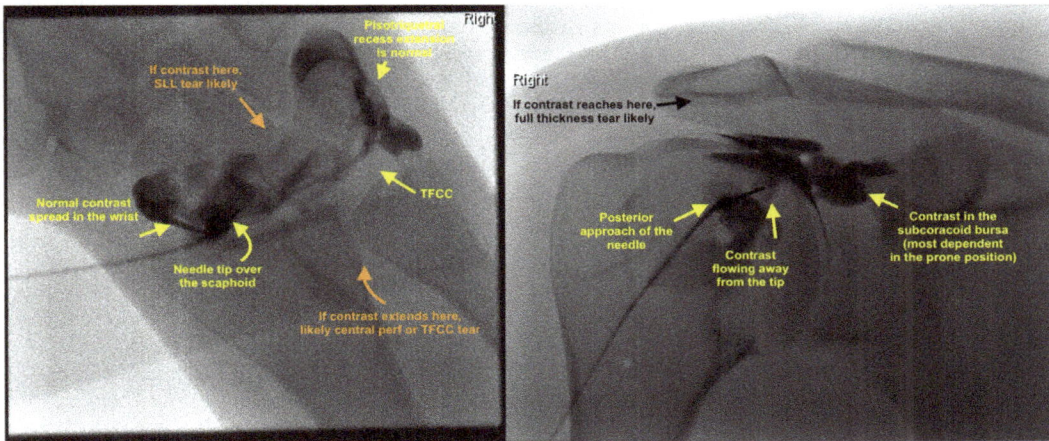

Figure 2.15.14 Normal contrast spread in wrist and shoulder on fluoroscopy and areas of abnormal areas of contrast spread in pathologies.

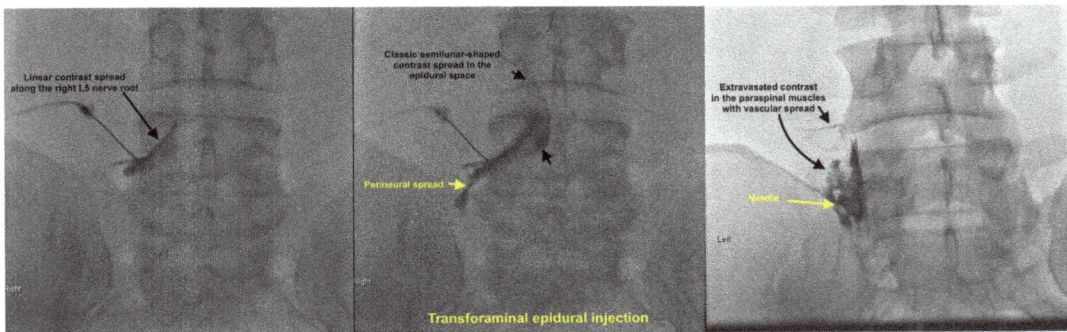

Figure 2.15.15 Fluoroscopy-guided neural block in different cases. Note differences in perineural, epidural, and paraspinal/vascular spread.

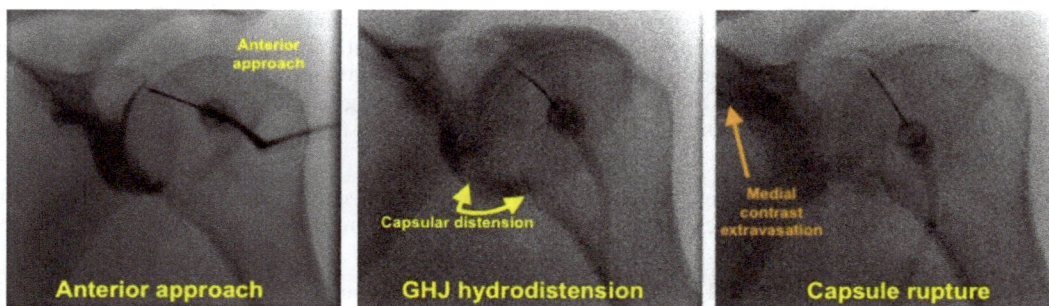

Figure 2.15.16   Fluoroscopy-guided shoulder hydrodistension and capsule rupture.

CONCLUSION

The accurate, minimally invasive, and effective nature of both diagnostic and therapeutic musculoskeletal procedures make them attractive options in the management of a wide range of pathologies. It is important for the practitioner to have a sound understanding of the advantages and limitations of all available modalities and to work collaboratively with their referring clinicians to ensure safe and effective treatment.

SUGGESTED READING

- O'Neill D, Asadi H. Musculoskeletal Intervention. In Kok H, Ryan E, Asadi H, Lee M. (eds) *Interventional Radiology for Medical Students*. Cham: Springer; 2018. https://doi.org/10.1007/978-3-319-53853-2_16

SBA QUESTIONS

1) A radiograph and MRI scan have been performed for a 20-year-old patient with left shoulder pain. The radiograph demonstrates a lesion with a sunburst periosteal reaction and cortical destruction with regions of disorganised osteoid matrix in the proximal humeral metaphysis. MRI confirms these findings with a large extra-osseous soft tissue component and extension of the mass into the surrounding musculature and distally along the medullary cavity into the mid diaphysis. You suspect an aggressive lesion such as an osteosarcoma. What is the most appropriate next course of action?

   A.   Ultrasound-guided biopsy of extraosseous soft tissue component via anterior approach

   B.   Discussion in the sarcoma MDT to agree on an appropriate diagnosis and treatment plan including appropriate biopsy track

   C.   CT-guided bone biopsy via lateral approach

   D.   Open surgical biopsy

   E.   Ultrasound-guided biopsy of extraosseous soft tissue component via posterior approach

2) An 18-year-old male patient with a 4-month history of left knee pain which is worse at night and relieved by aspirin. He has undergone a radiograph, CT, and MRI of the left knee and thigh region. The radiograph shows a small, lucent cortically based abnormality in the lateral femoral diaphysis with a combination of thick ossified and lamellated periosteal reaction overlying. A CT confirms the radiograph findings, and the MRI helps to better demonstrate the extent of periostitis. You suspect a diagnosis of an osteoid osteoma. What is the most appropriate first-line treatment option?

   A.   CT guided cryoablation

   B.   Amputation

   C.   CT-guided radiofrequency ablation

   D.   Conservative management

   E.   Curettage and bone grafting

3) A 75-year-old woman has a long-standing history of left hip pain which has been attributed to osteoarthritis by her orthopaedic consultant. She has been listed for a total hip replacement which is due to take place next month. Unfortunately, she has been admitted to the medical team due to a urinary tract infection. This has now been treated, but the patient's mobility is off her baseline due to worsening left hip pain. The medical team have asked for your assistance to help improve her pain to facilitate discharge. They feel a steroid injection into the left hip joint may be helpful. Which of the following options is the most appropriate next course of action?

A. Inject a steroid and local anaesthetic under fluoroscopic guidance

B. Inject steroid only under fluoroscopic guidance

C. Inject steroid and local anaesthetic under ultrasound guidance

D. Discuss with her orthopaedic consultant prior to performing any intervention

E. Inject local anaesthetic only under ultrasound guidance

Answers: (1) B, (2) C

(3) D: Because intra-articular injection of corticosteroid is a reasonable treatment option to reduce pain secondary to inflammation and a useful temporising measure prior to surgery in the treatment of hip joint osteoarthritis. Within 3 months of surgery; however, intra-articular steroid injection increases the risk of prosthetic joint infection, which could have disastrous consequences and discussion with the orthopaedic team would be the most appropriate option in this case to decide on the best course of action.

Chapter 2.16
Introduction to Sports Imaging—Common Pathologies

Nishika Bhatt, Siddharth Thaker, and Raj Bhatt

LEARNING OBJECTIVES

- To know common sports and activity-related pathologies for all major joints, which may present for musculoskeletal imaging
- To illustrate multimodality imaging appearances of various sports-related pathologies
- To understand biomechanics of various injuries and their effects on imaging appearances

---

INTRODUCTION

Sports imaging is central to diagnosing and managing musculoskeletal pathologies of the upper and lower limbs, which are particularly susceptible to trauma and overuse in athletic activities. Advanced imaging modalities such as MRI, CT, ultrasound, and X-rays provide critical insights into injury patterns, facilitating accurate diagnosis and treatment planning. This chapter explores the spectrum of limb pathologies in sports medicine and examines the diagnostic roles, strengths, and limitations of key imaging techniques in clinical practice.

This chapter depicts various common musculoskeletal pathologies one may encounter in the clinical practice. The core idea of the chapter is to make the reader understand pathogenesis and biomechanics behind injury and imaging appearances. Such cases may be a part of newly added short cases section or table viva.

LOWER LIMB PATHOLOGIES

KNEE PATHOLOGIES

Bone and soft tissue injuries around the knee are one of the most common injury patterns in any joints. Contact sports such as rugby and football usually result in bone and soft tissue injuries such as ligamentous and meniscal tears, traumatic patellar dislocations, or quadriceps tear, whereas track and field athletes usually suffer from repetitive microtrauma.

Knee Bone Marrow Oedema Patterns

Bone marrow oedema (BMO) in the knee is a key imaging finding in trauma-related injuries, such as anterior cruciate ligament (ACL) and posterior cruciate ligament (PCL) tears or patellar dislocation. It reflects trabecular microfractures, interstitial fluid accumulation, or reactive changes due to abnormal biomechanical stress. Common BMO mechanisms include:

- **Pivot shift injury** resulting in ACL injuries, with BMO at anterolateral femoral condyle—sulcus terminalis—and posterolateral tibial plateau depending upon knee flexion (Figure 2.16.1).

- **Dashboard injury** in motor vehicle collisions; associated with PCL tears.

- **Clip injury** in valgus stress leading to opening of the medial side; BMO in the lateral femoral condyle and tibial plateau; associated with MCL tears).

- **Hyperextension injury** from anterior tibial plateau and anterior femoral condyle BMO; associated with cruciate and meniscus tears.

- **Patellar dislocation**: BMO in the medial patellar facet and anterolateral femoral condyle, associated MPFL tears, and osteochondral injuries (Figure 2.16.2).

- MRI is the gold standard for assessing BMO, especially using high signal on STIR and T2W-fat suppressed images corresponding with low T1W signal.

DOI: 10.1201/9781003500247-25

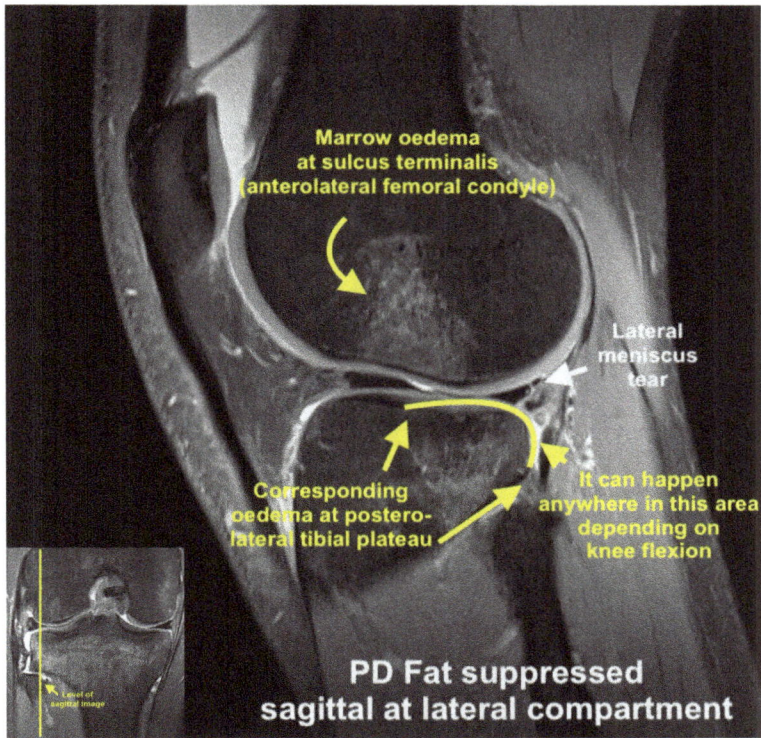

Figure 2.16.1 Typical pivot shift bone marrow on sagittal MRI image.

Osteochondral Defect

Osteochondral defects (OCDs) are characterised by focal injuries involving the articular cartilage and underlying subchondral bone (Figure 2.16.3), often due to trauma, repetitive microtrauma, or ischemic changes.

- In unstable lesions, there may also be detachment or displacement of cartilage and bone fragments, forming intra-articular loose bodies.

- BMO in the underlying native bone is a frequent finding, reflecting reactive hyperaemia, microfractures, or mechanical overload of the subchondral region.

- Inner medial femoral condyle—most common location in the knee.

Imaging

MRI is the gold standard modality for diagnosing and evaluating OCDs. It is performed to investigate the stability of the OCD.

- *Stable OCD*: Normal or low signal in the native bone underlying the OCD, bony bridging, lack of subchondral cyst, and maintained fatty marrow on T1W image.

- *Unstable OCD*: Fluid signal traversing between entire surface of OCD (Figure 2.16.3) and underlying native bone, fluid extending to the articular surface, large subchondral cyst; usually more than 5 mm, disrupted OCD and native bone interface, and focal articular defect.

MRI may also detect secondary features, such as joint effusion, synovitis, and intra-articular loose bodies—dislodged OCD fragment, further aiding in staging and treatment planning. MRI helps determining prognosis and guiding interventions, ranging from conservative management to surgical procedures like microfracture, osteochondral grafting, or chondroplasty.

267

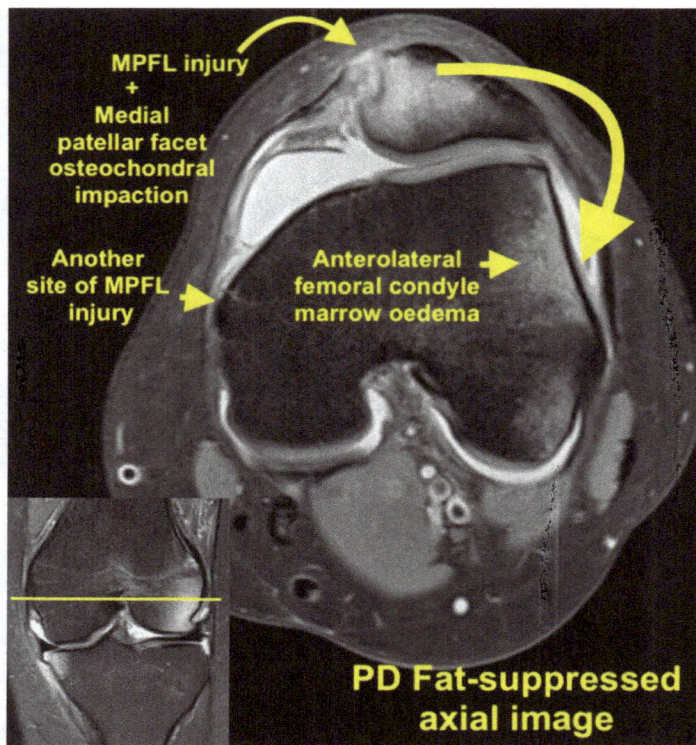

Figure 2.16.2 Bone marrow oedema pattern following acute lateral patellar dislocation event.

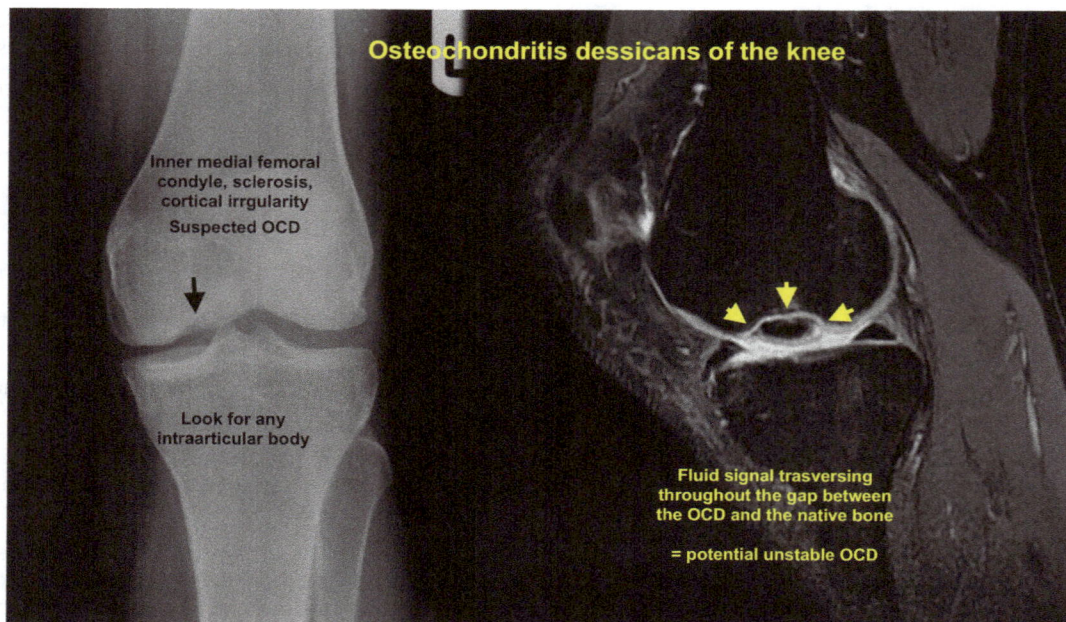

Figure 2.16.3 Osteochondral dessicans of the medial femoral condyle and its instability on MRI.

ACL and PCL Injuries

Cruciate ligament tears are common in high-energy trauma and sports involving sudden deceleration, hyperextension, or direct impact.

- ACL injuries can be partial or complete tears, often involving the proximal fibres near the femoral attachment; conversely, PCL injuries are typically caused by posterior tibial displacement due to hyperflexion or a direct blow, with tears often occurring at the mid-substance or tibial attachment.

- Associated findings include hemarthrosis, BMO, and concurrent injuries to the menisci, articular cartilage, or other ligaments.

  - MRI is the modality of choice for diagnosing and characterising ACL and PCL injuries.

- **Characteristic findings of ACL tear on MRI**: Ligament discontinuity, fibre-wavy contours, ligament falling away from Blumensaat's line, characteristic BMO patterns and ligament oedema and thickening, intra-articular fractures, and effusion (Figure 2.16.4).

- **Characteristic findings of PCL tear on MRI**: Thickened or oedematous PCL fibres, posterolateral corner damage, avulsion fractures, or effusions.

MCL and Posterolateral Corner Injuries

MCL and posterolateral corner (PLC) injuries represent significant disruptions to intrinsic stability of the joint. The MCL is critical to medial knee stability, resists valgus stress, and is frequently injured in athletic trauma or direct lateral impact. MCL injuries are classified into three grades (STIR or T2-FS MRI sequences are the best):

- **Grade I** involves microscopic fibre disruption and periligamentous oedema (seen as soft tissue oedema either superficial or deep to the MCL on MRI).

- **Grade II** reflects partial fibre tearing with ligament elongation (seen as partial width injury—axial images are better to assess on MRI).

- **Grade III** signifies complete rupture (seen as wavy and lax MCL, commonly at the femoral attachment, sometimes associated capsule injury causes joint fluid extravasating on superficial aspect of the MCL, tibial attachment MCL injuries—rare) (Figure 2.16.5).

- Chronic MCL injury at the femoral attachment shows linear calcification: Pellegrin–Stieda lesion (X-rays are better to assess them).

The PLC includes lateral collateral ligament, popliteus tendon, and arcuate complex (Figure 2.16.6), and is essential for varus and rotational stability.

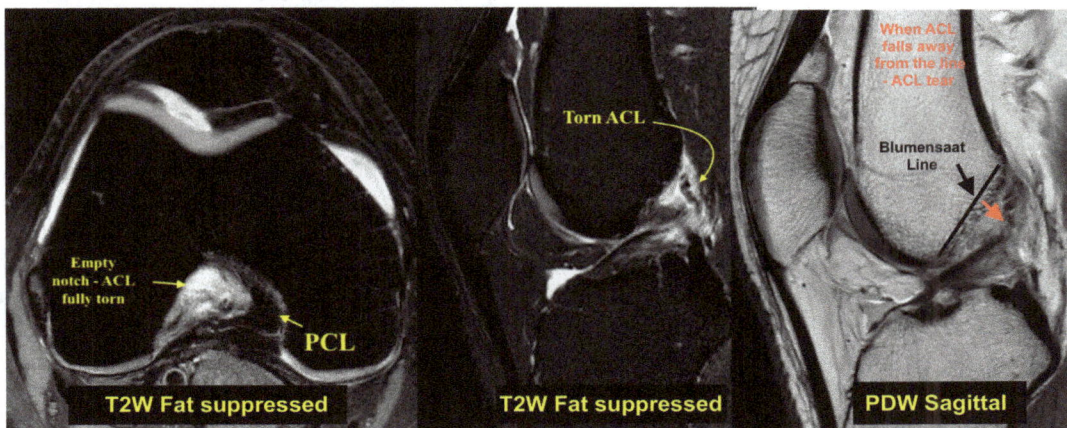

Figure 2.16.4   MRI features of ACL tear.

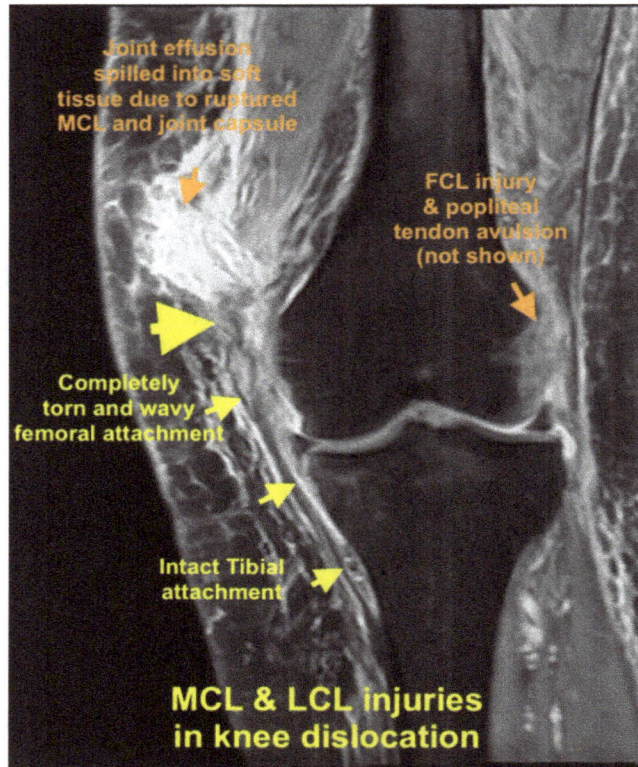

Figure 2.16.5 MCL and LCL tear in the knee dislocation.

- PLC injuries are typically associated with high-energy trauma or complex knee dislocations, associated with concurrent damage to the cruciate ligaments.

- Complications include ligament tears, avulsion fractures, and neural compromise, such as peroneal nerve injury.

- MRI is the diagnostic gold standard for these injuries showing soft tissue thickening, oedema, or discontinuity on coronal and axial images. MRI can show associated osteochondral injuries, BMO, and avulsions.

- Segond fracture is an indirect sign of underlying ACL injury. X-rays can better visualise it. It represents anterolateral ligament tibial attachment avulsion, which is not a part of posterolateral corner.

Meniscal Injuries

Meniscal injuries represent significant intra-articular knee pathologies, frequently encountered as acute traumatic tears and associated with knee osteoarthritis. Acute tears often present with pain, effusion, and mechanical symptoms such as joint locking, whereas degenerative tears manifest with chronic pain and episodic swelling, frequently accompanied by cartilage degeneration.

- The menisci, crescent-shaped fibrocartilaginous structures situated between the femoral condyles and the tibial plateau perform critical biomechanical functions, including load distribution, shock absorption, joint lubrication, and stabilisation.

- **Acute tears**: Due to rotational forces combined with axial loading, often seen in younger, active individuals (on MRI, it can happen in any part of the meniscus with any configuration).

- **Degenerative tears**: Due to chronic mechanical stress, seen in older populations with underlying osteoarthritic changes (on MRI, it usually seen as a radial tear at posterior root, degenerative maceration of the meniscus body or posterior horn-body junction, and extrusion).

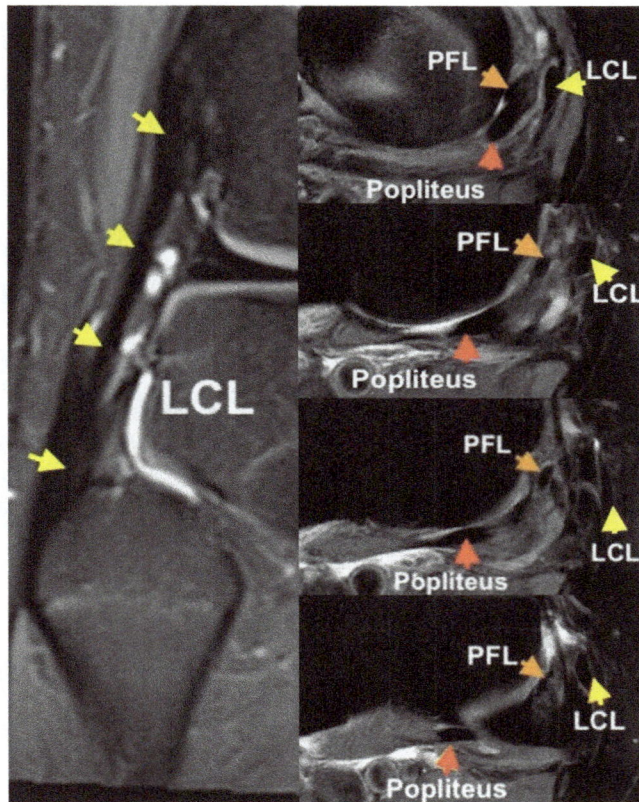

Figure 2.16.6 Normal posterolateral corner anatomy at multiple levels. (LCL—lateral collateral ligament, PFL—popliteofibular ligament.)

- Meniscal tears are classified according to their morphology (e.g. longitudinal, radial, horizontal, bucket-handle, flap, or complex), location (anterior horn, body, posterior horn, or junctions), and chronicity (acute versus degenerative).

- MRI in meniscal tears: The gold standard.

- Meniscal tears are identified as linear or complex high-signal abnormality on T2W/PDW-FS sequences extending to the one of the articular surfaces (Figure 2.16.7).

- Meniscus degeneration signal tends to be globular and usually presents at posterior horn-body junction.

- MRI can also detect the cross-sectional area of the meniscus involved in the tear. Such areas are described as—inner third (least vascular, white–white zone or white zone), middle third (more vascular, red–white zone or pink zone), and outer third/peripheral (most vascular, red–red zone or red zone).

- Additional findings on MRI: Subchondral oedema or ligamentous injuries.

- White zone tears are usually treated with meniscectomy due to poor healing potential, whereas pink or red zone tear can be treated with meniscus repair on patient-to-patient basis.

Patellar and Quadriceps Ruptures

- It presents as trauma, pain, feeling of a "pop" sensation, and extension lag.

- Quadriceps tendon ruptures commonly occur in individuals over age 40 due to chronic degenerative changes.

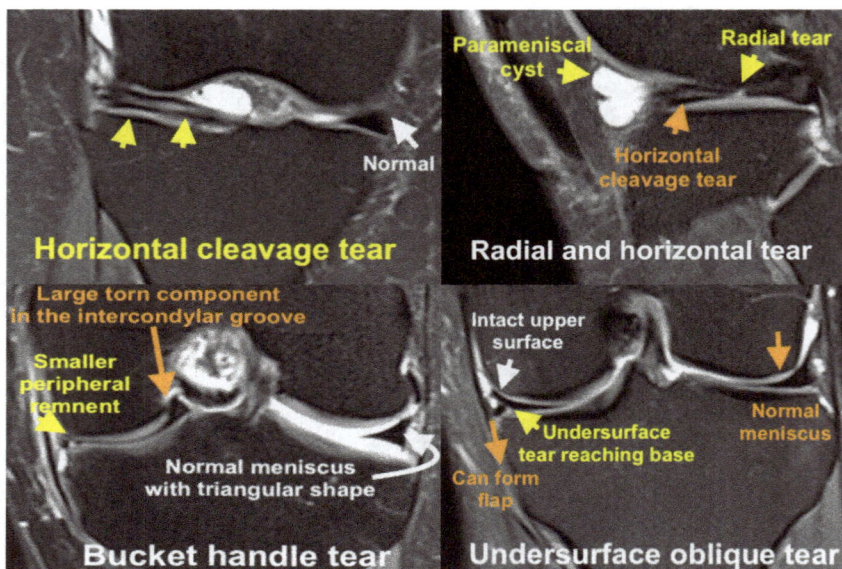

Figure 2.16.7 MRI appearances of various meniscus tears.

- Patellar tendon ruptures are more prevalent in younger populations and often result from high-energy trauma or athletic activities.

- The mechanism is the sudden eccentric loading of the extensor mechanism during forceful quadriceps contraction against resistance.

- Ruptures frequently occur at the tendon–bone interface or within the mid substance.

- Proximal migration of the patella (patella alta) in patellar tendon rupture.

- Distal migration of the patella (patella baja) in quadriceps tendon rupture.

- X-rays detect patellar sleeve avulsion fracture, soft tissue oedema around the injured tendon, obscured infrapatellar fat pad in patellar tendon rupture, and obscured quadriceps fat pad in distal quadriceps rupture without or with haemarthrosis (Figure 2.16.8).

- US provides fast and reliable imaging in A&E and fracture clinic settings.

- MRI is the most sensitive modality. Torn tendon appears as thickened, oedematous, and wavy structure with fluid/haematoma between two torn ends (Figure 2.16.9).

Medial Tibial Stress Syndrome

Medial tibial stress syndrome (MTSS), commonly referred to as shin splints, is an overuse injury frequently observed in athletes and military personnel, from cumulative microtrauma at the bone-muscle interface (Figure 2.16.10).

- Patients typically present with diffuse, activity-induced pain along the posteromedial tibial border, which gradually worsens with continued exertion.

- Differential diagnosis of MTSS: Tibial stress fracture (has similar clinical presentation, X-ray or MRI is usually requested to differentiate between the two) (Figure 2.16.11) or chronic exertional compartment syndrome (need compartment pressure measurement, non-radiological diagnosis).

- Radiographs are unremarkable in early stages or may demonstrate cortical thickening in chronic cases.

- MRI is the gold standard; MTSS (Fredericson) classification is based on periosteal and endosteal BMO on T2W-FS sequences and cortical thickening on T1W.

- CT and bone scintigraphy can provide additional diagnostic information when MRI is unavailable.

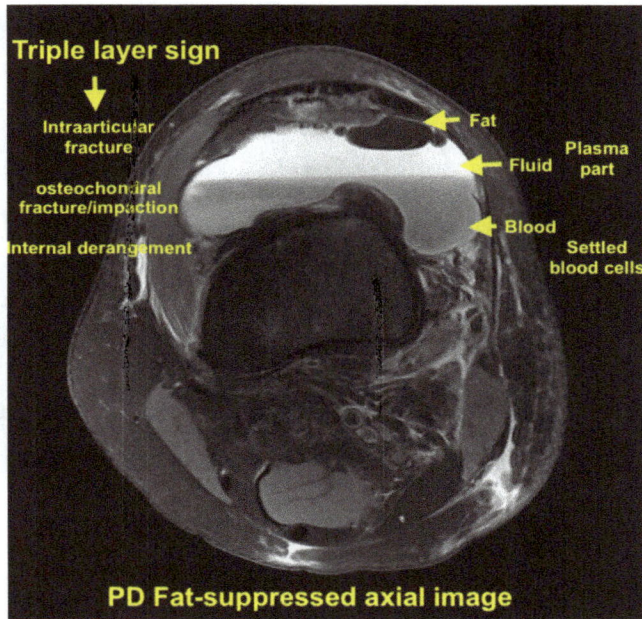

Figure 2.16.8 Triple layer sign in lipohaemarthrosis.

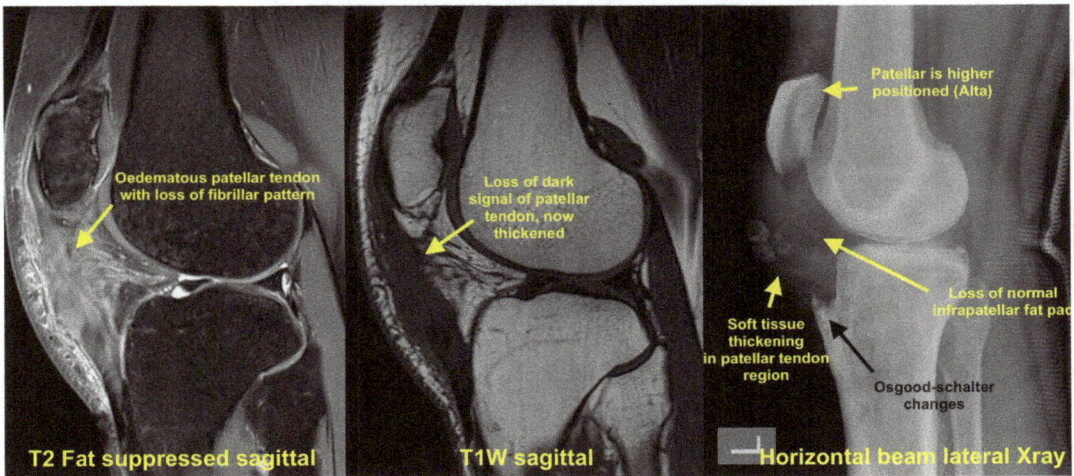

Figure 2.16.9 MRI and X-ray features of patellar tendon rupture.

FOOT AND ANKLE PATHOLOGIES
Osteochondral Lesions of the Talus

Osteochondral lesions of the talus are commonly caused by acute ankle trauma—inversion/dorsiflexion injuries or repetitive microtrauma sequelae. It results in persistent pain, mechanical instability, and progressive joint degeneration.

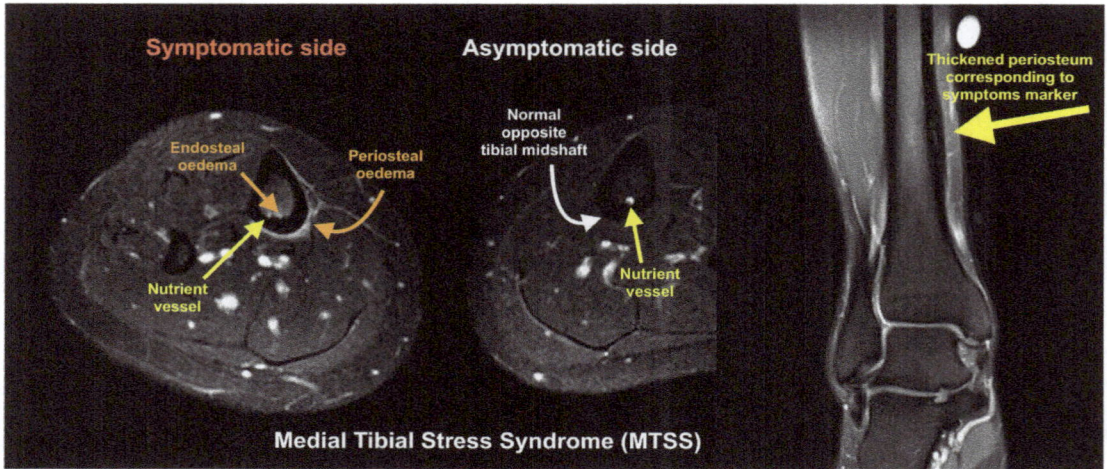

Figure 2.16.10   Medial tibial stress syndrome on MRI.

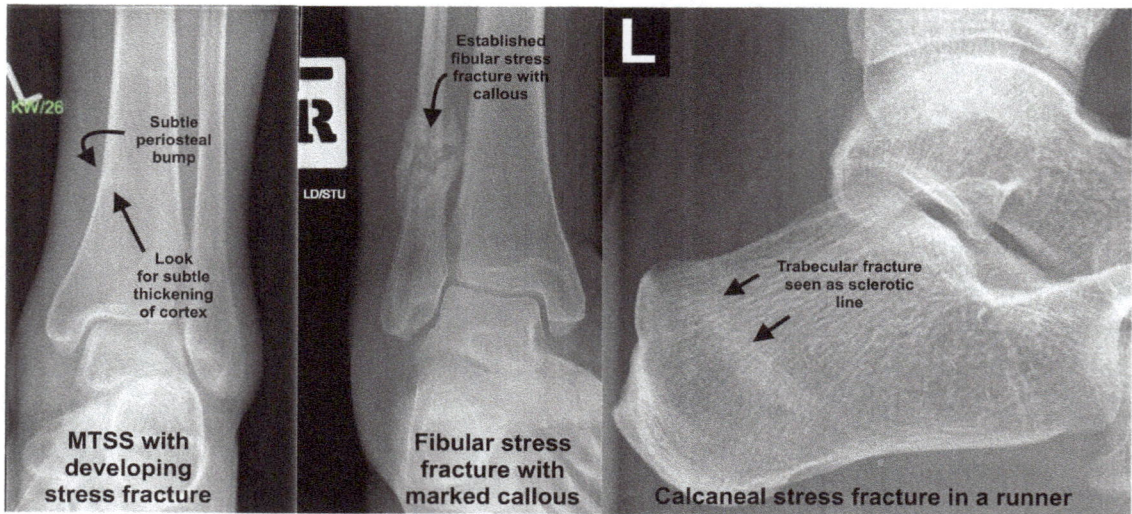

Figure 2.16.11   Stress fractures at various locations in the lower leg.

- Medial talar dome lesions are frequently deeper and associated with inversion and axial loading mechanisms, whereas lateral lesions tend to be more superficial and result from high-impact shear forces.

- Presenting symptoms include chronic ankle pain, effusion, stiffness, and mechanical symptoms such as catching or locking.

- Radiographs are a first-line modality (early lesions may be radiographically occult, advanced lesions may show subtle lucency or fragmentation) (Figure 2.16.12).

- CT reveals superior bony detail and readily assess lesion morphology and fragment stability.

- MRI is the gold standard, detects cartilage integrity, subchondral bone oedema, and lesion viability (MRI findings similar to knee OCDs).

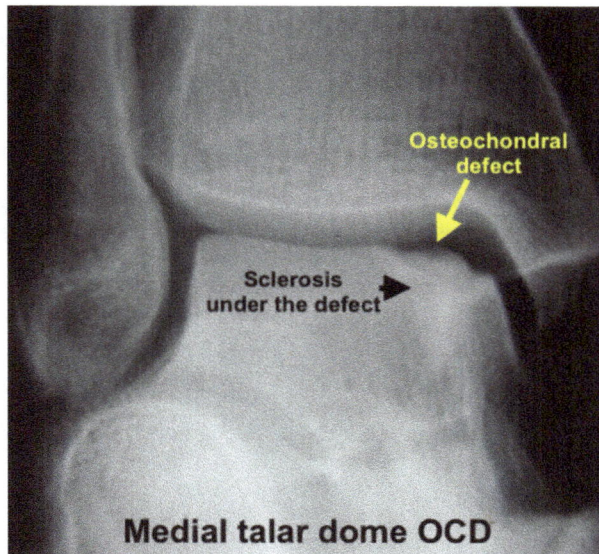

Figure 2.16.12 Talar dome OCD.

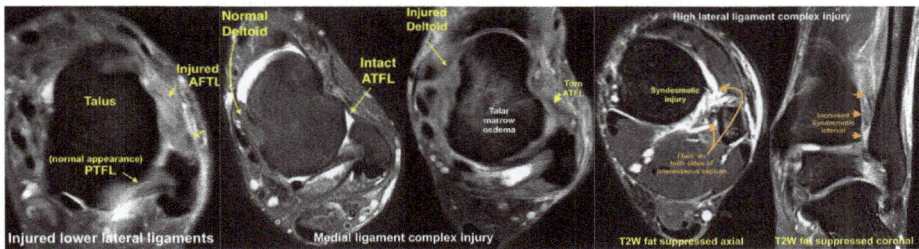

Figure 2.16.13 Injured low and high lateral and medial ligament complexes of the ankle.

■ Conservative management in stable lesions.

■ Surgical techniques in symptomatic and potentially unstable lesions such as microfracture, autologous chondrocyte implantation, or osteochondral grafting.

Lateral Ligament Complex Injuries of the Ankle

■ Common musculoskeletal injuries around the ankle.

■ Injuries to this complex are typically classified as high or low based on their anatomical location.

■ Low lateral ligament injuries primarily involve the ATFL (anterior talifibular ligament) and CFL (calcaneofibular ligament), occurring due to forced inversion. PTFL (posterior talofibular ligament) is robust and rarely ruptures.

■ High lateral ligament injuries extend to the syndesmotic structures, including the anterior inferior tibiofibular ligament (AITFL), interosseous membrane, and posterior inferior tibiofibular ligament (PITFL), often resulting from external rotation or dorsiflexion mechanisms.

■ MRI grading of lateral ligament complex injuries (Figure 2.16.13).

• Sprain (Grade I is most common, seen as mild oedema on MRI of the ATFL/CFL; commonly seen at the fibular attachment).

• Partial tear (Grade II, periligamentous oedema, one out of two bundles of ATFL is torn on MRI).

- Complete rupture (Grade III, loss of continuity and waviness of the ATFL, fluid signal traversing through the ATFL substance).

- Avulsion fracture at the ATFL fibular ligament (associated with small fracture at the fibular tip, some BMO at the distal fibula) in inversion injuries.

- Lateral ligament complex injuries can be complicated by osteochondral and tendon injuries.

Medial Ligament Injuries of the Ankle

The deltoid ligament complex is the most important structure. It consists of superficial and deep components. The superficial fibres (tibionavicular, tibiocalcaneal, and posterior tibiotalar ligaments) contribute to valgus stability, while the deep tibiotalar ligament is the primary stabiliser against external rotation forces.

- Medial ligament injuries typically result from excessive eversion or external rotation and are commonly associated with lateral ankle fractures, syndesmotic injuries, or posterior malleolar fractures.

- Chronic insufficiency can lead to valgus instability and progressive degenerative changes.

- X-rays show medial clear space widening (>4 mm) in syndesmotic injuries or associated fractures, such as medial malleolar or posterior malleolar fractures.

- Eversion stress views: Medial instability.

- US shows hypoechoic thickening or fibre discontinuity in acute deltoid injuries.

- MRI is the gold standard. Acute injuries appear as hyperintense signal changes on fluid-sensitive sequences. Partial tears show thickening and intrasubstance oedema (Figure 2.16.13). Complete ruptures demonstrate ligament discontinuity with surrounding fluid. Chronic injuries show soft tissue thickening and scarring with, sometimes, soft tissue nodule formation (which compresses anteromedial neurovascular bundle—anterior/anteromedial impingement).

- It also assesses associated osteochondral lesions, bone marrow oedema, and posterior tibial tendon dysfunction, which can contribute to medial instability.

Achilles Tendon Pathologies

- Achilles tendinopathy results from repetitive mechanical loading, microtrauma, and impaired tendon remodelling. It is commonly observed in athletes and individuals engaged in high-impact activities.

- Collagen disorganisation, tenocyte proliferation, neovascularisation, and mucoid degeneration cause imaging findings of tendon thickening and compromised mechanical properties.

Ultrasound

- Cost-effective and dynamic imaging modality.

- On grayscale imaging, tendinopathy manifests as tendon thickening (>7 mm), heterogeneous echotexture, and loss of the normal fibrillar pattern.

- Hypoechoic regions correspond to areas of collagen degeneration and increased water content (commonly mimics tendon tears).

- Power Doppler imaging shows neovascularisation within the Kager's fat pad, substance of the tendon or surrounding peritendinous tissues.

- Tendinopathy (Figure 2.16.14) is divided into two types depending upon the part of (Achilles tendon involved: Non-insertional is approximately 4–6 cm proximal to the calcaneal attachment), and insertional occurs (at the calcaneal tuberosity attachment, associated with Hagelund deformity, differentials include psoriatic arthritis/seronegative spondyloarthritis, gout, xanthomatous deposits).

- Achilles tendon tears (Figure 2.16.14): Watershed area (non-insertional tendinopathy) is most commonly involved. US assesses degree of tear, distance between torn ends on ankle dorsiflexion, neutral position and plantar flexion, healing response in form haematoma formation, organised haematoma and fibrogranular tissue, and fibrosis.

- Kager's fat invading into the torn ends of the tear suggests chronicity and may hamper tendon healing.

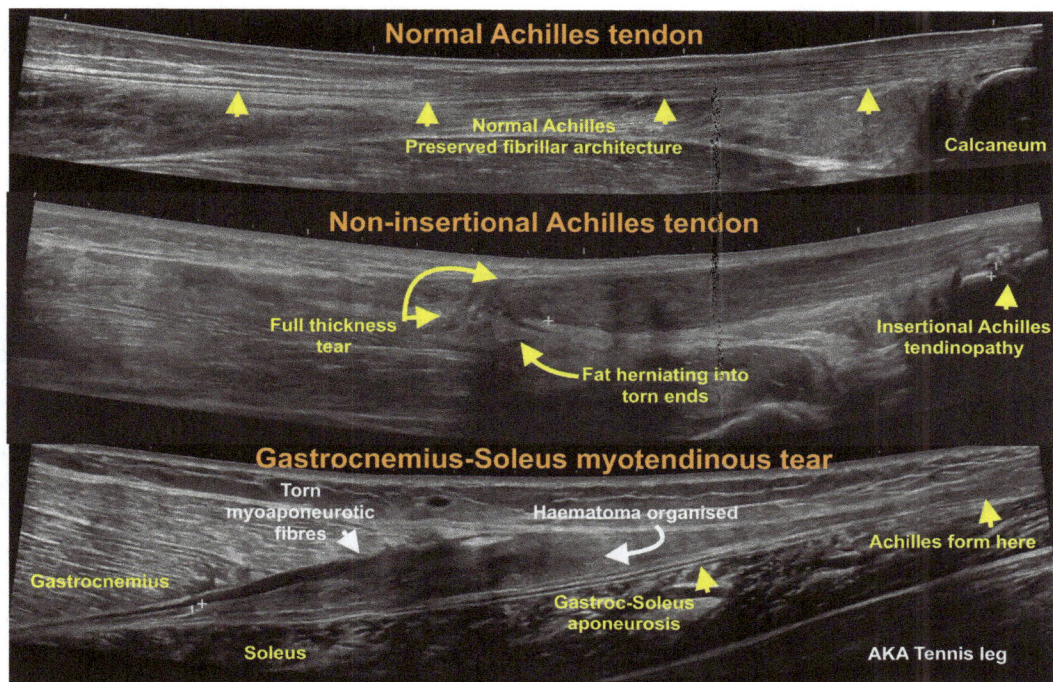

Figure 2.16.14 Various Achilles tendon pathologies on ultrasound.

- US is used in steroid injection and high-volume saline dissection in chronic Achilles tendinopathies.

- Medial gastrocnemius–Soleus aponeurosis tear (tennis leg) may mimic Achilles tendon tear (Figure 2.16.14), but it happens proximal to the formation of the Achilles tendon. Haematoma accumulates in the aponeurosis and may confound the exact length of the tear.

MRI: The Gold Standard

- On T1W sequences, tendon thickening with intermediate signal intensity (Figure 2.16.15).

- Fluid-sensitive sequences: Hyperintense intra-tendinous signal changes, reflecting fluid accumulation and degeneration.

- Associated MRI findings are paratenon inflammation, retrocalcaneal bursitis, and intra-tendinous tears.

- It differentiates tendinopathy from partial or complete ruptures and helps in surgical planning.

- It helps in the assessment of Achilles tendon re-tears.

Plantar Fasciitis

It predominantly involves the calcaneal attachment of the medial and central band and, uncommonly, the 5th metatarsal base attachment of the lateral band.

- Risk factors include excessive foot pronation, obesity, rheumatoid arthritis, diabetis, prolonged standing, and high-impact activities. Clinically, patients present with insidious-onset heel pain, typically worse with the first steps in the morning or after prolonged rest.

- US shows plantar fascia thickening (4–6 mm likely, >6 mm definitive), hypoechoic changes, associated calcaneal spur, increased plantar fascia vascularity and perifascial oedema. Doppler imaging may reveal increased vascularity in chronic cases.

- MRI shows plantar fascia thickening and oedema at the calcaneal attachment and adjacent bone marrow oedema.

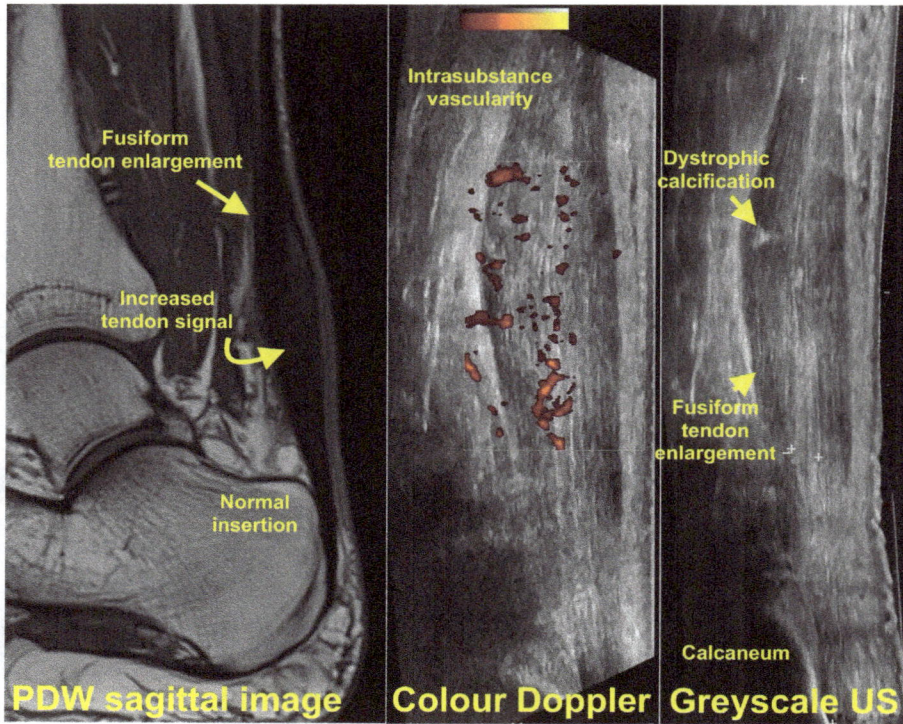

Figure 2.16.15 Non-insertional Achilles tendinopathy with mucoid degeneration and dystrophic calcification on MRI and ultrasound, respectively.

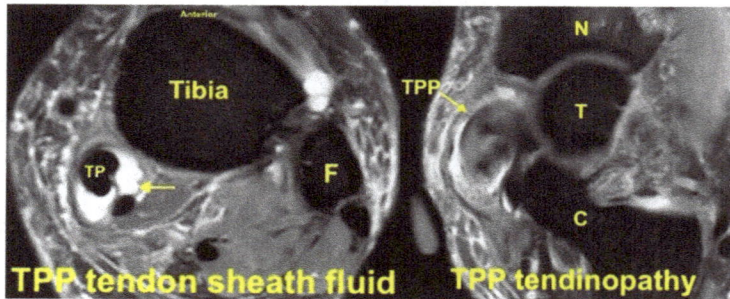

Figure 2.16.16 Tibialis posterior tenosynovitis and tendinosis.

Posterior Tibial Tendon Pathologies and Acquired Flatfoot

- The posterior tibial tendon (PTT) plays a crucial role in maintaining medial arch integrity and stabilising the foot during gait.

- Chronic mechanical overload, repetitive microtrauma, and degenerative changes contribute to tendon attenuation, particularly in middle-aged women and individuals with predisposing factors such as obesity, diabetes, and inflammatory arthropathies.

- PTT degeneration progresses from tenosynovitis to complete rupture (Figure 2.16.16) and rigid pes plano-valgus. It commonly involves navicular insertion. Sometimes, symptomatic accessory navicular (Os naviculare syndrome) mimic PTT tendinopathy.

- Clinically, patients present with medial foot pain, swelling, progressive arch collapse, and hindfoot valgus deformity.

- US: PTT tendon thickening, hypoechoic changes, intrasubstance tears, and potential discontinuity in complete rupture. PTT tenosynovitis presents as thickened synovial lining with tendon sheath effusion distending it with normal tendon encased within.

- Power Doppler imaging: Neovascularisation in early-stage disease of PTT tendinopathy and PTT tenosynovitis.

- MRI: Tendon thickening and oedema, partial-thickness tears, or complete discontinuity with tendon retraction.

- Associated MRI findings include sub-fibular impingement, sinus tarsi effusion, and spring ligament attenuation.

- Radiographs show secondary bony changes including loss of medial arch height, talar head uncovering, and hindfoot valgus.

Lisfranc Injuries and Metatarsal Stress Fractures

Lisfranc injuries result from acute trauma that disrupts the tarsometatarsal (TMT) joint complex.

- Lisfranc injuries involve damage to the Lisfranc ligament, which stabilises the medial cuneiform to the second metatarsal base.

- Mechanism: Axial loading on a plantarflexed foot, as seen in falls, motor vehicle accidents, and athletic activities.

- Clinically, patients present with midfoot pain, swelling, and an inability to bear weight.

- Radiographs (see Chapter 2.4) as first-line imaging show widening between the first and second metatarsal bases, joint incongruity, step off between the second metatarsal base and intermediate cuneiform, and the "fleck sign," indicative of ligamentous avulsion.

- CT when radiographs are inconclusive.

- MRI is used in selected cases for detecting ligamentous disruption and associated bone marrow oedema, improving diagnostic accuracy in subtle injuries.

Metatarsal stress fractures develop due to repetitive microtrauma exceeding the bone's remodelling capacity. It represents either fatigue or insufficiency fracture.

- Affects the 2nd and 3rd metatarsals due to their load-bearing function.

- Patients typically report progressive pain that initially resolves with rest but may worsen over time.

- Radiographs are normal in early cases, and periosteal reaction, cortical thickening, or fracture lines appear in later stages (Figure 2.16.17).

- MRI is the gold standard, detecting bone marrow oedema on fluid-sensitive sequences before structural disruption becomes apparent.

- Bone scintigraphy identifies early metabolic changes.

- CT is used to assess fracture healing and rule out complications such as non-union.

- Stable injuries can be managed conservatively with immobilisation and activity modification.

- Surgical intervention is often required in cases of significant instability, fracture displacement, or chronic non-union.

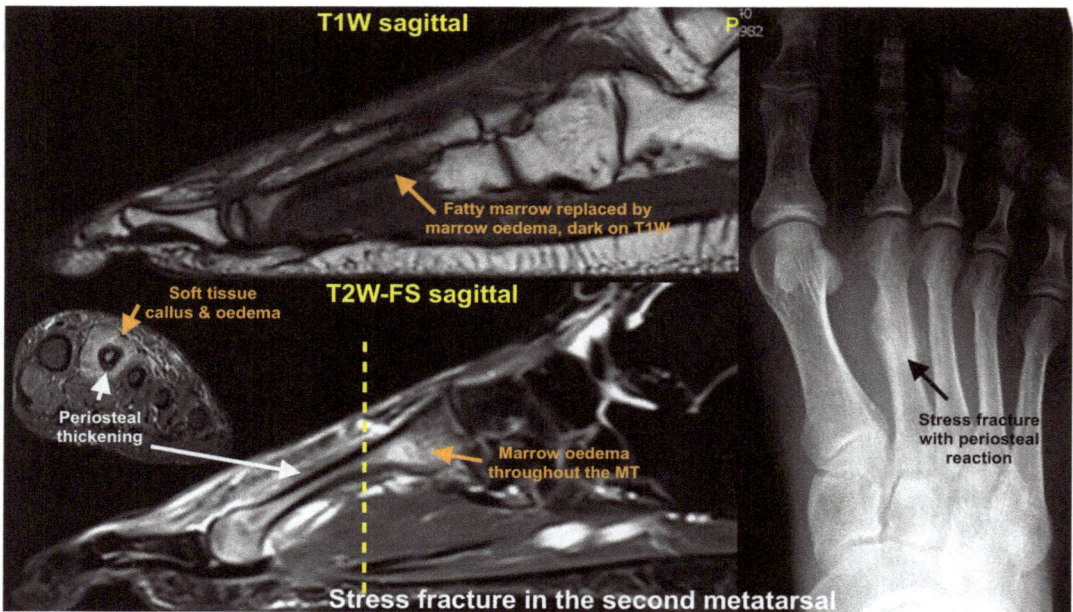

Figure 2.16.17   Metatarsal stress fracture on MRI and X-ray.

Morton's Neuroma and Intermetatarsal Bursitis

Morton's neuroma and intermetatarsal (IMT) bursitis (Figure 2.16.18) are common forefoot pathologies that can present with overlapping clinical symptoms, including forefoot pain, burning sensations, and paraesthesia. It is associated with mechanical overload, repetitive microtrauma, and improper footwear. It commonly involves the 2nd and 3rd web spaces.

Pathology	Morton's Neuroma	Intermetatarsal Bursitis
Mechanism	Misnomer reflecting perineural fibrosis and thickening of the common plantar digital nerve due to chronic entrapment between the metatarsal heads	Inflammation of the intermetatarsal bursa, often secondary to repetitive friction or mechanical stress
US	Shows a hypoechoic, noncompressible mass within the intermetatarsal space that may exhibit "Mulder's click" on dynamic assessment (forefoot squeeze)	An anechoic or hypoechoic fluid collection between the metatarsal heads Fully compressible on finger or probe pressure
MRI	Well-defined, low-to-intermediate signal intensity lesion on T1W Increased signal around the lesion on fluid-sensitive images due to perineural oedema Contrast enhancement	Follows fluid signal intensity Low on T1W and high on STIR or T2W-FS images Sometimes synovial thickening and surrounding inflamed tissue enhances

- Morton's neuroma and intermetatarsal bursa can co-exist.

- US is useful to perform steroid injection for both pathologies.

HIP AND PELVIS PATHOLOGIES
Occult Femoral Fractures

- They are "occult" on initial conventional radiographs and become apparent only on advanced imaging like CT or MRI, or close follow-up radiographs.

- Typical locations: Proximal femur, femoral neck, and intertrochanteric regions.

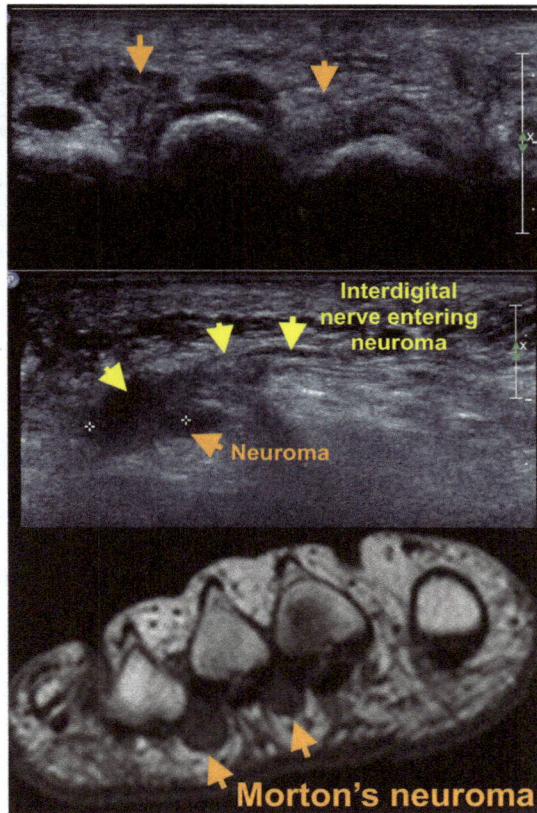

Figure 2.16.18 Morton's neuroma on ultrasound and MRI.

- Seen in elderly individuals with osteoporosis or younger patients subjected to high-impact trauma or repetitive stress (athletes with inadequate nutrition).
- If undiagnosed, occult femoral fractures can progress to complete fractures.
- Clinically, patients present with groin pain exacerbated by weight-bearing, often with no obvious history of trauma.
- Imaging is critical. Initial radiographs are negative or show subtle cortical irregularities.
- MRI is the gold standard; shows BMO as high signal intensity on fluid-sensitive sequences.
- CT shows subtle cortical disruptions and assessing fracture stability.
- Bone scintigraphy reveals increased metabolic activity in early stress fractures.
- Management ranges from protected weight-bearing to surgical fixation in high-risk cases.
- Bisphosphonate-related atypical femoral fracture is a special case that involves lateral cortex of the proximal third to midshaft of the femur (Figure 2.16.19). They can be bilateral. They require therapy modification and prophylactic intramedullary nailing.

Femoroacetabular Impingement

- FAI represents abnormal contact between the femoral head-neck junction and the acetabular rim, leading to progressive hip joint degeneration.

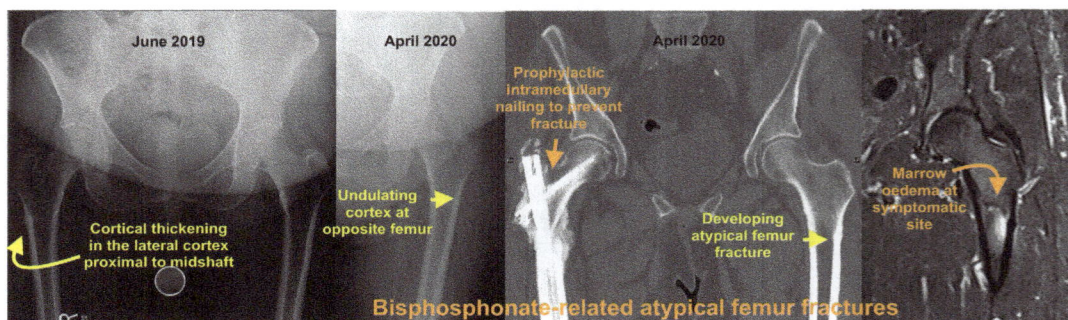

Figure 2.16.19 Temporal evolution of bisphosphonate-related atypical femoral fractures on both sides and utility of CT and MRI in them.

- It is classified into cam, pincer, and mixed-type impingement.

- Cam-type impingement: An aspherical femoral head or head-neck junction hypertrophy leading to abnormal femoral engagement with the acetabulum.

- Pincer-type impingement: Acetabular overcoverage causing premature impingement of the femoral neck against the acetabular rim.

- Mixed-type FAI involves features of both cam and pincer morphologies.

- FAI is associated with chondro-labral injury, subchondral cyst formation, and progressive cartilage degradation.

- X-rays are of the anteroposterior pelvis and Dunn views. Cam-type lesions show increased alpha angle (>55°) and pincer lesions appear as acetabular over-coverage (lateral centre-edge angle >40°) or a cross-over sign.

- MRI/MR arthrography assesses labral tears and articular cartilage damage.

- Management strategies include activity modification, physical therapy, and surgical intervention such as hip arthroscopy for labral repair and osteoplasty to correct bony abnormalities.

Avascular Necrosis

- Avascular necrosis (AVN) or osteonecrosis commonly affects weight-bearing joints, particularly the femoral head.

- Other involved sites: The humeral head, knee, talus, and scaphoid.

- AVN could be traumatic or non-traumatic.

- Traumatic AVN often follows fractures or dislocations that disrupt vascular integrity.

- Non-traumatic causes include corticosteroid use, excessive alcohol consumption, sickle cell disease, hypercoagulable states, and systemic conditions such as lupus and Gaucher's disease.

- Imaging is used to diagnose AVN and monitor the disease progression.

- Radiographs are normal in early stages and later show subchondral sclerosis and crescent sign indicative of subchondral collapse in advanced stages, and eventual joint destruction.

- MRI is the gold standard to diagnose and then monitor AVN. Common MRI appearances include geographic area, serpiginous linear signal or a characteristic double-line sign in established AVN. Subchondral collapse and evolving premature osteoarthritis are also best detected on MRI (Figure 2.16.20).

- Ficat–Arlet classification based on MRI is commonly used to assess the stage of the AVN and dictate further management.

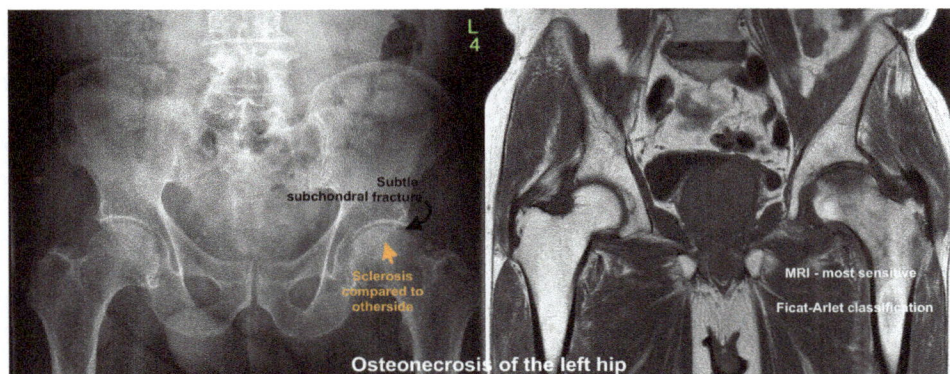

Figure 2.16.20   Hip AVN on X-ray and MRI.

■ More recently, percentage involvement of femoral head undergone AVN is calculated to help hip surgeons plan onwards management.

■ Differential diagnoses include transient osteoporosis (which lacks subchondral collapse), bone marrow oedema syndrome, osteomyelitis (which presents with marrow enhancement, joint effusion, soft tissue oedema, bone destruction, intraosseous abscess, and systemic signs), and stress fractures (which exhibit linear sclerosis without serpiginous margins).

■ Surgical management includes core decompression in early stages or joint arthroplasty in advanced cases.

MUSCULAR INJURIES OF THE RECTUS FEMORIS, ADDUCTORS, AND HAMSTRINGS

■ Muscle injuries involving the rectus femoris, adductors, and hamstrings are common in athletes and individuals engaged in high-intensity physical activities.

■ The rectus femoris is susceptible to strain injuries due to its role in both hip flexion and knee extension. The proximal myotendinous junction and the indirect head at the anterior inferior iliac spine (AIIS) are frequent sites of injury.

■ Adductor injuries, especially involving the adductor longus, are commonly seen in soccer and ice hockey players.

■ Hamstring injuries primarily affect the biceps femoris, often at the proximal myotendinous junction, are common in sprinters, cricket players, and high-speed sports.

■ US shows muscle fibre disruption, hematoma formation, and tendon retraction. It allows for real-time assessment of muscle contraction and healing progression.

■ MRI is the imaging of choice, particularly in athletes.

■ On MRI, acute muscle strains demonstrate oedema and haemorrhage on fluid-sensitive sequences with disruption of muscle fibres at the myotendinous junction. Partial tears exhibit focal discontinuity with adjacent hematoma, while complete ruptures show full-thickness tendon discontinuity with muscle retraction.

■ Chronic injuries may present with fibrosis and fatty infiltration, which are prognostic indicators for recurrent strain and prolonged recovery.

■ Multiple classifications are proposed to describe muscle injuries. BAMIC is most commonly used for hamstring injuries.

OSTEITIS PUBIS

It is commonly observed in athletes, particularly those engaged in sports requiring repetitive kicking, pivoting, or sudden directional changes, such as soccer and rugby.

■ Mechanism: Chronic microtrauma leading to subchondral bone marrow oedema, periostitis, and secondary degeneration of the fibrocartilaginous joint, ultimately resulting in pain and functional impairment.

- Radiographs show pubic symphysis widening, subchondral sclerosis, and irregular cortical margins in chronic cases.

- CT allows for detailed bony evaluation for erosions or reactive bone formation.

- MRI reveals bone marrow oedema (Figure 2.16.21), joint fluid, and soft tissue inflammation, while chronic cases may exhibit fibrosis and subchondral cyst formation.

- Differential diagnoses are pubic stress fractures, athletic pubalgia, and septic arthritis.

- Conservative treatment remains the mainstay, including rest, physiotherapy, and anti-inflammatory medications.

- Severe or refractory cases may require corticosteroid injections.

Looser's Zones

Looser's zones (pseudofractures)—cortical insufficiency fractures commonly associated with osteomalacia and, less frequently, other metabolic bone disorders such as rickets, renal osteodystrophy, and hyperparathyroidism.

- Typical locations: Medial femoral neck, pubic rami, lateral scapula, and ribs.

- Radiographs: Typically bilateral, symmetrical, lucent lines in transverse orientation, perpendicular to the cortex, often with sclerotic margins.

- CT: Detects subtle cortical disruptions.

- MRI: Reveals bone marrow oedema and adjacent soft tissue inflammation on fluid-sensitive sequences with low signal transverse line on T1W image (Figure 2.16.22).

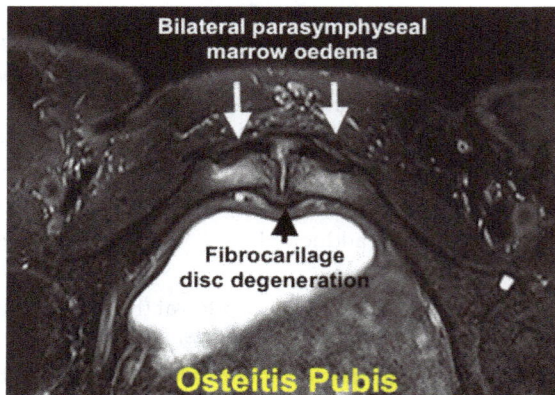

Figure 2.16.21　Osteitis pubis on axial MRI.

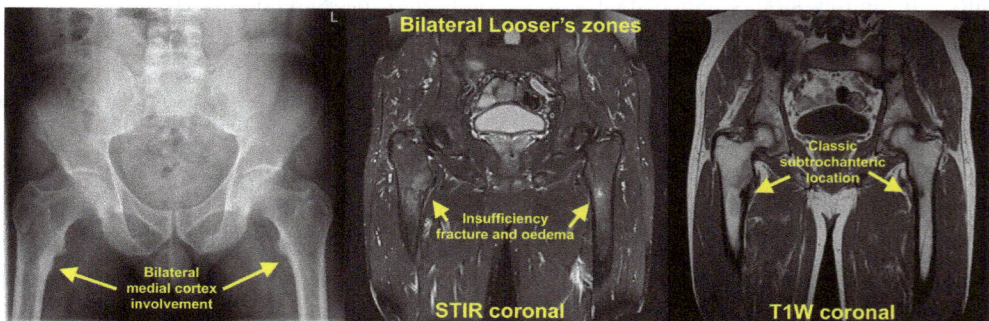

Figure 2.16.22　Looser's zones on X-ray and MRI.

284

- Bone scintigraphy: Increased radionuclide uptake due to active bone remodelling.

- Requires further investigations including dual-energy X-ray absorptiometry (DEXA) to detect reduced bone mineral density supporting an underlying metabolic disorder or osteoporosis and blood biochemistry including vitamin D level.

- Treatment involves correcting the underlying metabolic deficiency typically with vitamin D and calcium supplementation.

UPPPER LIMB PATHOLOGIES

SHOULDER PATHOLOGIES

Shoulder Instability

Shoulder dislocations, particularly anterior and posterior variants, are associated with osseous and soft tissue injuries that predispose patients to recurrent instability.

- Anterior dislocations, the most prevalent type, frequently result in Bankart lesions and Hill–Sachs defects.

- Posterior dislocations can lead to reverse Bankart and reverse Hill–Sachs lesions.

Imaging in Anterior Shoulder Instability

- Radiographs: Anteroposterior, axillary, and scapular-Y views are commonly used in dislocation and associated fractures. Stripped axial view is patient with severe shoulder movement restriction. The West Point and Stryker notch views can respectively improve glenoid and humeral head defects visualisation. Radiographs can detect bony Bankart's lesion, Hill–Sach's lesion (Figure 2.16.23), BHAGL (bony humeral avulsion of the inferior glenohumeral ligament), and associated rotator cuff avulsion fracture.

- MR arthrogram: Investigation of choice to assess glenoid bone loss, cartilage and labral injuries, rotator cuff assessment, and onwards management planning.

- Bipolar bone loss (anterior glenoid bone loss and Hill–Sach defects) requires assessment of "on-track" or "off-track" lesions.

- Labral injuries on MR arthrograms (Figure 2.16.24) vary according to the severity of previous subluxations. Following are common bone and labral lesions associated with anterior shoulder instability.

Pathology Name/Acronym	Description
Hill–Sachs lesion	Osteochondral defect at the posterosuperior humeral head
Bankart's lesion	Anteroinferior glenoid labrum avulsion associated with ruptured capsuloligamentous structures/periosteum
Bony Bankart's lesion	Bankart's lesion + anterior glenoid fracture
Perthe's lesion	Anteroinferior glenoid labrum injury with intact periosteum. Sometimes difficult to spot. Requires ABER position
ALPSA	Anteroinferior glenoid labrum is torn, medialised, and forms a small soft tissue nodule anteroinferiorly (most common)
GLAD	Glenoid labrum injury with articular cartilage defect
HAGL	Humeral attachment of inferior glenohumeral ligament is ruptured
BHAGL	HAGL + bony avulsion at the medial humerus
SLAP	Superior labral tear—various types

- In posterior dislocations, reverse Bankart lesions involve the posteroinferior labrum, whereas reverse Hill–Sachs defects (McLaughlin lesions) manifest as an anteromedial humeral head impaction injury.

- X-rays in posterior shoulder dislocation shows "trough sign."

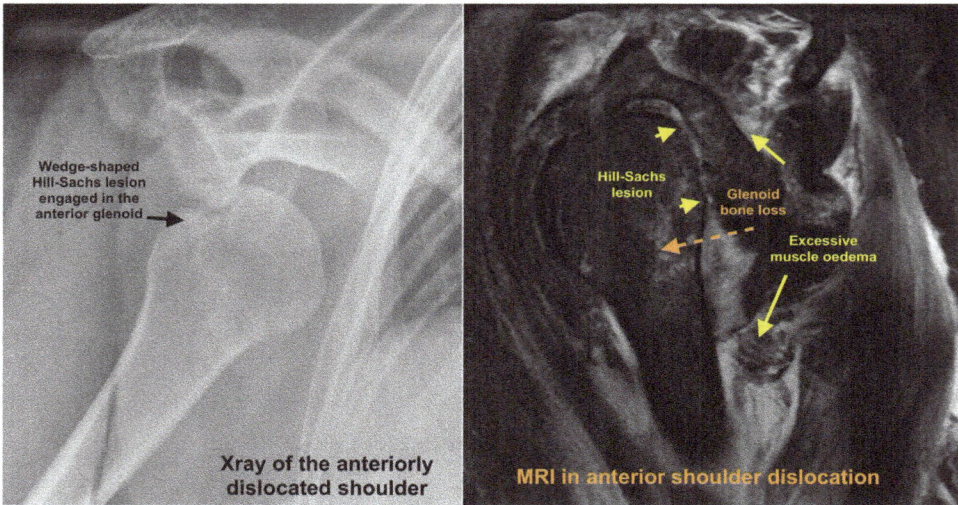

Figure 2.16.23 X-ray and MRI in persistent anteroinferior shoulder dislocation showing engagement of the humeral head and anterior glenoid.

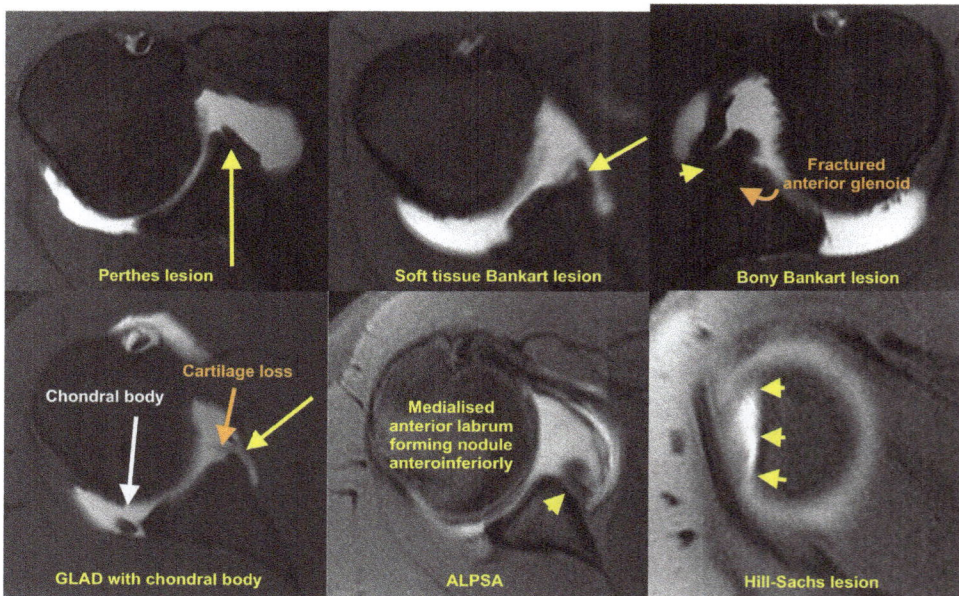

Figure 2.16.24 Various types of labral tears on shoulder MR arthrogram.

Rotator Cuff Tears

Rotator cuff tears are a common cause of shoulder pain and dysfunction, resulting from acute trauma or chronic degenerative changes.

- Supraspinatus tendon is most frequently affected. Larger tendon tears may involve infraspinatus and subscapularis.

- Cuff tear grading depends upon the location, dimensions of the tear, and involved thickness.

- Depending on size, cuff tears are classified as small (<1 cm), medium (1–3 cm), large (3–5 cm), and massive (>5 cm or involving 2 or more tendons).

- Depending on thickness, cuff tears can be classified as partial-thickness, full-thickness, or complete tears with tendon retraction.

- Chronic tears may exhibit fatty infiltration of cuff muscles (Goutellier classification), tendon atrophy, and secondary osteoarthritic changes in the glenohumeral joint (Rotator cuff arthropathy).

- **US**: Cost-effective. Features of a full-thickness tear include an anechoic defect within the tendon, non-visualisation of the tendon due to retraction, and dynamic abnormalities such as paradoxical movement during shoulder rotation.

- Partial-thickness tears appear as focal hypoechoic or anechoic defects, often best visualised with transducer compression.

- Secondary findings include cortical irregularities at the greater tuberosity and effusion within the subacromial-subdeltoid bursa.

- **MRI**: Gold standard for assessing rotator cuff tears and tendinopathy (Figure 2.16.25) and rotator cuff arthroapthy.

- Full-thickness tears: Hyperintense fluid-filled defects, with tendon discontinuity and potential retraction on fluid-sensitive sequences.

- Partial-thickness tears: Increased signal within the tendon without full disruption.

- Chronic tears: Muscle atrophy and fatty infiltration on T1W sequences.

Rotator Cuff Tendinopathy

- Degenerative condition.

- It commonly affects the supraspinatus tendon due to its high mechanical load.

- Infraspinatus and subscapularis tendons may also be involved.

- **US**: Tendinopathy is seen as tendon thickening, hypoechogenicity, and loss of fibrillar architecture. Intratendinous calcifications may be present, particularly in calcific tendinopathy.

- **Power Doppler imaging**: Increased vascularity.

- **Secondary findings**: Subacromial-subdeltoid bursitis and cortical irregularities at the greater tuberosity.

- US is also helpful in the image-guided steroid injection.

- **MRI**: Tendinopathy appears as increased intratendinous signal without complete fibre disruption on fluid-sensitive sequences and tendon thickening and mild atrophy on T1W images.

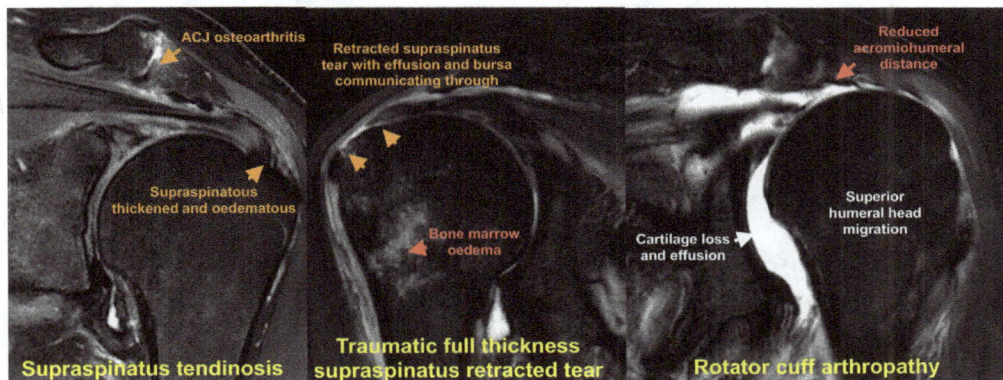

Figure 2.16.25 Evolution of supraspinatus tendinosis to rotator cuff arthropathy.

287

Acromioclavicular Joint (ACJ) Dislocations

- Due to fall onto the lateral shoulder or high-impact collisions.

- It involves disruption of the acromioclavicular and coracoclavicular ligaments.

- The Rockwood classification system grades ACJ injuries from type I (mild sprain) to type VI (severe inferior dislocation of the clavicle).

- **Radiographs**: First-line imaging, Standard anteroposterior (AP) shoulder, and Zanca views best assess ACJ alignment, while stress radiographs with weights can help differentiate higher-grade injuries. A widened ACJ space (>7 mm) and increased coracoclavicular distance (>13 mm) indicate ligamentous disruption.

- **CT**: Detecting subtle fractures or complex dislocations particularly in high-energy trauma.

- **MRI**: For assessment of ligamentous integrity, joint effusion, and associated injuries such as rotator cuff tears.

Parsonage–Turner Syndrome

- Parsonage–Turner syndrome (PTS) or neuralgic amyotrophy (Figure 2.16.26) is an idiopathic brachial plexopathy characterised by acute-onset shoulder pain followed by muscle weakness and atrophy, most commonly affecting the supraspinatus and infraspinatus muscles.

- Spinoglenoid cysts are ganglions arising from posterosuperior labral tears in the spinoglenoid notch. They can cause extrinsic compression on the suprascapular nerve, primarily affecting the infraspinatus muscle while sparing the supraspinatus due to the distal location of compression.

- Chronic nerve compression leads to denervation changes, including muscle atrophy and fatty infiltration.

- MRI: Preferred imaging technique.

- In PTS, MRI may show muscle oedema in affected muscles during the acute phase on fluid-sensitive sequences, followed by atrophy and fatty replacement in chronic cases on T1W images.

- In spinoglenoid cysts, MRI reveals a well-defined fluid-filled structure at the spinoglenoid notch, often associated with labral pathology (Figure 2.16.26).

- Accurate imaging differentiation is crucial, as PTS is managed conservatively, while spinoglenoid cysts may require surgical decompression if symptomatic.

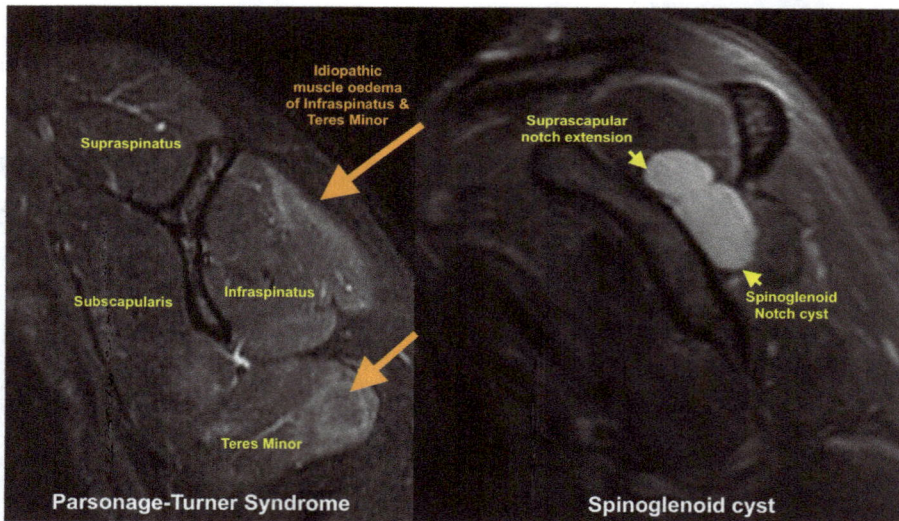

Figure 2.16.26 Parsonage–Turner syndrome and spinoglenoid cyst in two different MRIs.

Calcific Tendonitis of the Shoulder

- Calcific tendonitis is characterised by the deposition of hydroxyapatite crystals within the rotator cuff tendons, most frequently affecting the supraspinatus.

- Imaging features and stages of calcific tendinitis are described in Chapter 2.11 and relevant interventions are described in Chapter 2.15 in detail.

ELBOW PATHOLOGIES

Distal Biceps Tendon Injuries

- They range from tendinosis and partial tears to complete ruptures.

- Traumatic distal biceps ruptures affect the dominant arm in middle-aged males and are often associated with predisposing factors such as smoking, corticosteroid use, and repetitive mechanical stress.

- Partial tears may lead to pain and weakness, whereas complete ruptures cause a visible deformity, often described as the "Popeye sign," with significant loss of supination and flexion strength.

- US: Preferred imaging in acute setttings. A normal distal biceps tendon appears as a hyperechoic, fibrillar structure, inserting onto the radial tuberosity. In tendinosis, the tendon may appear thickened and hypoechoic. Partial tears manifest as focal hypoechoic defects with associated fluid (Figure 2.16.27), while complete ruptures show tendon discontinuity, retraction, coiling of the tendon at the distal arm level.

- Cobra position of the hand is useful in detecting partial tear near the radial tuberosity attachment and bicipitoradial bursa.

- MRI: Gold standard, it shows tendon discontinuity, retraction, and surrounding oedema.

- Axial images best visualise radial tuberosity involvement.

- Complete ruptures often requiring surgical repair to restore function.

Common Extensor Origin (CEO) and Common Flexor Origin (CFO) Tendinopathy

- Common overuse injuries in athletes engaged in racquet sports, golf, and throwing activities.

- CEO tendinopathy (lateral epicondylitis/tennis elbow) results from repetitive wrist extension and forearm supination, leading to microtears, collagen disorganisation, and neovascularisation, primarily affecting the extensor carpi radialis brevis (ECRB).

- CFO tendinopathy (medial epicondylitis/golfer's elbow) arises from repetitive wrist flexion and pronation, with pathology predominantly involving the pronator teres and flexor carpi radialis.

- Chronic cases may progress to partial or full-thickness tendon tears, resulting in persistent pain and functional impairment.

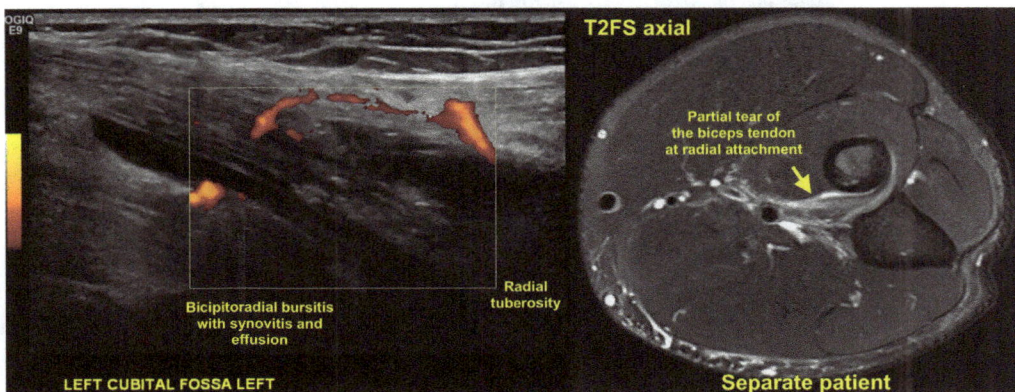

Figure 2.16.27   Bicipitoradial bursitis on US and partial-thickness distal biceps tear on MRI.

- US: Highly effective imaging modality. Tendinopathy manifests as tendon thickening, hypoechogenicity, and loss of the normal fibrillar pattern associated with cortical irregularities, dystrophic calcification, and increased intratendinous and soft tissue vascularities. Partial tears appear as focal hypoechoic defects, while complete ruptures demonstrate tendon discontinuity, retraction, and associated haematoma.

- MRI: Provides better contrast resolution with similar features better visualised (Figure 2.16.28).

Osteochondritis Dissecans (OCD) of the Elbow

- OCD of the elbow is a common condition in young athletes, particularly those involved in throwing sports and gymnastics.

- The capitellum is the most frequently affected site.

- Its radiographic and MRI features are comparable to those described for the OCD of the knee.

Ligamentous Injuries of the Elbow

- Ligamentous injuries of the elbow, particularly involving the radial collateral ligament (RCL), ulnar collateral ligament (UCL), and lateral ulnar collateral ligament (LUCL), are significant concerns in athletes.

- They are crucial to elbow stability.

- The UCL resists valgus stress, the RCL stabilising against varus forces, and the LUCL preventing posterolateral rotatory instability (Figure 2.16.29).

- Repetitive stress, particularly in throwing sports, can lead to ligamentous attenuation, microtears, and eventual rupture, predisposing athletes to chronic instability and functional impairment.

- US: Cost effective and dynamic assessment.

- In acute injuries, partial or full-thickness ligament tears appear as hypoechoic or anechoic defects with fibre discontinuity, often accompanied by joint effusion.

- Stress manoeuvres under US can further evaluate ligament laxity.

- Chronic injuries may demonstrate ligament thickening, hypoechogenicity, and calcification, indicative of soft tissue remodelling.

- MRI provides similar details with greater sensitivity than US.

- In chronic injuries, ligament thickening, mucoid degeneration, and secondary findings such as valgus overload changes or posterolateral rotatory instability may be evident.

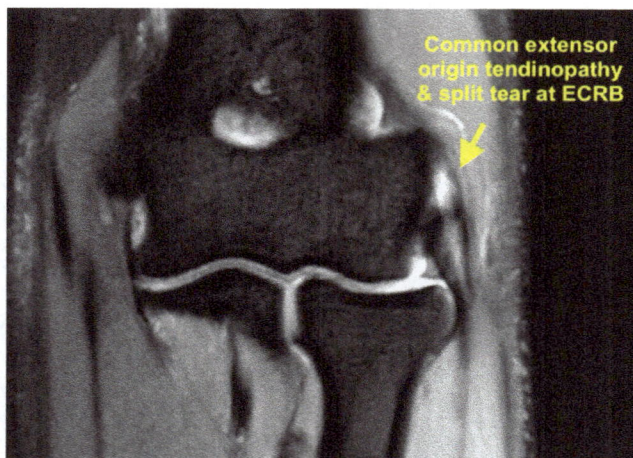

Figure 2.16.28 Partial-thickness common extensor origin tear on MRI.

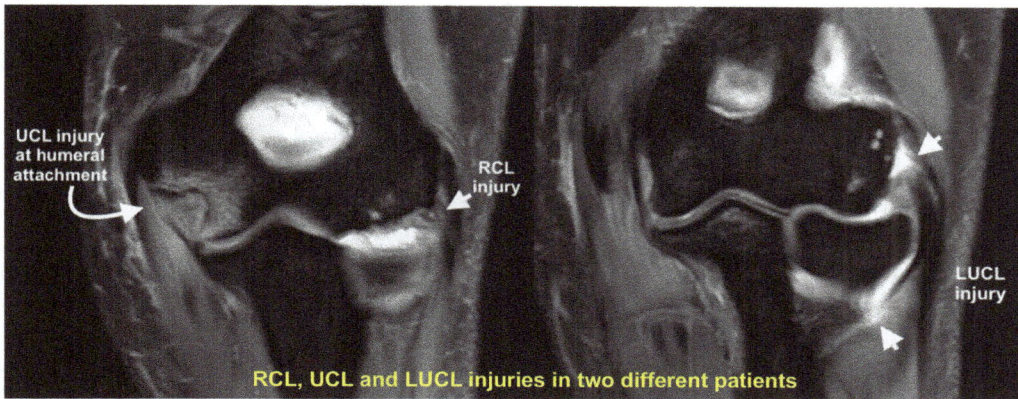

Figure 2.16.29   Internal derangements of the elbow on MRI.

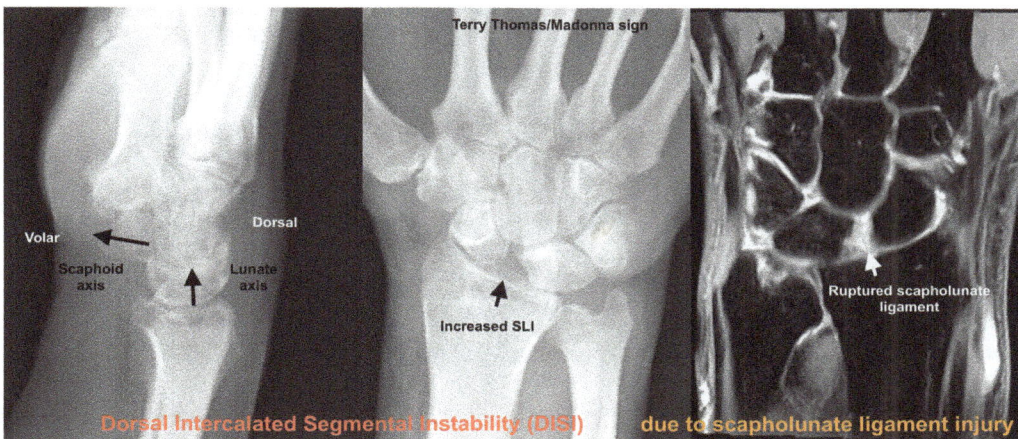

Figure 2.16.30   Dorsal intercalated segmental instability in scapholunate ligament tear.

WRIST PATHOLOGIES
Ligamentous Injuries of the Wrist

- Ligamentous injuries of the wrist are common in athletes, particularly in gymnastics, tennis, and football.

- These injuries can lead to wrist instability including scapholunate advanced collapse (SLAC), volar intercalated segment instability (VISI), and dorsal intercalated segment instability (DISI), which, if undiagnosed, may progress to degenerative changes.

- Scapholunate ligament (SLL) disruption: Causes scapholunate dissociation and DISI (Figure 2.16.30).

- Lunotriquetral ligament (LTL) injury: Results in VISI, where the lunate tilts volarly due to unopposed flexor forces (Figure 2.16.31).

- Chronic instability causes SLAC wrist: Scapholunate widening, scaphoid flexion, and radiocarpal osteoarthritis (Figure 2.16.32).

- MRI: Gold standard, partial tears appear as focal thinning or discontinuity, while complete ruptures show fluid-filled gaps.

- Dynamic fluoroscopy or stress radiographs can detect dissociative injuries.

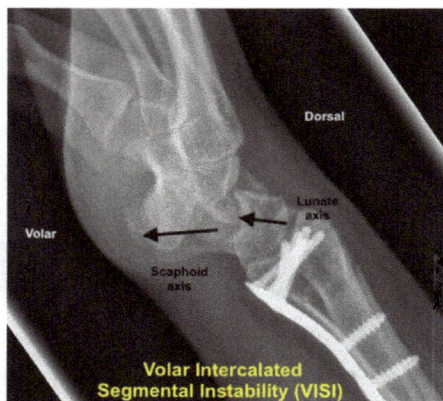

Figure 2.16.31 Volar intercalated segmental instability in lunotriquetral ligament tear.

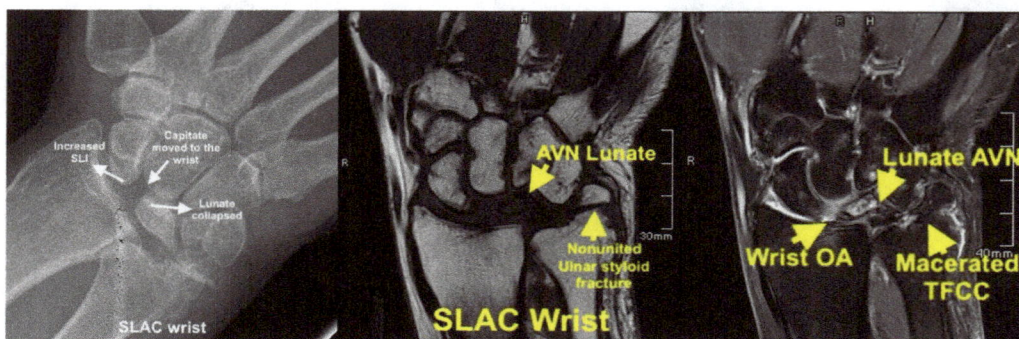

Figure 2.16.32 Scapholunate advanced collapse and lunate AVN in chronic SLL injury.

De Quervain's Tenosynovitis

- Overuse injury affecting the first dorsal compartment of the wrist, particularly in athletes engaged in repetitive wrist and thumb movements, such as racquet sports, rowing, and golf.

- Thickening and inflammation of the extensor pollicis brevis (EPB) and abductor pollicis longus (APL) tendon sheath as they pass through the fibro-osseous tunnel at the radial styloid.

- Chronic friction leads to synovial hypertrophy, stenosis, and eventual tendon degeneration, resulting in pain, swelling, and crepitus along the radial wrist.

- US: Tendon sheath thickening, hypoechogenicity, and fluid distension.

- Power Doppler imaging: Increased vascularity.

- US-guided corticosteroid injection is commonly prescribed treatment. Anatomic variations, such as a septate first dorsal compartment, may contribute to persistent symptoms.

- MRI: Tendon sheath effusion, peritendinous oedema, tendon degeneration, and thickening of the retinaculum (Figure 2.16.33).

Triangular Fibrocartilage Complex Injuries

- Triangular fibrocartilage complex (TFCC) injuries commonly cause ulnar-sided wrist pain in athletes, particularly those involved in racquet sports, gymnastics, and weightlifting.

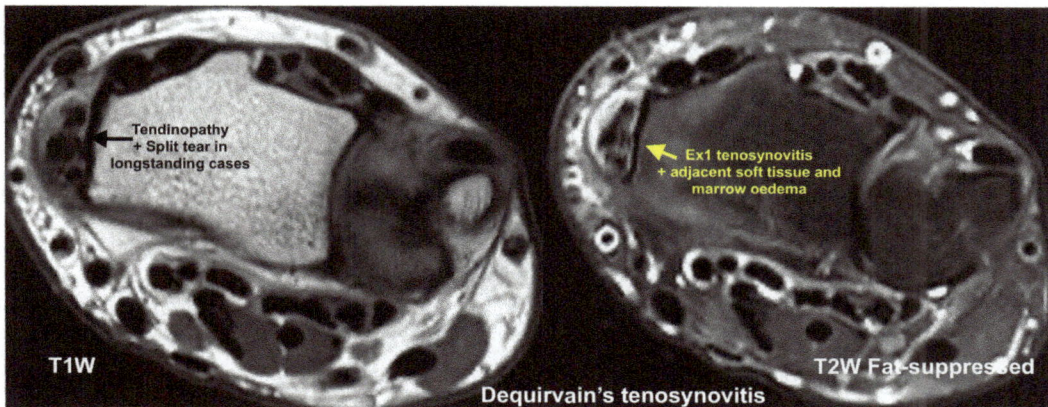

Figure 2.16.33 MRI appearances of De Quervain's tenosynovitis.

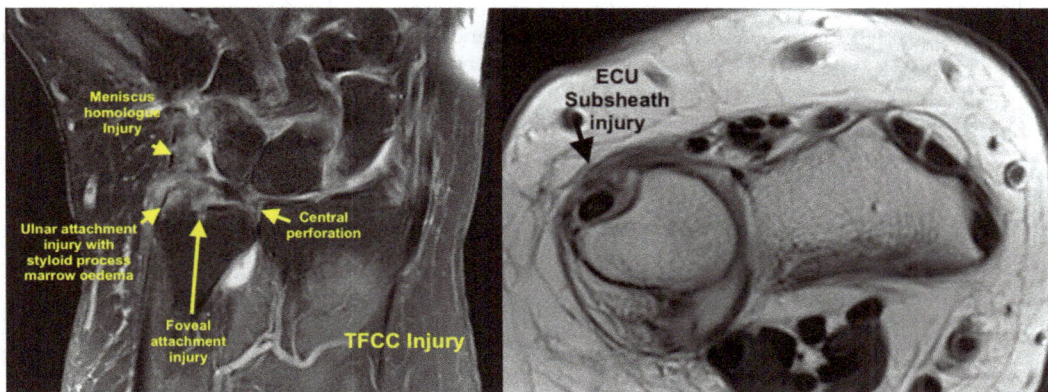

Figure 2.16.34 MRI in high-grade TFCC injury showing multiple injuried components.

- The TFCC provides stability to the distal radioulnar joint (DRUJ) and acts as a load-bearing structure between the ulna and carpus.

- Injuries can be traumatic or degenerative (associated with ulnar variance).

- MR arthrography: Gold standard, hyperintense signal or fluid undercutting within the fibrocartilage with discontinuity indicating a tear (Figure 2.16.34).

- Central perforations are common in degenerative cases, while traumatic injuries often involve the periphery.

- Splinting and physiotherapy in stable injuries to arthroscopic debridement or repair in high-grade tears are usual management strategies.

Pulley Injuries

- Pulley injuries are common in athletes involved in climbing, gymnastics, and sports requiring forceful grip.

- The A2 and A4 pulleys are critical in maintaining tendon apposition to the phalanges, preventing bow-stringing and ensuring efficient force transmission.

- Pulley injuries typically result from sudden overload, leading to partial or complete rupture, with associated pain, swelling, and reduced grip strength.

- US: A normal pulley appears as a hyperechoic band encircling the flexor tendons, while disruption results in tendon bowstringing, best demonstrated during resisted finger flexion.

- Partial tears appear as hypoechoic thickening or focal defects, whereas complete ruptures show discontinuity with increased tendon excursion from the phalangeal surface.

- MRI: Shows pulley disruption, tendon displacement, and peritendinous oedema.

- Management: Splinting and rehabilitation in partial tears to surgical repair in high-grade ruptures, optimising functional recovery and return to sport.

Trigger Finger

- Trigger finger, or stenosing tenosynovitis, is a common condition in athletes who engage in repetitive gripping activities, such as climbers, golfers, and racquet sports players.

- It arises from inflammation and thickening of the flexor tendon sheath, most commonly at the level of the A1 pulley.

- Clinically, athletes may experience painful clicking, locking, or catching of the affected digit, which can impair grip strength and performance.

- US: Thickened A1 pulley appears as a hypoechoic band overlying the flexor tendons (Figure 2.16.35), with associated tenosynovitis presenting as fluid distension and increased Doppler vascularity. The triggering mechanism can be reproduced by dynamic US assessment.

- MRI: Less commonly used but provides detailed evaluation of associated soft tissue changes such as peritendinous oedema and flexor tendon thickening.

- Corticosteroid injections to surgical release in refractory cases are usual management.

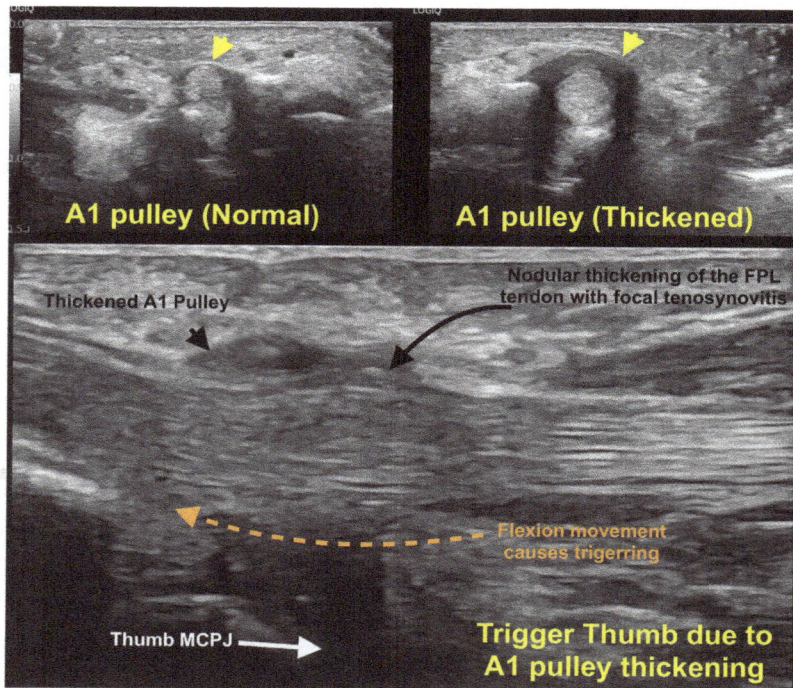

Figure 2.16.35 US in trigger thumb with A1 pulley thickening.

CONCLUSION

Sports and activity-related injuries are common presentations to A&E, fracture clinics, trauma hubs, orthopaedic and sports departments. Such injuries require a logical imaging approach and robust knowledge of biomechanics and injuries patterns to reach to a correct diagnosis. X-rays and ultrasound are commonly performed initial imaging investigations to detect bone and soft tissue injuries respectively. MRI is performed when clinical or radiological dilemma persists or management altering decisions are to be made.

SUGGESTED READING

- Stoller DW, ed. *Magnetic Resonance Imaging in Orthopaedics and Sports Medicine*. Lippincott Williams & Wilkins; 2007.

SBA QUESTIONS

1) A 23-year-old rugby player presented with acutely swollen knee and anterior knee pain following a tackle injury. Clinical history suggests no similar previous episodes, and clinical assessment reveals no patellar laxity. X-rays of the knee demonstrate a small fracture fragment in the intercondylar region. To investigate it in detail, a clinical decision to proceed with an MRI was made. Which is the least expected finding on the MRI?

   A. Bone marrow oedema in the medial patellar facet

   B. Bone marrow oedema in the anterolateral femoral condyle with cartilage loss

   C. ACL tear

   D. Injured femoral attachment of MPFL ligament

   E. Convex femoral trochlea with vertical medial patellar facet

2) A 19-year-old kick-boxer presented with ulnar-sided wrist pain following a traumatic event. X-rays of the wrist shows no bony injury. MRI was performed as a next imaging to assess for potential soft tissue injuries. Which would be least common soft tissue injury responsible for the patient's symptoms?

   A. Extensor carpi ulnaris subsheath injury

   B. Dorsal radioulnar ligament injury

   C. TFCC foveal attachment injury at the distal ulna

   D. Lunotriquetral ligament injury

   E. Meniscal homologue injury

3) Which of the following glenoid lesions is NOT associated with anterior shoulder instability?

   A. Bankart's lesion

   B. Perthe's lesion

   C. Hill–Sach's lesion

   D. ALPSA lesion

   E. GLAD lesion

Answers: (1) E, (2) D, (3) C

Index

Note: Page numbers in *italics* indicate a figure and page numbers in **bold** indicate a table on the corresponding page.

For Product Safety Concerns and Information please contact our EU representative GPSR@taylorandfrancis.com
Taylor & Francis Verlag GmbH, Kaufingerstraße 24, 80331 München, Germany